W9-DCM-902

NURSING PHOTOBOOK™

Carrying Out Special Procedures

NURSING83 BOOKS™
INTERMED COMMUNICATIONS, INC.
SPRINGHOUSE, PENNSYLVANIA

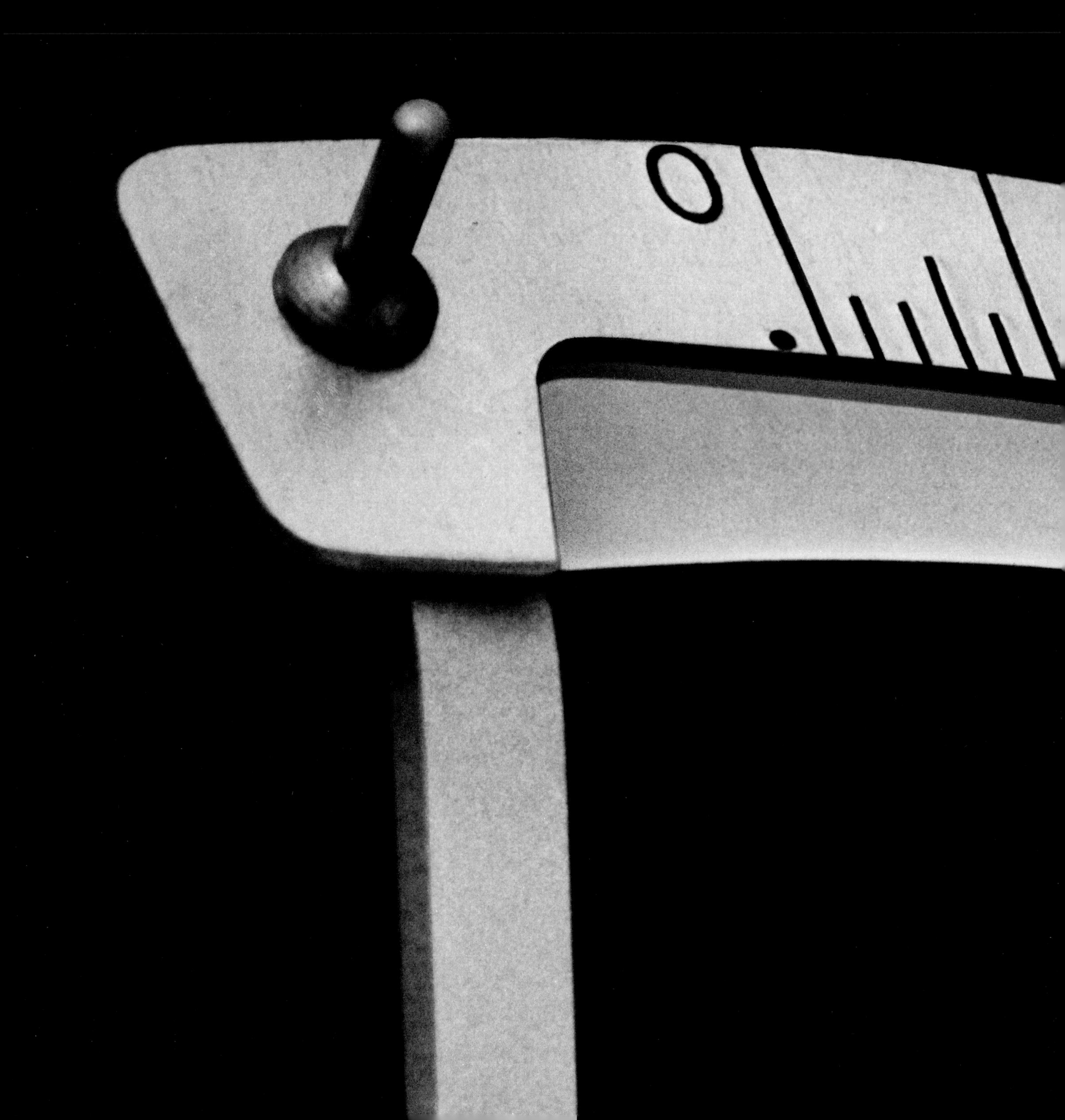
0

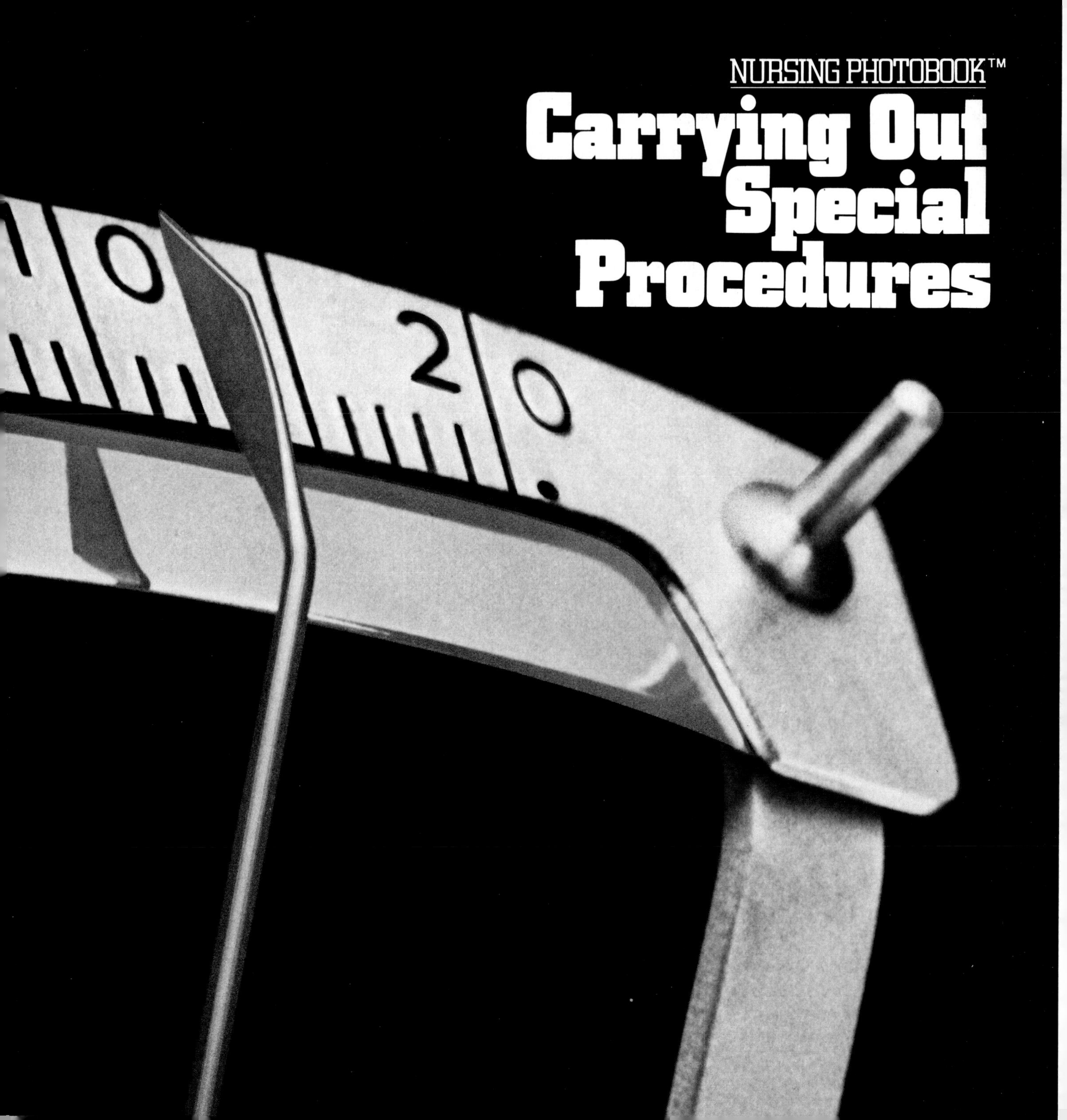
NURSING PHOTOBOOK™
Carrying Out Special Procedures
10
20

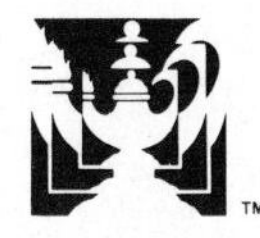

NURSING83 BOOKS

NURSING PHOTOBOOK™ SERIES
Providing Respiratory Care
Managing I.V. Therapy
Dealing with Emergencies
Giving Medications
Assessing Your Patients
Using Monitors
Providing Early Mobility
Giving Cardiac Care
Performing GI Procedures
Implementing Urologic Procedures
Controlling Infection
Ensuring Intensive Care
Coping with Neurologic Disorders
Caring for Surgical Patients
Working with Orthopedic Patients
Nursing Pediatric Patients
Helping Geriatric Patients
Attending Ob/Gyn Patients
Aiding Ambulatory Patients
Carrying Out Special Procedures

NURSING SKILLBOOK® SERIES
Dealing with Death and Dying
Reading EKGs Correctly
Managing Diabetics Properly
Assessing Vital Functions Accurately
Helping Cancer Patients Effectively
Giving Cardiovascular Drugs Safely
Giving Emergency Care Competently
Monitoring Fluid and Electrolytes Precisely
Documenting Patient Care Responsibly
Combatting Cardiovascular Diseases Skillfully
Coping with Neurologic Problems Proficiently
Nursing Critically Ill Patients Confidently
Using Crisis Intervention Wisely

NURSE'S REFERENCE LIBRARY® SERIES
Diseases
Diagnostics
Drugs
Assessment
Procedures

***Nursing83* DRUG HANDBOOK™**

NURSING PHOTOBOOK™ Series

PUBLISHER
Eugene W. Jackson

EDITORIAL PROJECT DIRECTOR
Jean Robinson

CLINICAL DIRECTOR
Barbara McVan, RN

ART DIRECTOR
Lisa A. Gilde

EDITORIAL MANAGER
Patricia R. Urosevich

Intermed Communications Book Division

DIRECTOR
Timothy B. King

DIRECTOR, RESEARCH
Elizabeth O'Brien

DIRECTOR, PRODUCTION AND PURCHASING
Bacil Guiley

Staff for this volume

BOOK EDITOR
Katherine W. Carey

CLINICAL EDITOR
Mary L. Clements, RN, CCRN

ASSOCIATE EDITORS
Dario F. Bernardini
Paul Vigna, Jr.

PHOTOGRAPHER
Paul A. Cohen

ASSOCIATE DESIGNERS
Scott M. Stephens
Carol Stickles

ASSISTANT PHOTOGRAPHER
Thom Staudenmayer

EDITORIAL/GRAPHIC COORDINATOR
Doreen K. Stowers

ADMINISTRATIVE ASSISTANT
Cynthia A. O'Connell

COPY EDITORS
Barbara Hodgson
David R. Moreau

EDITORIAL STAFF ASSISTANT
Katharine G. Morris

ART PRODUCTION MANAGER
Robert Perry

ARTISTS
Diane Fox
Donald G. Knauss
Sandra Sanders
Louise Stamper
Joan Walsh
Robert Walsh
Ron Yablon

RESEARCHER
Vonda Heller

TYPOGRAPHY MANAGER
David C. Kosten

TYPOGRAPHY ASSISTANTS
Janice Haber
Ethel Halle
Diane Paluba
Nancy Wirs

PRODUCTION MANAGERS
Wilbur D. Davidson
Robert L. Dean, Jr.

PRODUCTION ASSISTANT
Terry Cooney

ILLUSTRATORS
Michael Adams
Robert Jackson
Bob Jones
Bud Yingling

SERIES GRAPHIC DESIGNER
John C. Isely

COVER PHOTO
Photographic Illustrations

Clinical consultants for this volume

Marie I. Piovoso, RN, BSN
Staff Nurse, Acute Hemodialysis Unit
Wilmington Medical Center
Wilmington, Del.

Susan Ruppert, RN, BSN, MSN
Practitioner/Teacher
Department of Nursing Education
University of Texas Health Science Center
San Antonio, Tex.

PB-010283

Library of Congress Cataloging in Publication Data

Main entry under title:

Carrying out special procedures.

(Nursing photobook)
Bibliography: p.
Includes index.
1. Nursing. 2. Diagnosis, Laboratory. I. Intermed Communications, Inc. II. Series.
RT48.C38 1983 616 82-25846
ISBN 0-916730-45-X

Contents

Contributors

At the time of original publication, these contributors held the following positions.

Leland J. Green, an allergist in the Lansdale (Pa.) Medical Group, received his MD degree from the University of Minnesota in Minneapolis. He is a member of the American Society for Clinical Hypnosis and the Society of Neuro-Linguistic Programming.

Patricia A. Hong, a captain in the U.S. Air Force Nurse Corps, is on the staff in the Special Care Unit at the U.S. Air Force Hospital, Elmendorf Air Force Base in Anchorage, Alaska. She received a BSN degree from the University of Maryland in Baltimore and an MA degree from the University of Washington in Seattle. Ms. Hong is a member of the American Association of Critical-Care Nurses.

Molly McKenney is a nutrition support nurse at the Wilmington (Del.) Medical Center. She earned a BSN degree from the University of Delaware in Newark.

Pamela S. Messer is a nursing supervisor at the Bryn Mawr Rehabilitation Hospital in Malvern, Pennsylvania. She earned her BSN degree from Widener University in Chester, Pennsylvania and is currently working toward an MSN/MBA degree. Ms. Messer is a member of the American Nurses' Association, the Pennsylvania Nurses' Association, and the Association of Rehabilitation Nurses.

Carlene R. Peat, a pulmonary nurse specialist, is supervisor of the Respiratory Care Department at the Kaiser Foundation Hospital in Walnut Creek, California. Ms. Peat earned a nursing diploma from the St. Francis School of Nursing, Hamtramek, Michigan; a BSN degree from Holy Names College, Oakland, California; and certification as a respiratory therapist from Pruitt College, Concord, California.

Marie I. Piovoso, an advisor for this PHOTOBOOK, is a staff nurse in the Acute Hemodialysis Unit at the Wilmington (Del.) Medical Center. She received a BSN degree from the University of Delaware in Newark.

Susan Ruppert, also an advisor for this book, is a practitioner/teacher in the Department of Nursing Education at The Methodist Hospital in Houston. Ms. Ruppert holds an associate degree in nursing from the Illinois Valley Community College in Oglesby, a BSN degree from Northern Illinois University in DeKalb, and an MSN degree from the University of Texas Health Science Center in San Antonio.

Ellen Sitton is a radiotherapy nurse specialist IV at the M.D. Anderson Hospital in Houston. She earned a nursing diploma from Cook County Hospital School of Nursing in Chicago and a BSN degree from the University of Illinois, also in Chicago.

Deborah Smolka is a home peritoneal dialysis nurse coordinator at the Wilmington (Del.) Medical Center. Ms. Smolka was graduated with a BSN degree from the University of Delaware in Newark.

Introduction

Chances are, you're already a highly competent nurse. And this means you're always looking for opportunities to refine your skills. This PHOTOBOOK's designed for nurses like you. Use it to learn about some procedures that may not be part of your daily routine. By mastering them, you can give each patient the best care, no matter what his particular health problems are.

Consider diagnostic testing, for instance. Are you accustomed to collecting blood and urine specimens—and then seeing them whisked away to the lab for analysis? If so, you may be surprised to learn that you can easily perform many routine diagnostic tests yourself, right in your unit. We show you how. In addition to blood and urine testing, you'll learn how to assess nutritional status, determine gastric pH, and identify cerebrospinal fluid drainage. We also provide detailed information on glaucoma screening using either an indentation (Schiøtz) tonometer or a noncontact tonometer.

Now, think about all the new equipment and techniques that seem to appear almost daily. For your patient, these advances can be invaluable—as long as you know how to put them to good use. This book's second section will help. In it, you'll learn about pumps designed to deliver cardiovascular medications, tube feedings, and insulin. You'll also find out about specific I.V. administration equipment that'll make your job easier and other equipment, such as the Hickman catheter, that can make your patient's *life* easier.

Next, we shift our focus to the patient with a special problem. Has he suffered traumatic injuries? Does he have kidney disease? Cancer? Disseminated intravascular coagulation? Learn new approaches to these health problems in the third section. In it, you'll find information on such procedures as autotransfusion, compartment syndrome monitoring, peritoneal lavage, and continuous ambulatory peritoneal dialysis. You'll also learn about radiation therapy precautions and special care considerations for a comatose patient.

The final section of this book deals with problems you've probably faced many times but may not have known how to handle. Suppose, for example, your patient has a trach tube in place. How can the two of you communicate with minimal frustration? We have some practical suggestions you'll find helpful. Ever attempted to help a patient put on a brace or prosthesis—and felt inept doing so? After reading the chapter on braces and prostheses, you'll be prepared to assist with confidence. Does your patient have questions about alternate pain control methods, such as acupuncture and hypnosis? We supply information that'll enable you to discuss the pros and cons of each. We also provide details on postmortem care and outline your responsibilities when organ donation is anticipated.

We think you'll be impressed with the wide range of procedures we cover. What do they have in common? They all help you give your patients the care they deserve—which we all agree is the very best.

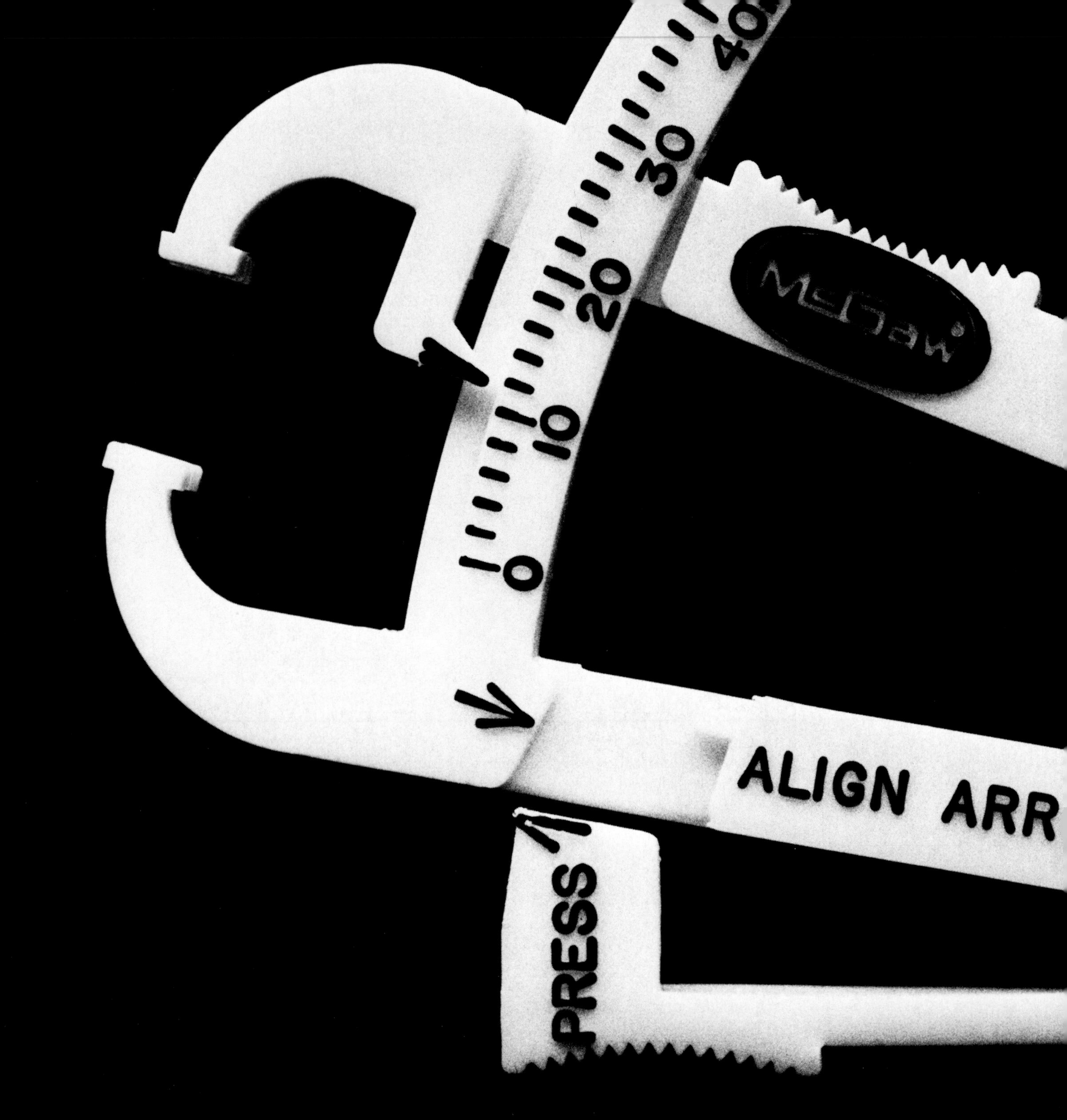

0
10
20
30
40
ALIGN ARR
PRESS

Performing Diagnostic Procedures

Urine tests

Blood tests

Nutritional tests

Special tests

Urine tests

Urine testing can provide valuable information about your patient's condition. By following the procedures shown on the next few pages, you can assess your patient's urine quickly, easily, and with a minimum of equipment.

Why are these tests so valuable? Because their results can help the doctor decide whether to order more extensive tests or change your patient's treatment plan. And because they're easy to perform, you can include them in your nursing routine.

In the following pages, you'll learn how to:

- collect a urine specimen.
- use such tablets as Clinitest and Acetest to check for urine glucose and ketones.
- use reagent strips.
- measure urine's specific gravity.

In addition, we provide you with a list of medications that can alter urine test results. To learn more, study this section carefully.

How the kidneys produce urine

As a prelude to urine testing, let's briefly review kidney function. Your patient should have two kidneys, one on either side of his spine. These red-brown, bean-shaped organs are about the length and width of an adult's fist and are situated at the back of the abdominal cavity, between the thoracic and lumbar regions.

As you know, the kidneys serve as the body's filtering units. When functioning properly, they:

- excrete excess water and nitrogenous waste products of metabolism (chiefly creatinine and urea).
- conserve and reabsorb essential substances in the blood; for instance, sugars, sodium, and potassium.
- regulate the acid-base balance, volume, and electrolyte concentration of blood plasma.
- secrete hormones essential to blood flow and arterial pressure, including renin (a potent hypertensive) and erythropoietin, which stimulates red blood cell production.

Understanding kidney function

Blood enters each kidney through the renal artery and passes through progressively smaller vascular channels. The blood then enters the nephrons, the kidney's principal filtering units. Read the story at right to better understand how nephrons work.

The kidneys return to the body about 99% of the water filtered from the blood. The remaining water and most of its solutes are excreted as urine.

Urine composition and volume

Urine always includes water, urea, uric acid, and sodium chloride. In addition, it usually contains other nonprotein nitrogen compounds, citric acid and other organic acids, and sulfur-containing compounds. If the kidneys aren't functioning properly for any reason, urine may also contain such substances as protein, glucose, ketones, hemoglobin, lipids, bacteria, pus, urobilinogen, calculi, white blood cells, and red blood cells.

Normally, urine ranges in color from pale yellow to dark amber. It should be clear, with only a mild odor. But its appearance and odor may be affected by diet, physical activity, and emotional stress.

The kidneys closely regulate urine volume, which depends on fluid intake, solute concentration in the filtrate, cardiac output, hormonal influences, and fluid loss through the lungs, large bowel, and skin. Although an adult's urine volume may range from 800 to 2,000 ml/day, the average is 1,200 to 1,500 ml/day. A child's volume ranges from 300 to 1,500 ml/day.

When your patient's urine volume exceeds 2,000 ml/day, document the problem as polyuria. Document urine volume below 500 ml/day as oliguria and urine volume below 125 ml/day as anuria. If your patient develops any of these problems, investigate quickly to determine the cause.

Following the nephron pathway

Each kidney contains more than 1 million nephrons, a complicated collection of ducts and blood vessels that filter metabolic wastes, excess water, electrolytes, and other substances from the blood. Each day, the nephrons filter about 200 qt (189 liters) of blood.

Here's how the nephron pathway works:

- The afferent arteriole brings blood to the glomerulus, a vascular ultrafilter that's enfolded in Bowman's capsule. The glomerulus removes some water and all solutes, except colloids (large molecules, such as proteins and certain starches).
- The efferent arteriole then carries the filtered blood away from the glomerulus and returns it to the renal artery.
- From the glomerulus, the filtered fluid (glomerular filtrate) travels through the proximal convoluted tubule, Henle's loop, the distal convoluted tubule, and the collecting tubule. As the fluid travels, the kidney begins reabsorbing many of the filtered substances, according to the body's needs, by either *passive transport* or *active transport.*

Passive transport occurs when a substance is transported without any energy expenditure by cells. Take water, for example. When water concentration inside the tubules is greater than it is in the bloodstream, water's *passively* transported by osmosis and diffusion from the tubules back into the bloodstream.

Other substances (such as potassium, glucose, and sodium) are *actively* transported when a cell releases energy to capture and absorb them. Depending on its needs, the cell may then use the substances, return them to the tubule, or expel them into the bloodstream.

A cell may also actively excrete substances (for example, hydrogen and urate ions) into the tubules. Some passive secretion also occurs. All these mechanisms help the body conserve substances it needs and dispose of those it doesn't need.

- The final waste product—urine—drains from the collecting tubule into the kidney pelvis.
- Finally, the urine travels from the kidney pelvis through the ureter to the bladder, which excretes it.

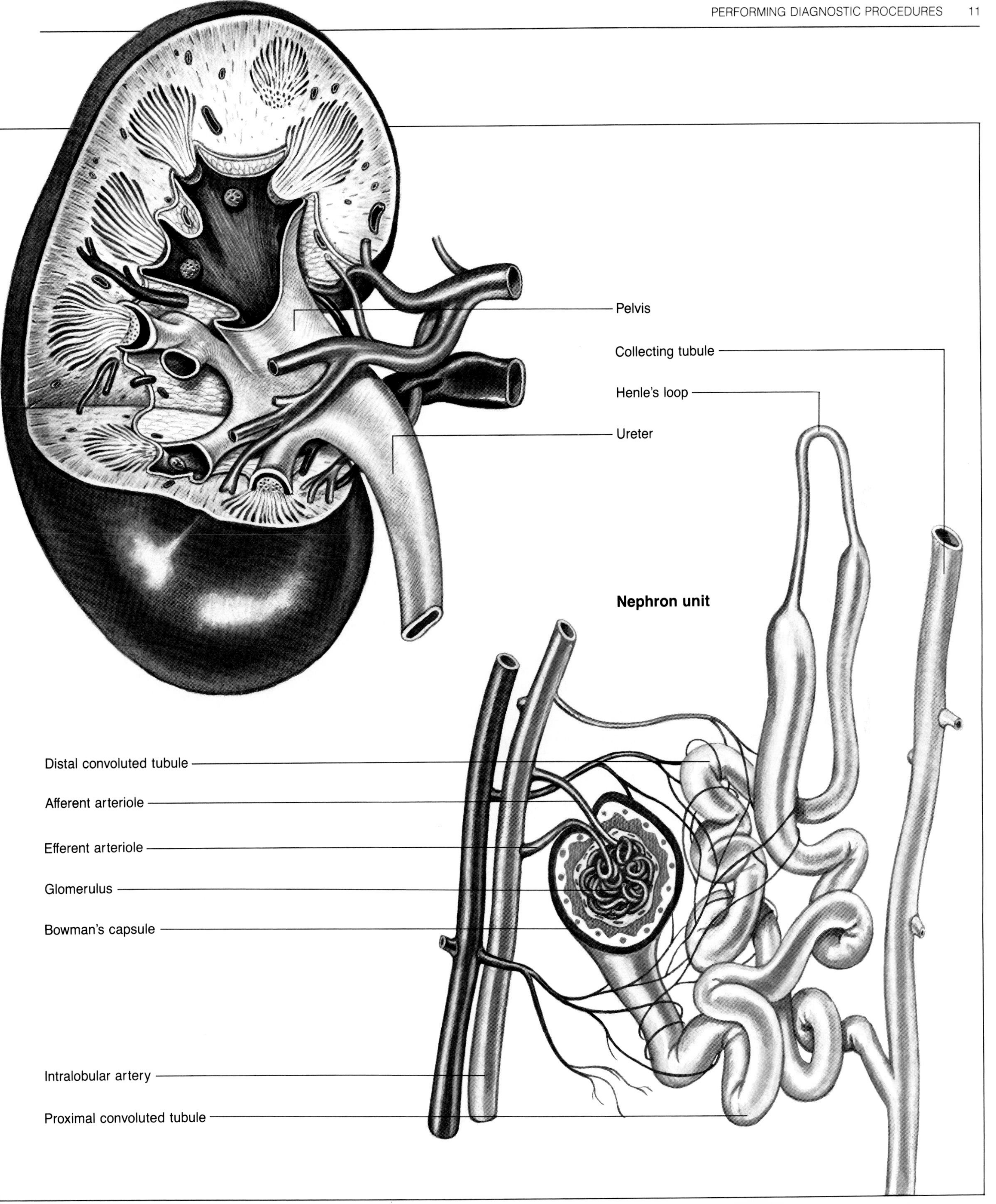
Pelvis
Collecting tubule
Henle's loop
Ureter
Nephron unit
Distal convoluted tubule
Afferent arteriole
Efferent arteriole
Glomerulus
Bowman's capsule
Intralobular artery
Proximal convoluted tubule

Urine tests

Learning about urine specimen types

When you ask your patient for a urine specimen, you'll request one of the following six types.

- *Random.* Patient simply urinates into a specimen container. Because a random specimen is easy to collect, test results can be available quickly. But test results are generally less reliable than those obtained with other specimen types.
- *Second voided.* Patient urinates and discards the urine. Thirty minutes later, he urinates into a specimen container.
- *Clean catch (midstream).* Patient carefully cleans his penis (a female patient cleans her perineum), urinates a small amount into a bedpan or toilet, and stops. Then, he uses a sterile specimen container to catch the urine in midstream.
- *First morning.* Patient urinates and collects a specimen immediately after waking in the morning. This specimen type contains the day's most concentrated urine, so it's especially suitable for nitrate, protein, and sediment analyses.
- *Fasting.* Patient fasts overnight and collects a first-morning specimen. The fasting specimen is used for glucose testing.
- *Timed.* The most common timed specimen is a 24-hour collection. The timed specimen determines the urinary concentration of such substances as proteins and creatinine, permitting a comparison with the total output over a specified period. *Note:* Certain tests require that the 24-hour specimen be collected in a special container or that it be refrigerated. Check your lab manual.

Aspirating a urine specimen

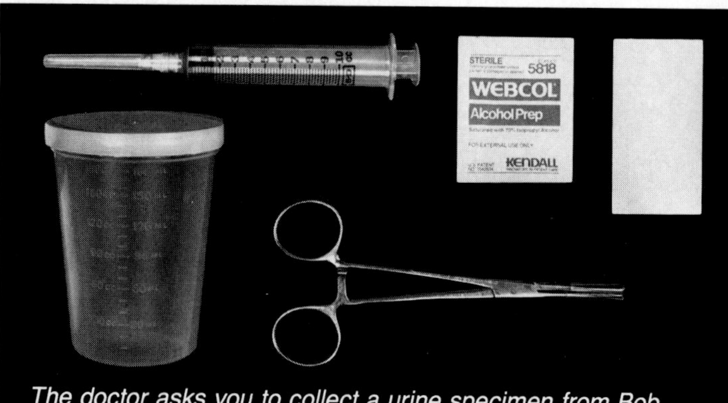

The doctor asks you to collect a urine specimen from Bob Schaffer, a 36-year-old diabetic with an indwelling (Foley) catheter.

Because the Foley catheter is a closed system, don't disconnect the catheter from the drainage tubing to take a specimen. Doing so can introduce bacteria into the patient's urinary tract. Instead, aspirate urine from the drainage tubing aspiration port. Here's how.

First, gather the following equipment: sterile 10-ml syringe, 21G or 22G needle, alcohol swab, sterile specimen container with cap, label, and guarded hemostat or toothless clamp.

Note: *Don't use a needle with a bore larger than 21G. Repeated use of larger needles may cause the port to leak, contaminating the system.*

Wash your hands. Then, tell your patient what you're going to do.

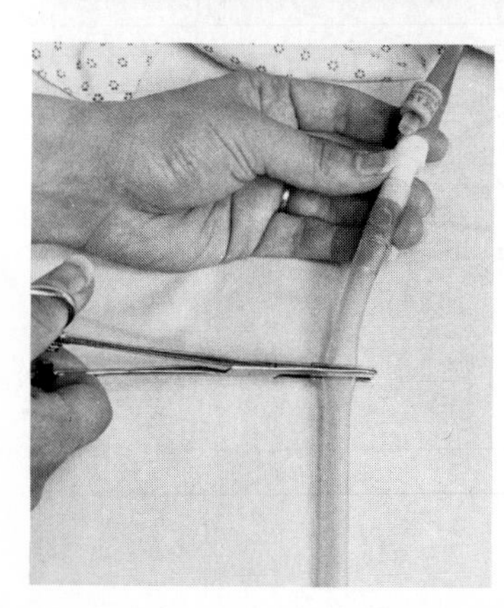

1 If urine is already flowing through the drainage tubing, a specimen is readily available. But if urine isn't flowing, clamp the tubing 3″ (7.6 cm) distal to the aspiration port, as shown. Then, check the tubing every 5 to 10 minutes for sufficient urine accumulation. *Caution:* Leaving the tubing clamped for longer than 10 minutes may cause urine to pool in the bladder, which may lead to infection.

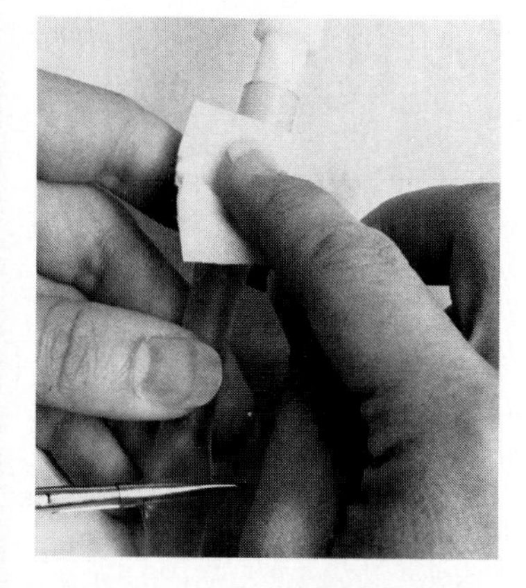

2 When enough urine's collected in the tubing, prepare to aspirate the specimen. First, clean the aspiration port with an alcohol swab, as the nurse is doing here.

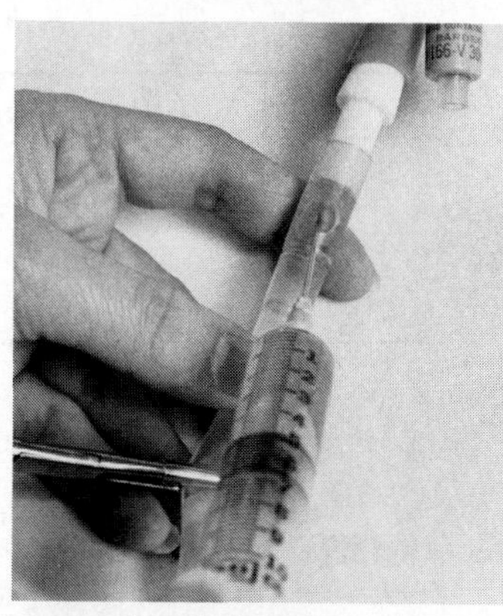

3 Uncap the needle. Then, insert the needle in the aspiration port and aspirate the specimen, as shown.

Note: If the catheter tubing is rubber and self-sealing, you can aspirate the specimen from the distal end of the catheter. But remember, this works only with rubber catheters. Silastic, silicone, and plastic catheters aren't self-sealing.

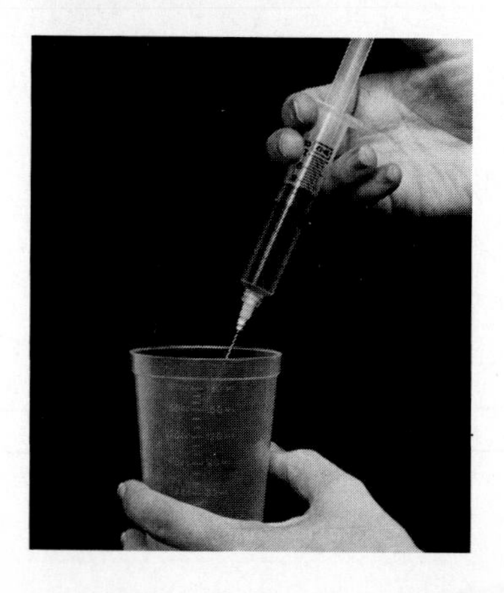

4 Next, withdraw the needle, and expel the urine into the specimen container. Then remove the clamp from the drainage tubing. Cap the container and label it. If you can't test the urine immediately, refrigerate it.

Document on your patient's intake/output record the amount of urine aspirated.

Interpreting urine test results

Is your patient taking medications? If so, they may affect urine test results. Some medications, for example, cause positive results through a local effect on the kidneys; however, these results don't reflect a systemic disorder. Other medications cause false-positive results. Can you identify these medications and anticipate their effects on urine testing? Read this chart for guidance.

	Clinistix	Clinitest tablet	Diastix	Ketostix	Acetest tablet	Tes-Tape	Specific gravity
Albumin							○
Ammonium chloride	–	–	–			–	
Ascorbic acid (large doses)	▲	+	▲			▲	
Asparaginase	–	–	–			–	
Carbamazepine	–	–	–			–	
Cephalosporins		+					
Chloramphenicol		+					
Corticosteroids	–	–	–			–	
Dextran							○
Dextrothyroxine	–	–	–			–	
Ether				#	#		
Glucose (concentrated)							○
Insulin (excessive doses)				#	#		
Isoniazid		+		#	#		
Isopropyl alcohol				#	#		
Levodopa	▲	+				▲	
Lithium carbonate	–	–	–			–	
Mannitol							○
Metaxalone		+					
Methyldopa	+					+	
Nalidixic acid		+					
Nicotinic acid	–	–	–			–	
Phenazopyridine	+		+	*		+	
Phenothiazines (long-term)	–	–	–			–	
Probenecid		+					
Radiopaque contrast media							○
Salicylates (large doses)	▲	+	▲	*	*	▲	
Sulfobromophthalein (BSP dye)				*	*		
Tetracycline		+					
Tetracycline with ascorbic acid buffer		+					
Thiazide diuretics	–	–	–			–	

Key
+ causes false-positive glycosuria
– causes true glycosuria
▲ causes false-negative glucose results
* causes false-positive ketonuria
# causes true ketonuria
○ increases specific gravity

Urine tests

Testing for ketones

Now that you have Mr. Schaffer's urine specimen, you can begin testing it. First, test for ketones, which appear in urine only when fat metabolism increases; for example, in starvation or uncontrolled diabetes mellitus. To detect ketones, you'll perform an Acetest. The white Acetest tablet, which contains glycine, reacts to ketones present in urine by turning lavender-purple.

Prepare for the test by obtaining a bottle of Acetest tablets with accompanying color chart, urine specimen, medicine dropper, and paper towel. Remember, make sure you test the specimen within 60 minutes after collecting it. Otherwise, refrigerate the specimen, and then allow it to warm to room temperature before testing it.

Explain the procedure to your patient. Important: *For accurate results, perform the test in a well-lighted area.*

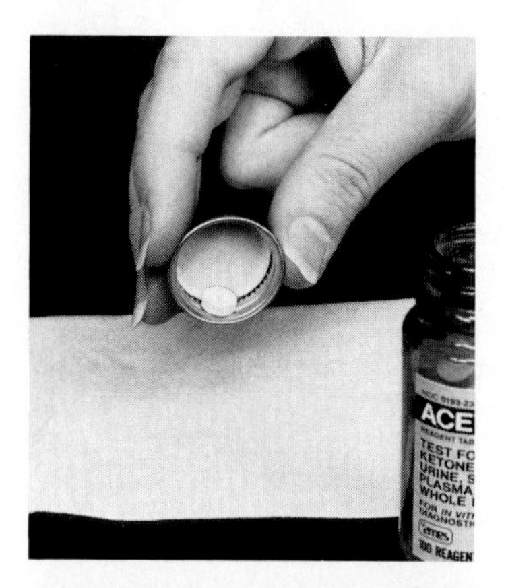

1 First, check the expiration date on the Acetest bottle to make sure its contents are fresh. Next, transfer a single tablet to the bottle cap. Then, gently drop it onto the paper.

Note: Make sure the tablet is white. If it's darkened or discolored, discard it.

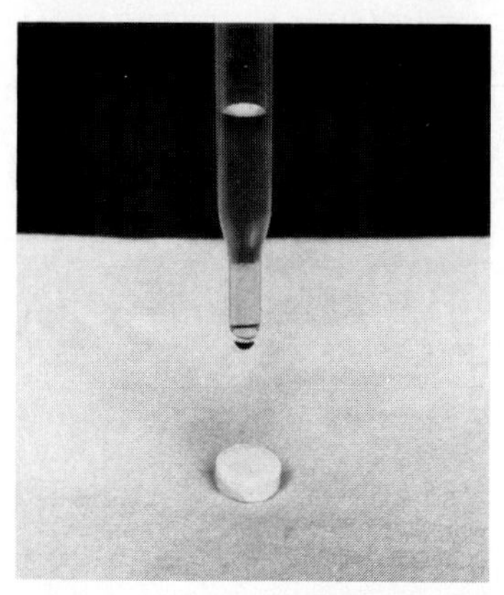

2 Next, place one drop of urine on the tablet. Wait 30 seconds and then compare the tablet's color with the color chart.

Important: Make sure you read the test result at exactly 30 seconds. After 2 minutes' exposure to urine, Acetest tablets turn purple, regardless of the urine's ketone content.

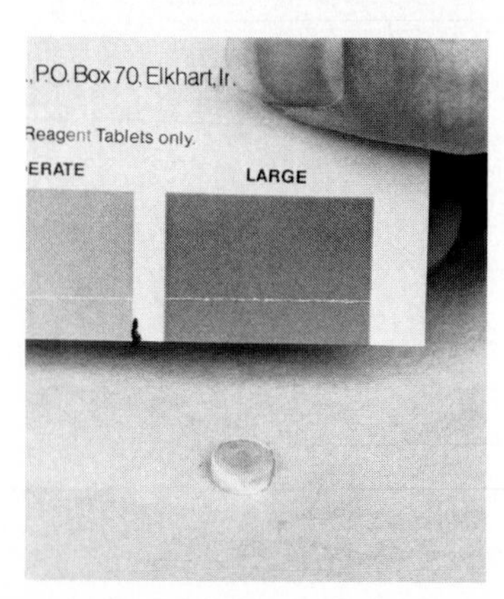

3 After determining which chart color most closely matches the tablet's color, record the test result. Identify the result as negative, trace, moderate, or large, depending on the tablet's color change.

Inform the doctor if ketones are detected in Mr. Schaffer's urine. Finally, document the results on the appropriate form.

Using a Clinitest reagent tablet

Sixty-two-year-old Mildred Copenhaver has diabetes. The doctor orders glucose oxidase testing to monitor her urine glucose levels during insulin therapy. You'll use a Clinitest reagent tablet, as shown below. Here's how it works:

When you drop a Clinitest tablet into a urine and water solution, a chemical reaction occurs. As the tablet dissolves, the solution changes color. By observing this color change, you can determine the amount of sugar in your patient's urine.

First, obtain the following: urine specimen, medicine dropper, water, 10-ml test tube, bottle of Clinitest tablets, Clinitest color chart, and a watch with a second hand. Check the tablet bottle's expiration date before proceeding.

Caution: *Perform this test with special care. Because a Clinitest tablet can cause a caustic burn when it reacts with moisture, try to avoid touching it.*

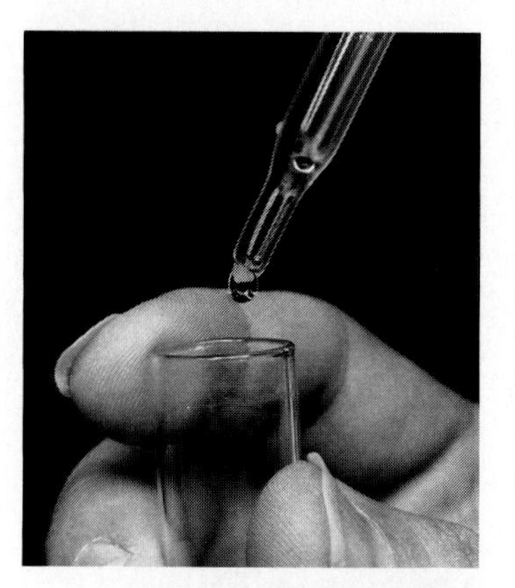

1 Fill the medicine dropper with urine. Then, squeeze 5 drops of urine into the test tube, as the nurse is doing here.

Note: If you suspect more than 2% glucose in your patient's urine, use the Clinitest 2-drop method, as shown in step 7.

Next, thoroughly rinse out the medicine dropper with water, and add 10 drops of water to the test tube.

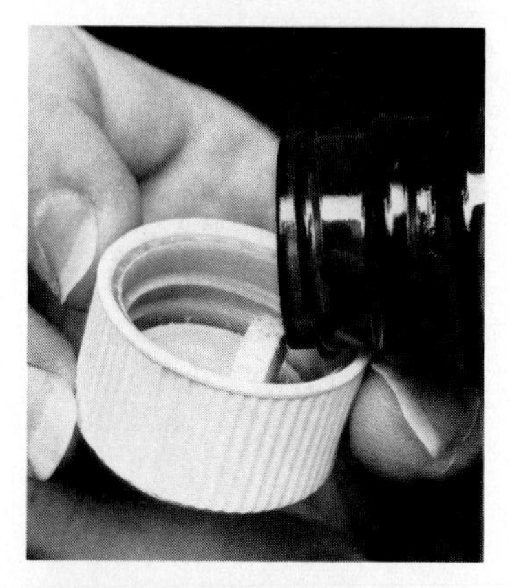

2 Now, unscrew the Clinitest bottle cap and allow a tablet to fall into the cap. Check to be sure the tablet's a mottled blue-white color. If it's dark blue, discard it and obtain a fresh one.

Remember: Avoid touching the tablet. If you must handle it, make sure your hands are dry.

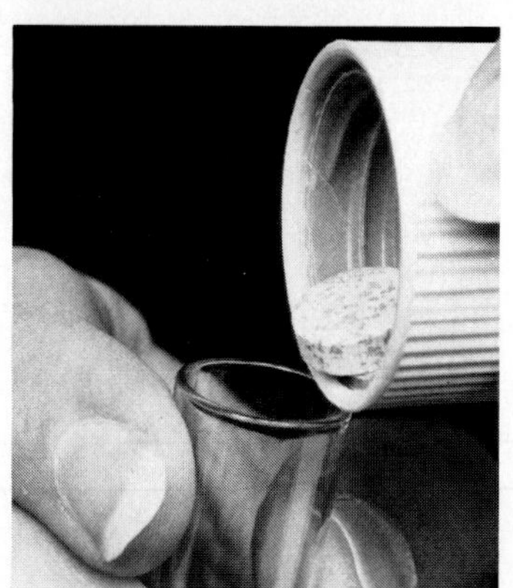

3 Place the test tube in a rack or hold the tube close to the top. This'll prevent thermal burns from the tablet's reaction to the urine. Then, drop the tablet into the test tube. When the tablet effervesces, the mixture becomes boiling hot.

Immediately recap the bottle, to keep the remaining tablets fresh.

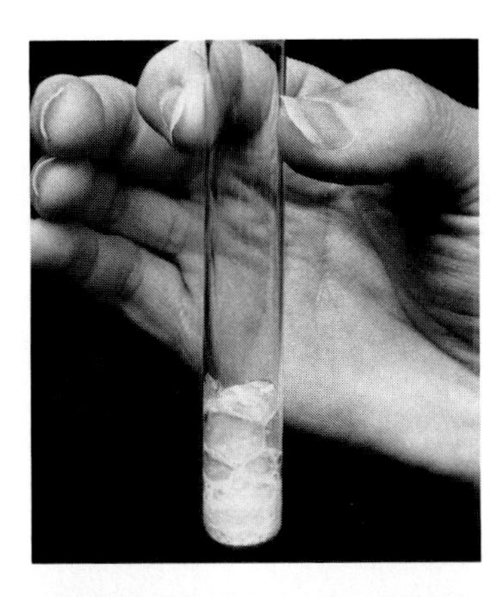

4 You may see an immediate, rapid color change from blue-green to orange to green-brown. This rapid reaction, called the pass-through phase, signifies a high urine glucose level. Document the results as over 2% (2 g/dl or more).

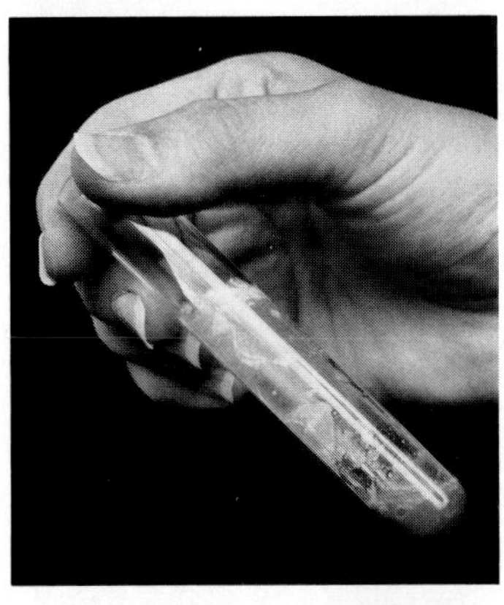

5 If the pass-through phase doesn't occur, allow the effervescence to subside. Then, wait 15 seconds and gently agitate the mixture in the tube.

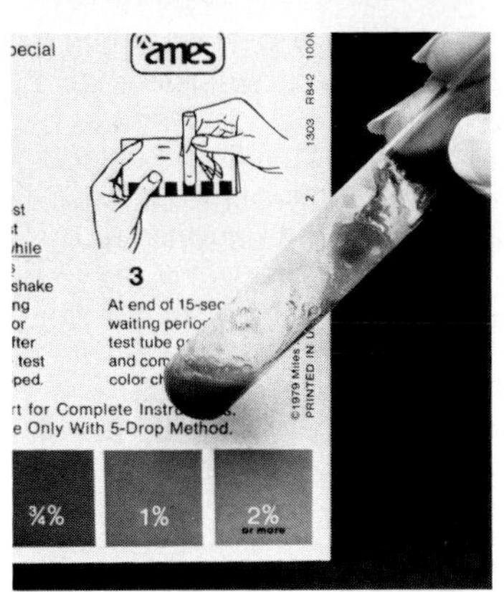

6 If you observe immediate color changes, hold the test tube against the Clinitest color chart. Make sure you perform the comparison in a well-lighted area. Document the results.

Note: Ignore any color changes that occur after 15 seconds.

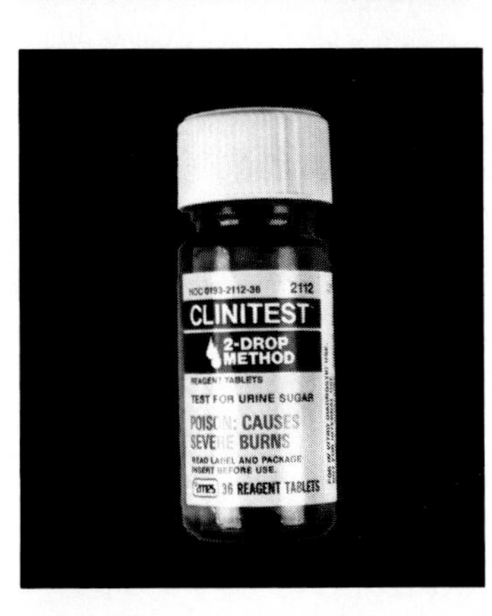

7 The Clinitest 2-drop method can help you identify up to 5% glucose in the urine. Obtain Clinitest 2-drop–method tablets and proceed as above, with this exception: Use only 2 drops of urine instead of 5. Be sure to use the special color chart for the 2-drop method.

Finally, document the results on the appropriate form.

Learning about reagent strips

You may use a reagent strip to test your patient's urine for hemoglobin, glucose, ketones, pH, and protein. Most types are firm plastic strips with reagent blocks affixed to one end. These blocks change color when they come in contact with the urine contents you're testing for.

Note: One exception is Tes-Tape (see page 17). This strip has no block affixed to it. During a test, the section of the strip that is immersed changes color.

Tests using reagent strips can be performed quickly and easily. All you need is the strip, a corresponding color chart, a fresh urine specimen, and a watch with a second hand. After recording your results, immediately dispose of the strip.

Ensuring accurate results

For accurate test results, follow these guidelines:

- Collect the urine in a clean, dry container. (If the container's reusable, remove all soap residue before using it.) Then, perform the test as quickly as possible.
- Use a fresh urine specimen. If you can't perform the test within an hour after collecting the specimen, refrigerate it. Prolonged exposure of unpreserved urine to room temperature may result in microbial contamination and bacterial consumption of urine glucose. This causes false-negative test results. *Note:* Allow a refrigerated specimen to warm to room temperature before testing it.
- Avoid touching the strip's reagent blocks with your fingers. If you do, discard the strip and use a fresh one.
- Follow the test directions carefully, and observe the color of the test blocks at exactly the time specified; for instance, after 30 seconds. *Important:* Always compare the test blocks with the color chart under a bright light. Have a co-worker make the comparison if you're color blind.

Storage tips

Store the bottles of reagent strips in a dry, dark location, at a temperature below 86° F. (30° C.). But don't store them in a refrigerator. Dispose of a bottle and its contents after the expiration date marked on the label has passed or if its contents have been exposed to heat, moisture, or excessive air. Also, discard any strip with darkened or discolored reagent blocks.

When you open a new bottle of reagent strips, mark the date on the bottle's label. If you don't use all the strips within 4 months of this date, dispose of the bottle and its remaining contents.

To preserve each strip's sensitivity, never remove one until you plan to use it. Then, replace the bottle cap.

Urine tests

Using reagent strips

Let's assume you're caring for 41-year-old Hugh Wynn, who was admitted to your unit with possible kidney trauma. As part of the diagnostic workup, his doctor orders thorough urine testing to monitor ketones, glucose levels, and blood pigment levels. Do you know how to proceed?

Of course, you'll measure blood pigment with a Hemastix reagent strip. But you can measure ketones and glucose level in one of several ways. For convenience and accuracy, use Keto-Diastix, if possible; this strip measures both *ketones and glucose level. If Keto-Diastix isn't available, measure the glucose level with either Diastix or Clinistix. Then, measure ketones with Ketostix. In this photostory, we'll show you how to use all these reagent strips.*

After obtaining bottles of the strips you need, explain the procedure to your patient. Because you'll need a second-voided specimen, tell him how to collect one.

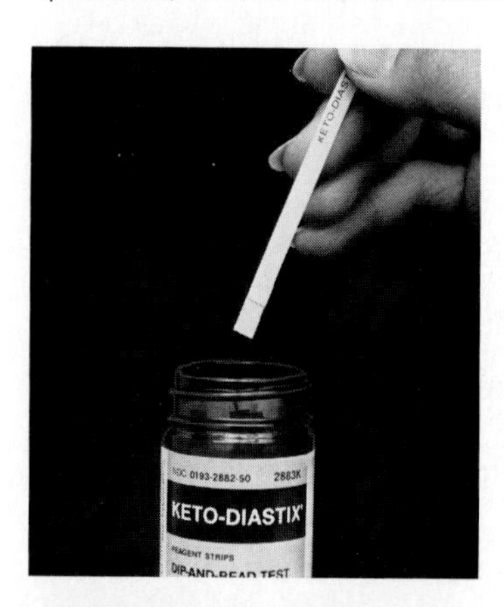

1 After obtaining the urine specimen, prepare to test it for ketones and glucose with a Keto-Diastix strip. Remove a strip from the bottle and immediately recap the bottle.

As you know, the strip has two test blocks affixed to one end. The ketone test block is buff-pink; the glucose test block is green. *Important:* Don't use the strip if its blocks are darkened or discolored.

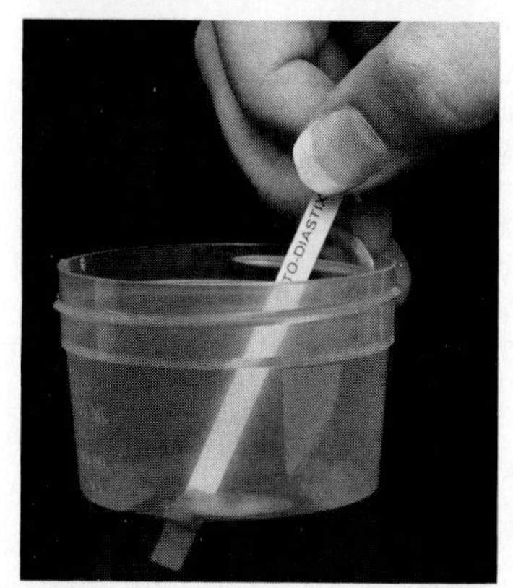

2 Immerse the test blocks in the urine specimen for 1 second.

Then, remove the reagent strip from the specimen and tap the strip against the specimen container to shake off excess urine. Wait 15 seconds, and compare the ketone test block color with the ketone color chart on the bottle label.

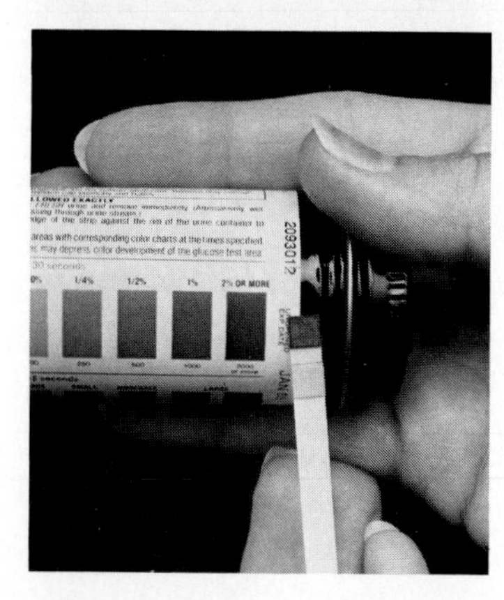

3 Then, wait 15 seconds longer and compare the glucose block with the label's glucose color chart, as the nurse is doing here.

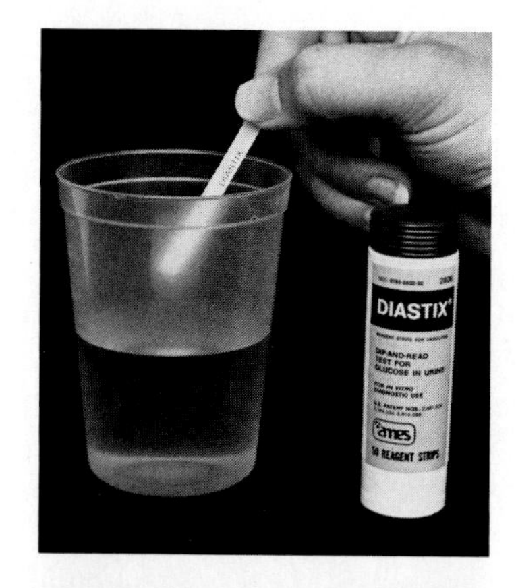

4 Now, suppose you're testing only glucose levels with a Diastix strip.

Dip the strip in the specimen. Remove it immediately and note the time. Then, remove the excess urine by tapping the strip against the container.

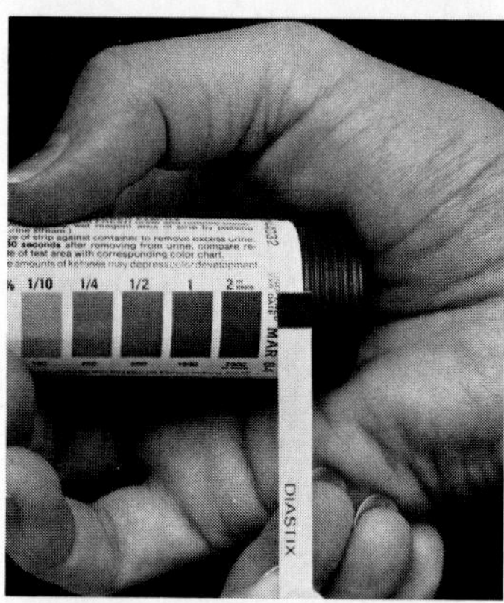

5 Exactly 30 seconds after removing the strip, compare the test block with the bottle's color chart, as shown. Ignore any color changes that develop after 30 seconds.

Document the results.

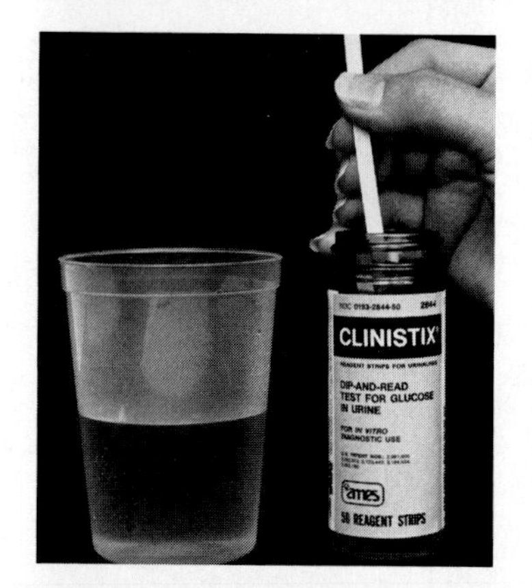

6 If you prefer, use a Clinistix reagent strip instead of Diastix to measure glucose. Keep in mind, however, that Clinistix test results are less precise than Diastix results.

To use a Clinistix strip, immerse its test block in the urine specimen. Remove the strip, and note the time. Remove any excess urine by tapping the strip against the container.

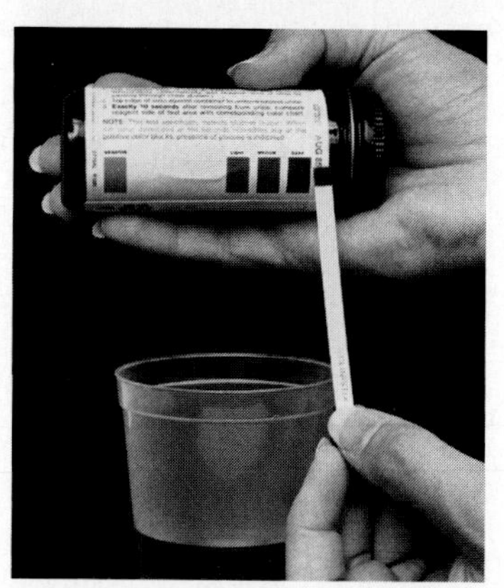

7 Exactly 10 seconds after taking the strip out of the urine, compare the test block's color with the bottle's color chart. Ignore any color changes that develop after 10 seconds.

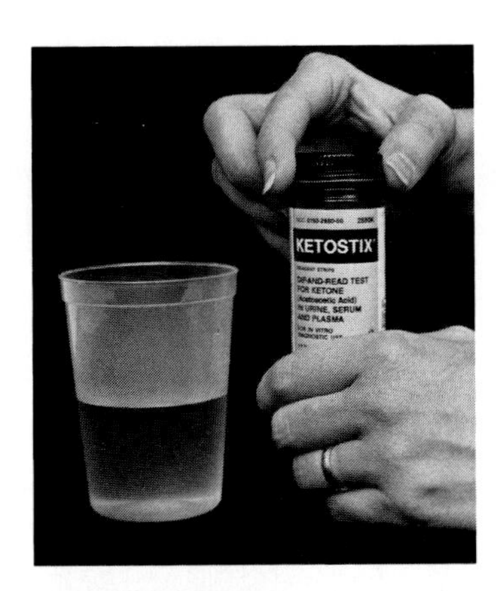

8 Testing strictly for ketones? If so, use a Ketostix reagent strip.

First, dip the strip into the second-voided urine specimen and immediately remove it. Remove excess urine by tapping the strip against the container.

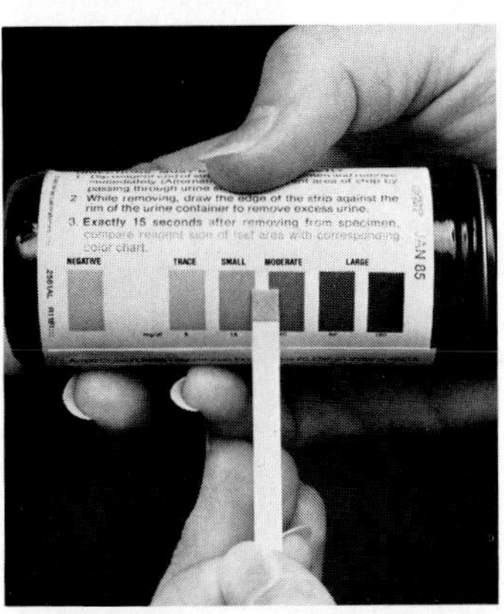

9 Exactly 15 seconds after removing the strip, compare the test block's color with the chart on the label. Then, record your results as negative, trace, small, moderate, or large, depending on your finding.

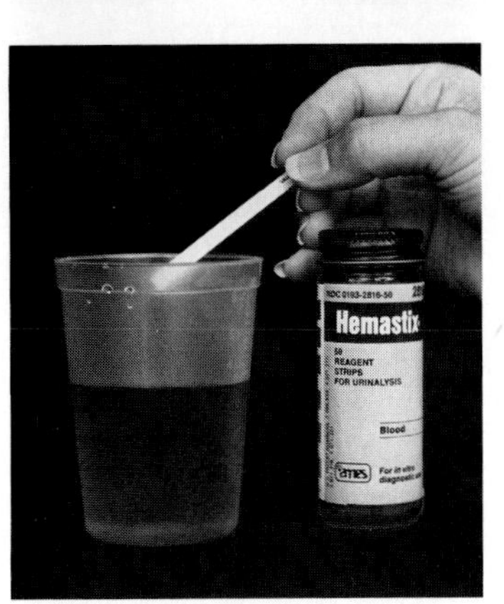

10 To test for blood pigment in the urine, use a Hemastix reagent strip. *Note:* You can use a random urine specimen to perform this test.

To begin, dip the test strip into the urine specimen and immediately withdraw the strip. Note the time. Then, tap the strip against the container to remove excess urine.

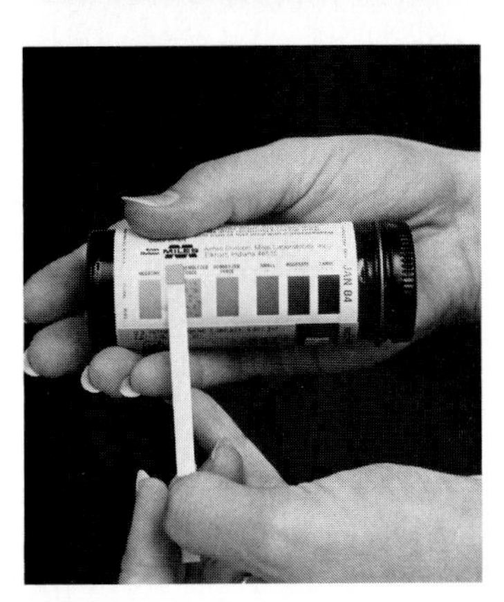

11 Exactly 40 seconds after removing the strip, compare the test block's color with the label's color chart. Consider the test result positive if the block turns blue. A positive result could indicate excessive hemolysis, anemia, or red blood cells in the urine. *Note:* Nephrotoxic drugs and anticoagulants may cause positive results; vitamin C may cause a false-negative result.

Document all results.

Monitoring glucose with Tes-Tape

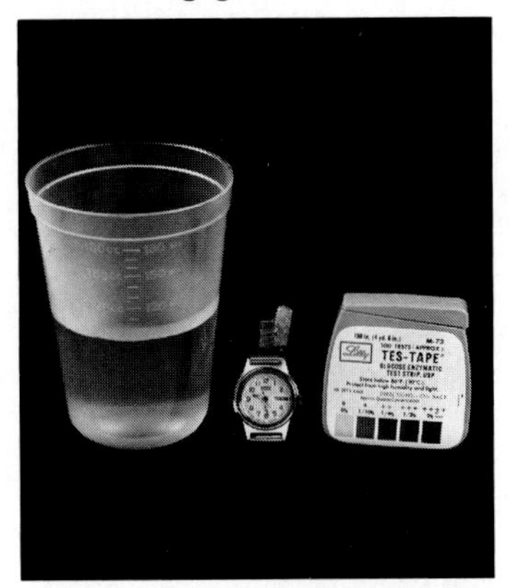

1 Remember Mrs. Copenhaver? You used a Clinitest tablet to determine her urine glucose level (see pages 14 and 15). Let's say the results indicated an unusually high glucose level. You decide to double-check the results with a Tes-Tape reagent strip.

Gather a second-voided specimen, Tes-Tape dispenser, and watch with a second hand. (If it's still fresh, use the same specimen you collected for the Clinitest procedure.)

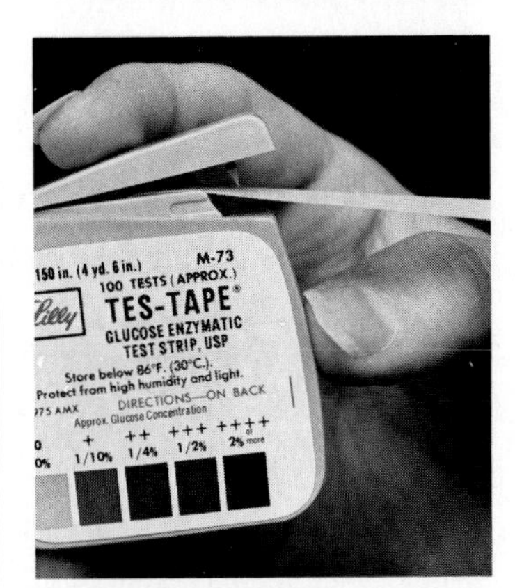

2 To remove a Tes-Tape strip from its dispenser, pull out about 1½" (3.8 cm) from the roll as shown, and snap down the lid. Tear off the strip by pulling it straight out.

Dispose of the strip if it's dark yellow or yellow-brown or if the dispenser's expiration date has passed. Obtain another dispenser before proceeding.

If the strip's OK, use it immediately. Excessive handling may cause false test results.

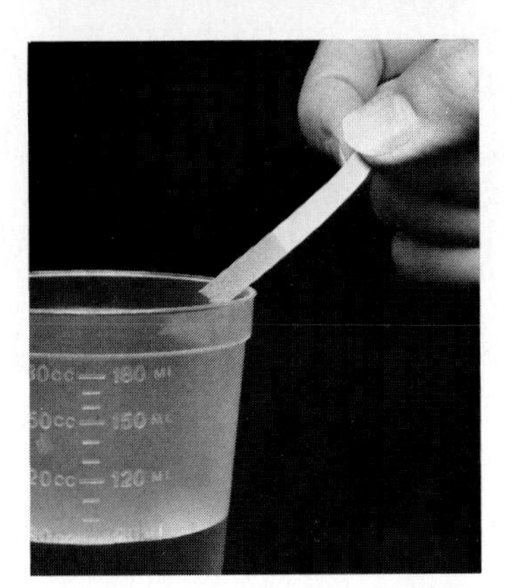

3 Now, immerse ¼" (6 mm) of the strip in the specimen and hold it there for 2 seconds. Then, remove any excess urine by tapping the strip against the side of the container, as the nurse is doing here. Note the time and hold the strip in the air.

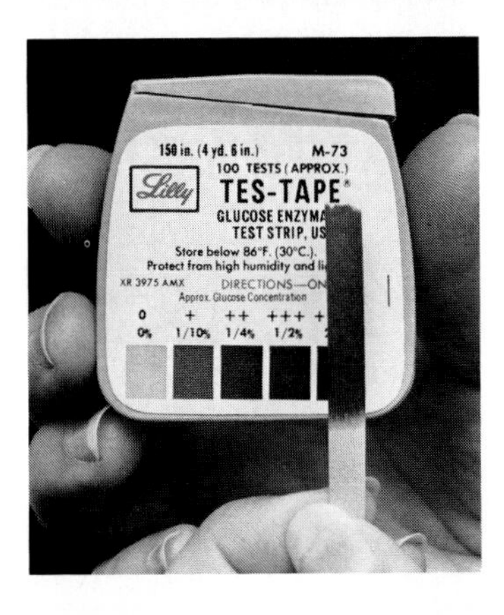

4 Exactly 60 seconds after removing the strip from the urine, examine it under a bright light and compare the darkest part of the strip with the color chart.

If the strip indicates a glucose concentration of ½% (0.5%) or higher, wait an additional 60 seconds and make another comparison.

Finally, document the results on the appropriate form.

Urine tests

Understanding specific gravity

As you know, the kidneys filter out the bloodstream's waste products. But that's not all they do. In addition, they excrete water to maintain the body's fluid balance. The amount of water they excrete depends on the body's needs. When the body's overhydrated, the kidneys excrete more water than they do when the body's dehydrated. The proportion of water to urine waste products determines the urine's concentration.

This proportion is called *specific gravity.* Although specific gravity can range from 1.001 to 1.040, it usually falls between 1.010 and 1.025.

When fluid intake and output are low, expect specific gravity to be high. (For example, specific gravity's usually highest in the morning from lack of fluid intake during sleep.) Conversely, expect specific gravity to be low when fluid intake and output are high.

You can measure specific gravity in urine with a refractometer or a urinometer. By determining specific gravity, these instruments help you evaluate the kidneys' capacity to concentrate urine in response to fluid intake.

For more information on testing for specific gravity and interpreting the results, carefully read the next few pages.

Using a refractometer

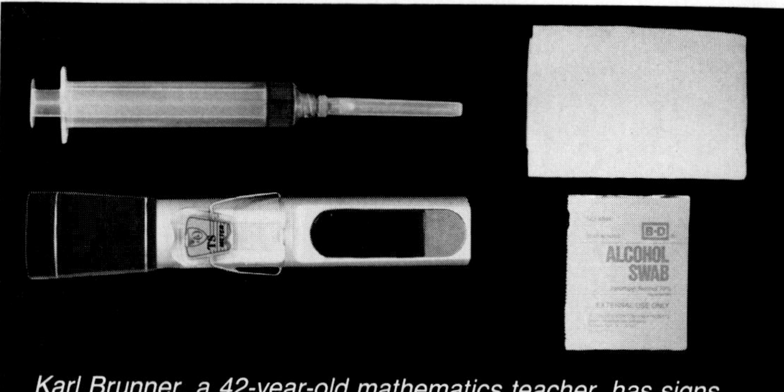

Karl Brunner, a 42-year-old mathematics teacher, has signs of acute kidney failure. His daily urinary output is less than 350 ml, while his blood urea nitrogen, serum creatinine, and serum potassium levels are elevated. To obtain the most accurate output measurements, the doctor has ordered the insertion of an indwelling (Foley) catheter. As part of your assessment, you'll measure the specific gravity of Mr. Brunner's urine.

Because Mr. Brunner's urinary output is low, perform this test with a refractometer, which requires only three drops of urine. The cylindrical refractometer determines the refraction index of urine. This measurement correlates closely to specific gravity.

Before proceeding with the test, collect the equipment shown above: 10-ml syringe with 21G needle, alcohol swab, refractometer, and tissue or lens paper. Then, explain the procedure to your patient.

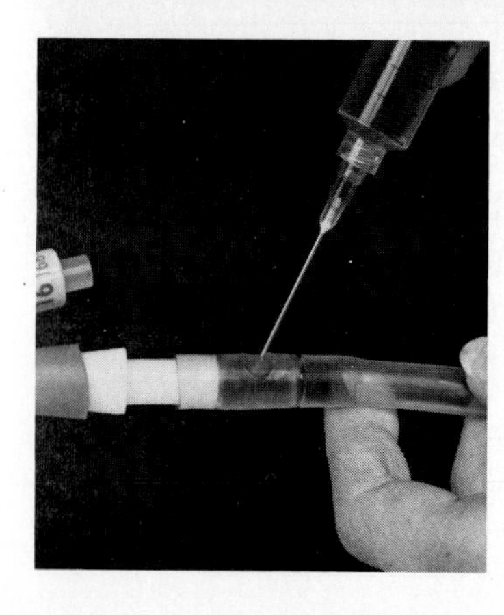

1 Next, clean the catheter's aspiration port with the alcohol swab. Then, use the needle and syringe to aspirate urine from your patient's catheter.

Note: Because the refractometer requires only three drops, use the remaining urine for other testing procedures; for instance, to measure ketones and glucose.

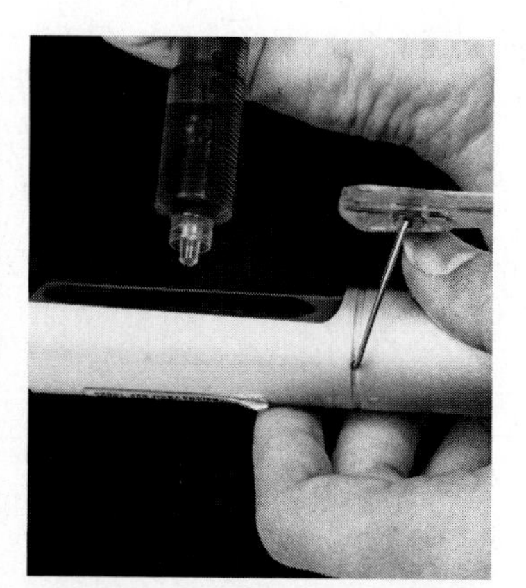

2 Lift the plastic coverslip attached to the tapered end of the refractometer. Then, place three drops of urine on the tapered end. To trap the urine between the coverslip and the refractometer's scale, slowly replace the coverslip.

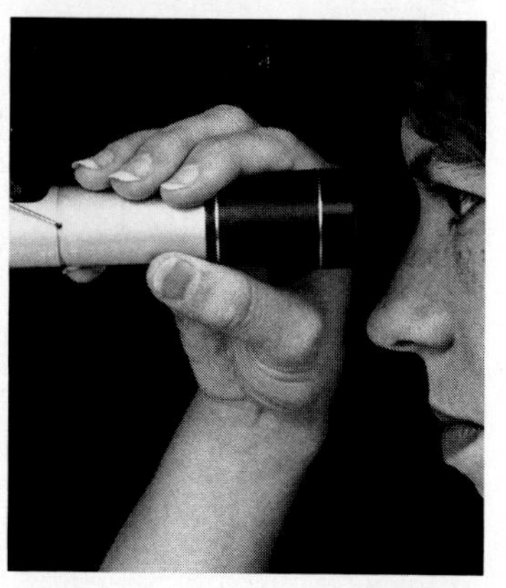

3 Now, hold the instrument horizontally and look into the eyepiece, as shown. Direct the refractometer's tapered end toward a light. *Caution:* Avoid holding the refractometer vertically; for example, to look toward a ceiling light. The urine will run down the instrument's side.

Looking through the eyepiece, you'll see a scale with a shadow over it. Specific gravity is indicated by the shadow's edge on the scale.

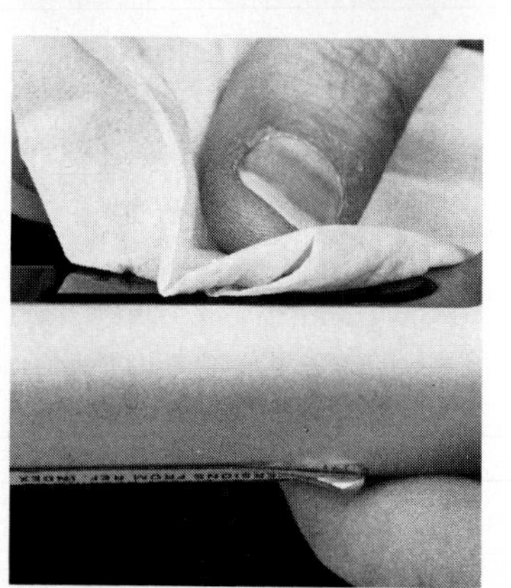

4 Document the results on the appropriate form.

Clean the refractometer's coverslip and the tapered end with tissue or lens paper. Finally, store it in its case (if it has one).

Using a urinometer

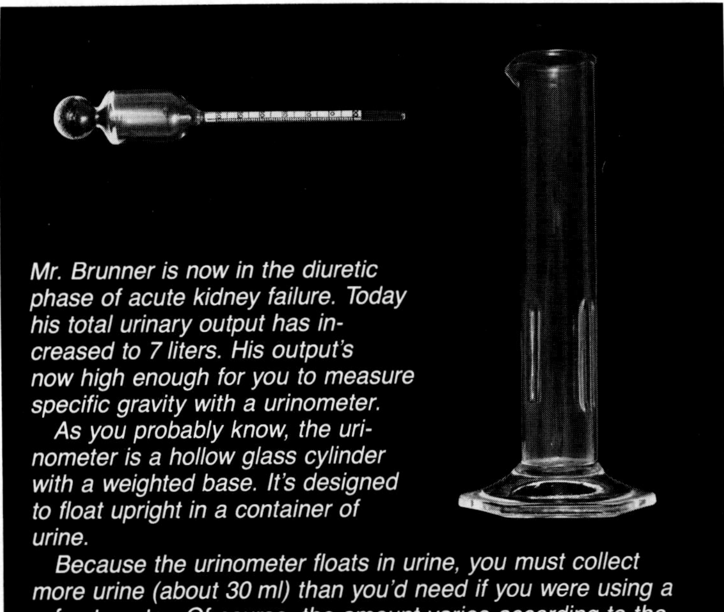

Mr. Brunner is now in the diuretic phase of acute kidney failure. Today his total urinary output has increased to 7 liters. His output's now high enough for you to measure specific gravity with a urinometer.

As you probably know, the urinometer is a hollow glass cylinder with a weighted base. It's designed to float upright in a container of urine.

Because the urinometer floats in urine, you must collect more urine (about 30 ml) than you'd need if you were using a refractometer. Of course, the amount varies according to the size of the container holding the urine. For example, if you place the specimen in a small container, such as a syringe case, you'll need less urine. But no matter what size container you use, make sure the urinometer floats freely.

To begin the procedure, obtain a urinometer and a urine specimen container. Fill the container with a urine specimen.

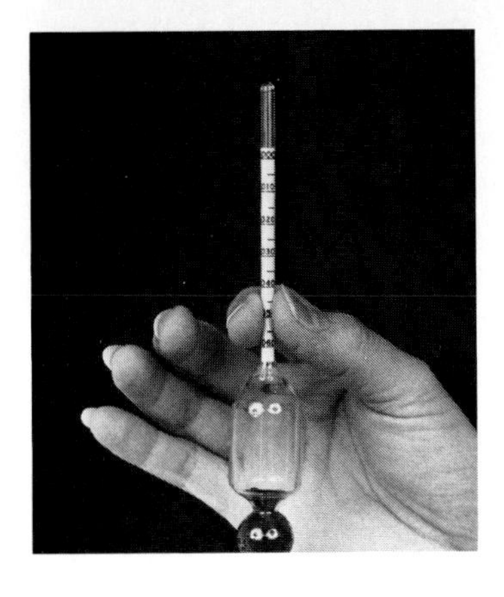

1 Next, carefully inspect the urinometer for chips or cracks. If you see any, get another urinometer.

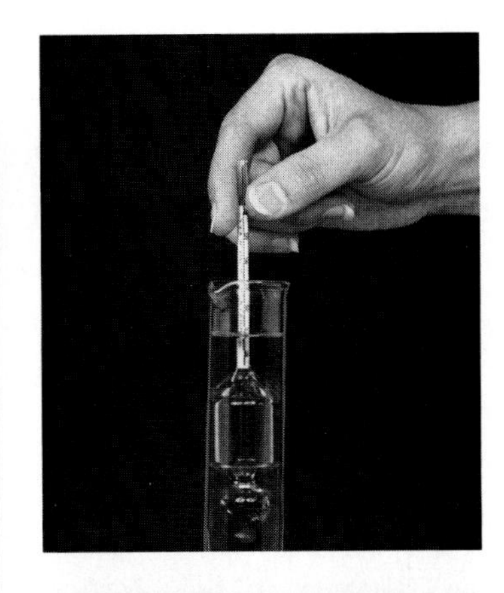

2 Now, place the urinometer in the urine, and turn it slightly to make sure it's floating freely.

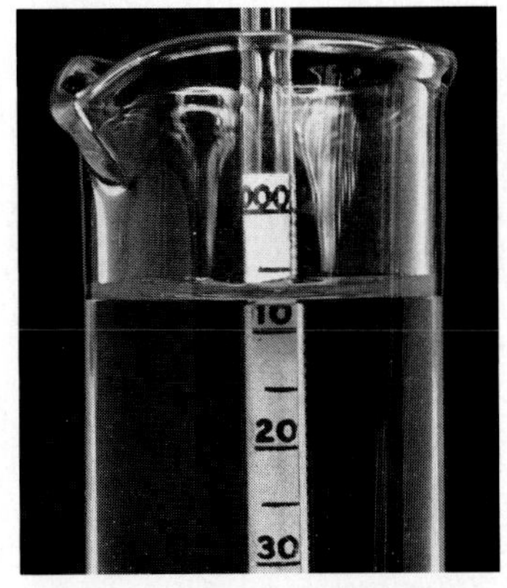

3 After the urinometer stops bobbing, determine specific gravity by locating the urine level on it. Take care to read the level at the bottom of the meniscus.

Important: When you take the reading, make sure the urinometer isn't touching the container's sides.

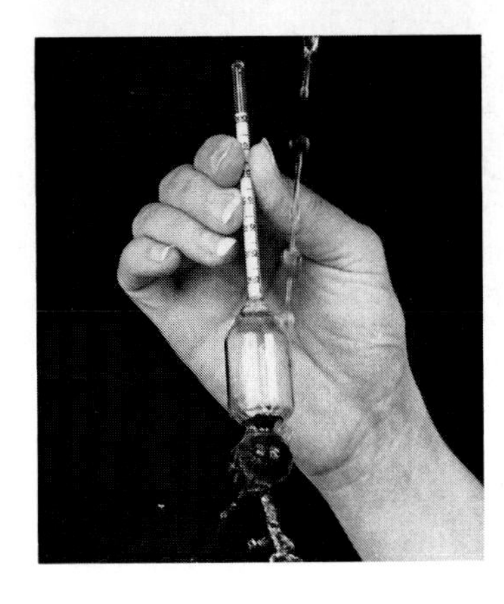

4 Document the results on the appropriate form. Then, rinse the urinometer and the glass cylinder.

Periodically, test the urinometer's accuracy by measuring the specific gravity of distilled water. The result should be 1.000. If it's not, adjust your urine test results to reflect the difference. If the difference is extreme, use another urinometer.

Evaluating specific gravity test results

Have you tested your patient's urine for specific gravity? If so, this chart will help you interpret the results and assess their implications.

Value	Interpretation	Implication
1.010 to 1.025	Normal	• Results are inversely proportional to volume. *Note:* In chronic kidney failure, the specific gravity may become fixed at 1.010, regardless of urine volume.
1.001 to 1.003	Low	• Usually associated with high urinary volume • Causes for high urinary volume include diabetes insipidus, glomerulonephritis, pyelonephritis, excessive drinking, and use of diuretics • May result from kidneys' attempt to reduce volume overload
1.025 to 1.040	High	• May result from liver disease, congestive heart failure, diabetes mellitus, or dehydration caused by reduced fluid intake or increasing fluid loss. *Note:* Be aware that false-positive results may be caused by albumin, dextran, concentrated glucose, radiopaque contrast media, and osmotic diuretics.

Urine tests

Learning about urine pH

The kidneys normally excrete strong, nonvolatile acids (sulfuric and phosphoric) and excess alkali. This combination determines the urine's pH. Urine pH normally ranges from 4.5 to 8.0. Diet, medications, and changes in body metabolism, however, can cause wide variations in pH.

Alkaline pH (above 7.0) causes turbidity and the formation of phosphate, carbonate, and amorphous crystals. Acid pH (below 7.0) also causes turbidity, as well as the formation of oxylate, amorphous urate, and uric acid crystals.

What factors affect urine pH? Consider the following information.

Alkaline pH may result from:

- vegetarian diet
- Fanconi's syndrome
- urinary tract infection
- metabolic or respiratory alkalosis
- chronic cystitis
- acute and chronic kidney failure
- ingestion of citrus fruit
- such medications as acetazolamide (Diamox*), amphotericin B (Fungizone), mafenide, and sodium bicarbonate.

Conversely, your patient's urine may become acidic from:

- high meat intake
- tuberculosis of the kidney
- pyrexia
- phenylketonuria
- respiratory or metabolic acidosis
- fever
- diarrhea
- dehydration
- fasting or a diet that fails to provide adequate nutrition
- cranberry juice
- such medications as ammonium chloride, ascorbic acid, diazoxide (Hyperstat*), methenamine hippurate, methenamine mandelate (Mandelamine*), and metolazone (Zaroxolyn*).

Assessing pH

To assess urine pH levels, dip a pH reagent strip into a urine specimen. The strip changes color according to the level of urine pH. Then, compare the strip with an accompanying color chart. Read the following photostory for details.

For accurate results, always test a fresh urine specimen. Also, keep in mind that the pH level of the first specimen voided each day may be lower than normal because of respiratory acidosis during sleep.

*Available in both the United States and Canada

Testing urine pH

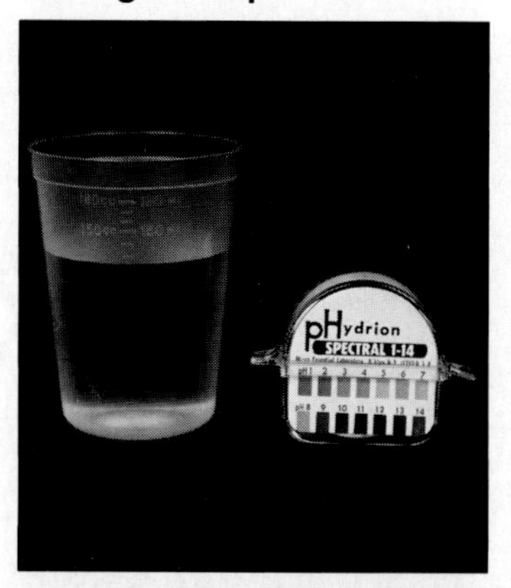

1 Elke Flataker, a 42-year-old clerk typist, is in your hospital undergoing tests for a suspected urinary tract infection. As part of your assessment, you'll be testing her urine pH level. Here's what to do.

Obtain a dispenser of pH reagent paper with a color chart, and a fresh urine specimen. Because the first-voided specimen is more acidic than normal, use a specimen voided later in the day, unless ordered otherwise.

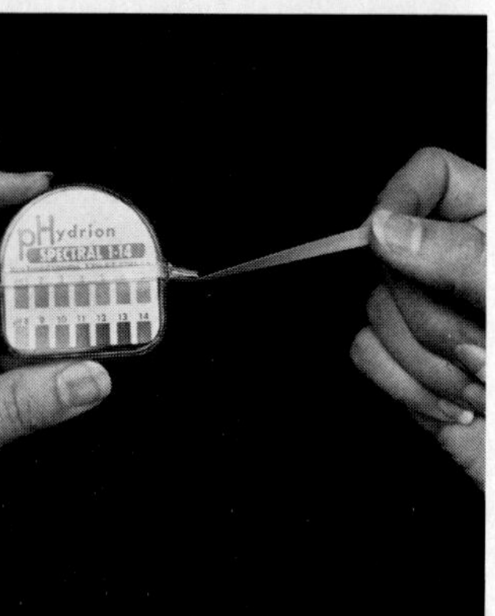
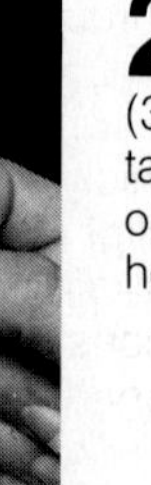

2 Tear off a strip of reagent paper that's about 1½" (3.8 cm) long. To prevent contaminating the paper with skin oils, hold only its end, as shown here.

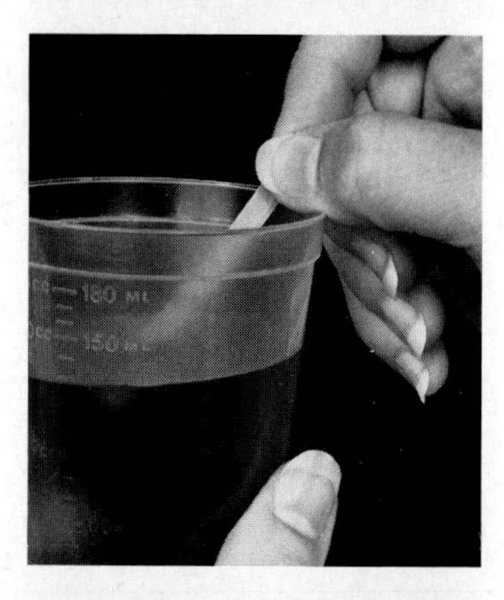

3 Next, dip 1" to 1¼" (2.5 to 3.2 cm) of the strip into the specimen. Then, remove the strip and tap it against the side of the container to remove excess urine.

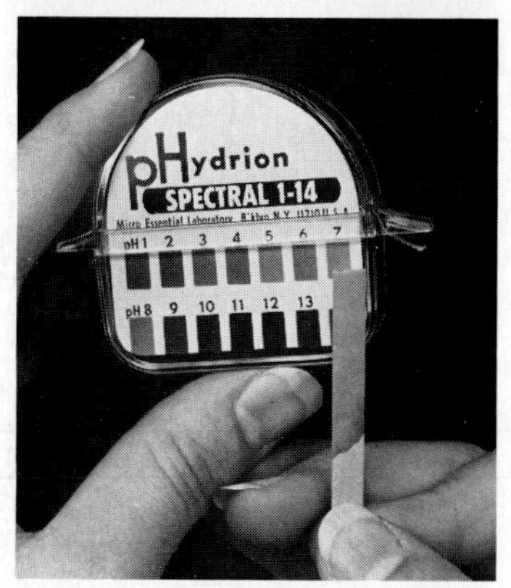

4 Immediately compare the strip's color with the dispenser's color chart.

Finally, document the result on the appropriate form.

Blood tests

As a nurse, you know that blood tests provide valuable insight into your patient's condition. But you may *not* know that you can easily perform many of these tests in your own unit. In this section, we acquaint you with blood tests you can do yourself.

For example, we show you several techniques for measuring blood glucose levels. You'll also learn how to perform a spin hematocrit test to determine the volume percentage of red blood cells in your patient's blood.

Of course, all these tests require a blood specimen. To help you obtain one with confidence, we review two easy collection methods. And we introduce you to the Autoclix lancet, which your patient can use at home to collect blood specimens.

To help you understand how blood coagulates, we identify and describe each factor that's essential to the clotting process. In addition, we teach you a way to assess blood clotting time.

Sound like helpful information? Read the following pages to learn more.

Learning about blood

As you know, blood delivers oxygen to the body's tissues and returns carbon dioxide to the lungs. But that's not all it does. Blood also:

- produces and transports antibodies
- maintains hemostasis by transporting platelets and clotting factors. (For details on clotting factors, see pages 30 and 31.)
- repairs tissue injuries
- regulates body temperature
- moves nutrients and regulatory hormones to body tissues
- disposes of metabolic wastes through the kidneys, lungs, and skin.

Healthy blood is three times thicker than water, tastes slightly salty, and maintains an alkaline pH of 7.35 to 7.45. It consists of four components: erythrocytes (red blood cells), leukocytes (white blood cells), thrombocytes (platelets), and plasma (a clear, straw-colored liquid). For now, let's focus on red blood cells.

Red blood cells: Performing a vital role

Red blood cells are vital for transporting oxygen and carbon dioxide. Normal cells are biconcave disks, ranging in color from pale pink at the center to deep pink at the edges. On the average, their life span is 120 days. As these cells age, they become fragile. After they rupture and decompose, the spleen removes them from the bloodstream.

Hemoglobin, an oxygen-carrying protein, is the main element in a red blood cell. It constitutes about 90% of the mature cell's dry weight.

To thoroughly evaluate blood, you need a complete blood count (CBC), a series of tests designed to count both red and white blood cells and measure hematocrit and hemoglobin. But you can quickly and accurately evaluate red blood cell volume alone by using the micromethod, as shown on page 25. The results can help you identify a variety of disorders, such as fluid imbalance, polycythemia, and anemia.

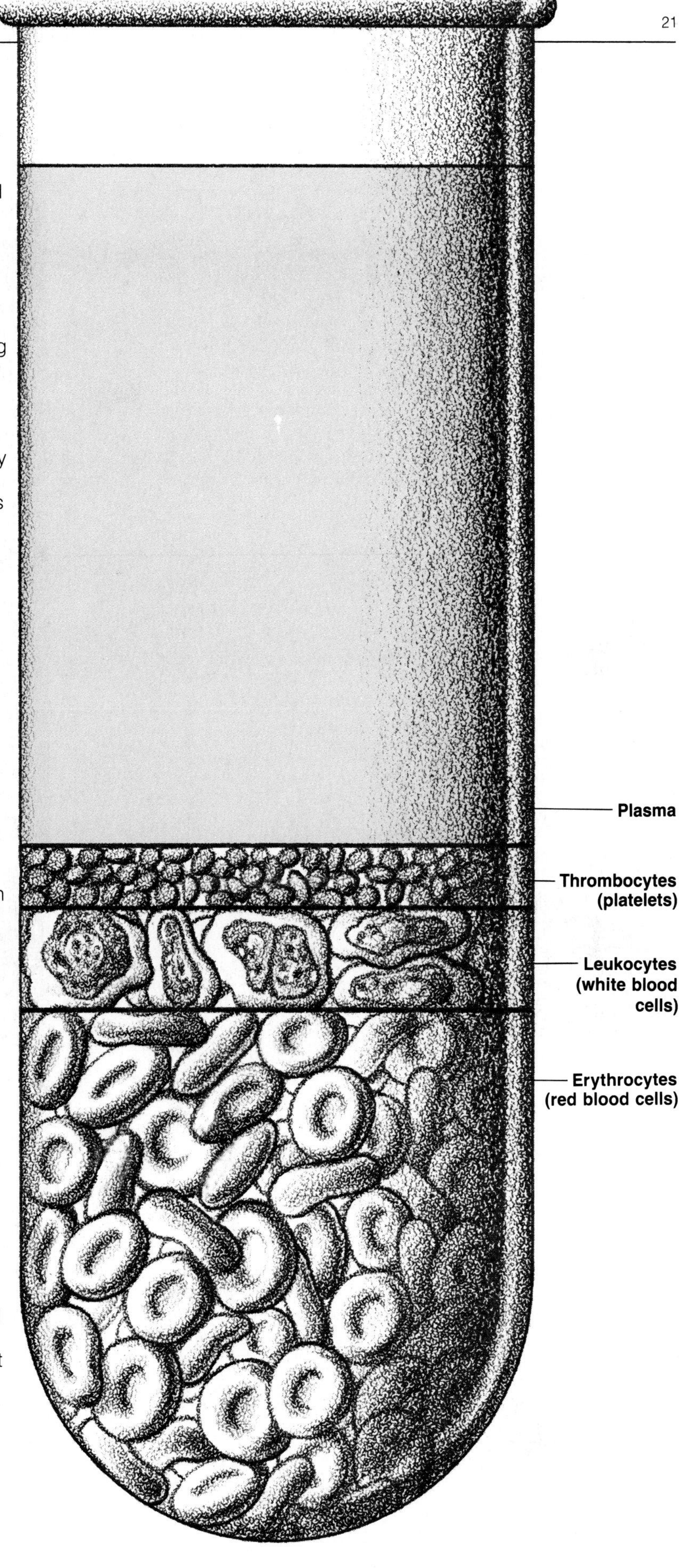

Blood tests

Performing a fingerstick: Some guidelines

Although performing a fingerstick for a blood specimen should be an easy procedure, you can become frustrated by not doing it correctly. Worse yet, you may increase your patient's discomfort. To help you attain quick and accurate results with a minimum of pain for your patient, review these guidelines. Then, read the following photostory for more details.

Before the procedure

- Make sure you have enough capillary collection tubes to collect the number of specimens the test requires.
- Place all the equipment you'll need within easy reach. Consider keeping everything together in a basket or container, in a specific spot.
- To help speed the procedure, organize the equipment in the order you'll use it; for example, alcohol swab, lancet, gauze pad, capillary tubes, putty, and so on.
- Explain to your patient what you're doing, and answer all his questions.
- When choosing a puncture site, select a finger that your patient doesn't use frequently; for instance, the middle finger of his nondominant hand. Be sure the finger you've chosen isn't swollen; fluid from a swollen finger will dilute the specimen.
- If the finger you select is dirty, wash it with soap and warm water before cleansing it with alcohol. In addition to helping cleanse the finger, warm water increases the finger's capillary blood flow.

Nursing tip: Wrapping the patient's hand in a warm towel also increases capillary blood flow.

- Keep your patient's finger below his heart level to further promote capillary blood flow.

During the procedure

- Stick the finger toward the outer edge. Avoid sticking the tip.
- Each time you collect a specimen from the same patient, choose a different puncture site. Avoid repeatedly sticking the same finger.
- To prevent air bubbles from forming in the capillary tube, keep its tip immersed in the blood drop.

After the procedure

- As you withdraw the tube, use a dry gauze pad to apply direct pressure to the puncture site. Doing so helps stop the bleeding and discourages the patient from sticking this finger in his mouth.
- If you're collecting specimens from several patients consecutively, correctly label all the tubes for one patient before proceeding to the next patient.

How to perform a fingerstick

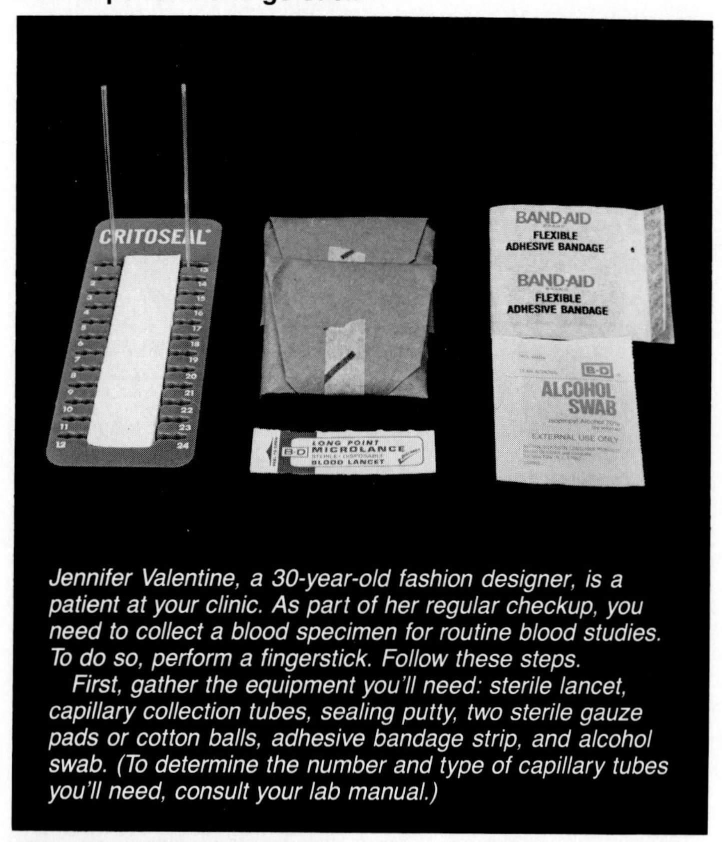

Jennifer Valentine, a 30-year-old fashion designer, is a patient at your clinic. As part of her regular checkup, you need to collect a blood specimen for routine blood studies. To do so, perform a fingerstick. Follow these steps.

First, gather the equipment you'll need: sterile lancet, capillary collection tubes, sealing putty, two sterile gauze pads or cotton balls, adhesive bandage strip, and alcohol swab. (To determine the number and type of capillary tubes you'll need, consult your lab manual.)

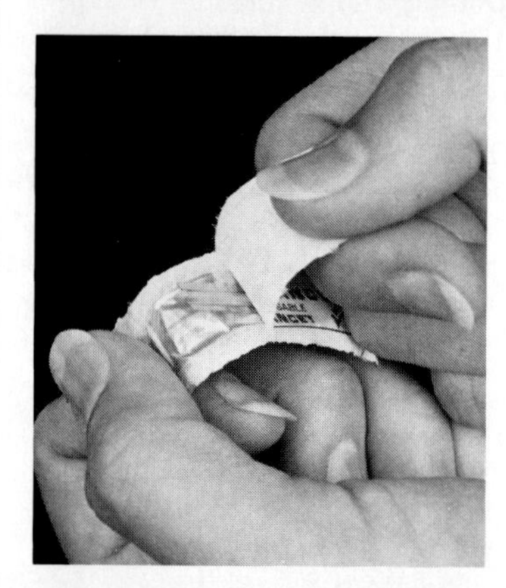

1 Now, place the equipment on a nearby clean surface. Open the lancet's wrapper. To keep the lancet sterile, leave it in the wrapper until you're ready to use it.

Next, prepare Ms. Valentine for the procedure. Explain what you'll be doing, and answer all her questions. Then, instruct her to thoroughly wash and dry her hands as you do so yourself.

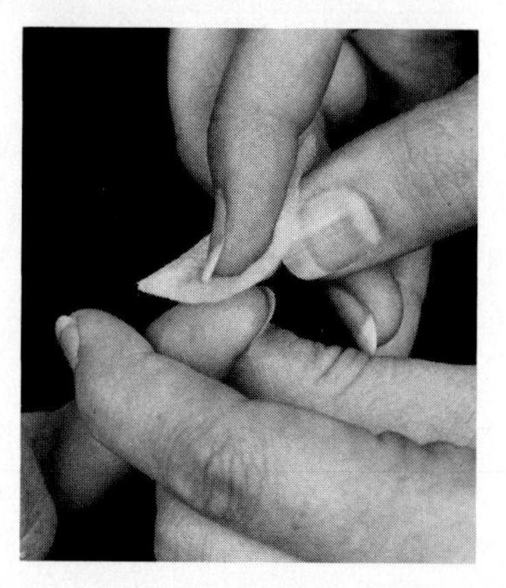

2 To minimize the risk of such postprocedure complications as bruising, choose the middle finger of her nondominant hand as the puncture site. (Because she uses her nondominant hand less frequently than her other hand, she'll be less likely to injure the site while it heals.)

Using a circular motion, cleanse the puncture site with an alcohol swab, as shown here.

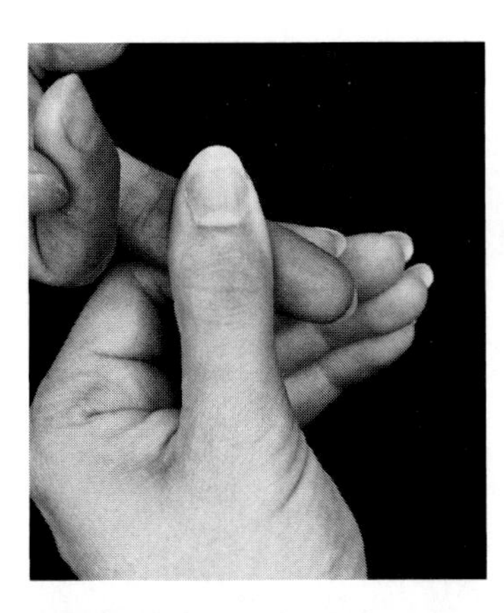

3 To engorge the capillaries, firmly grasp your patient's finger near its tip. But don't touch the puncture site, or you'll contaminate it. To increase blood flow to the tip, position her finger below heart level.

Nursing tip: If you have trouble engorging the fingertip, plan to make the stick with two lancets placed together, side by side. This produces a larger puncture and increases bleeding.

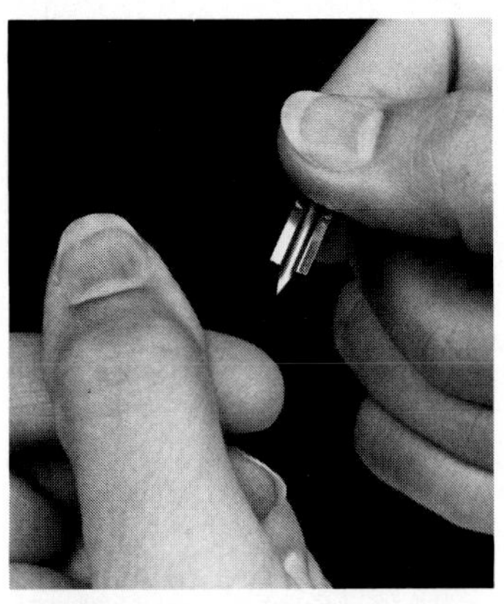

4 Now, grasp the lancet between the thumb and forefinger of your dominant hand. At the same time, stabilize your patient's fingertip with your nondominant hand, as the nurse is doing here. Continue applying firm pressure to maintain flushing.

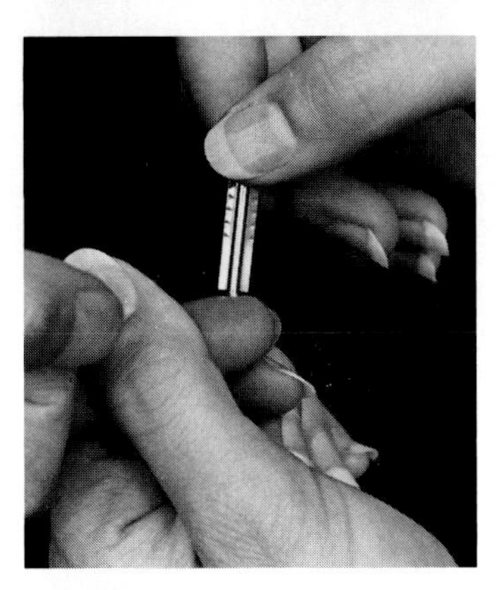

5 Position the lancet about 2" (5.1 cm) from the side of her fingertip.

With one quick, firm motion, move the lancet in a short arc so it penetrates the fingertip at a 90° angle. Then, immediately withdraw the lancet.

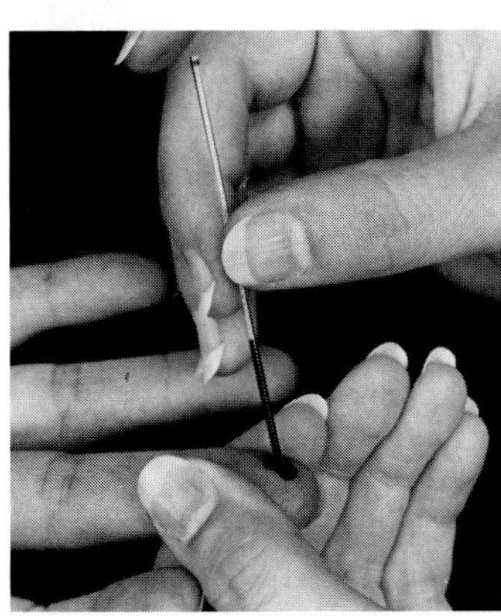

6 To prevent specimen dilution with tissue fluid, absorb the first blood drop with a gauze pad. When another drop forms, place the capillary tube's tip in it.

Important: Leave the top of the tube open so capillary action draws blood up the tube.

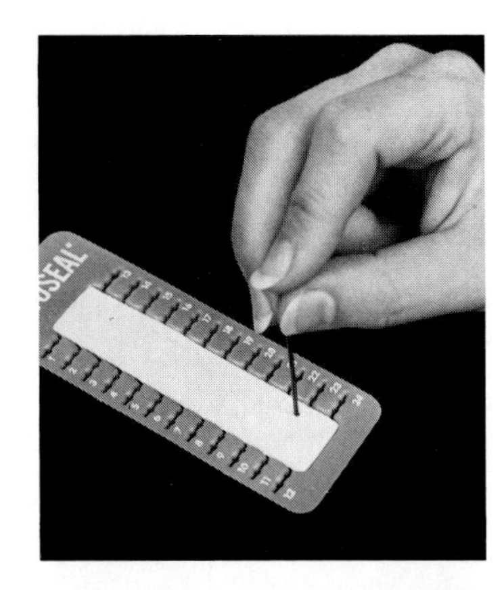

7 When the tube's filled with blood, place your fingertip over the top and carefully remove the tube from the site. Then, press the tube's bottom in sealing putty, as shown here. This prevents the blood from spilling when you take away your fingertip.

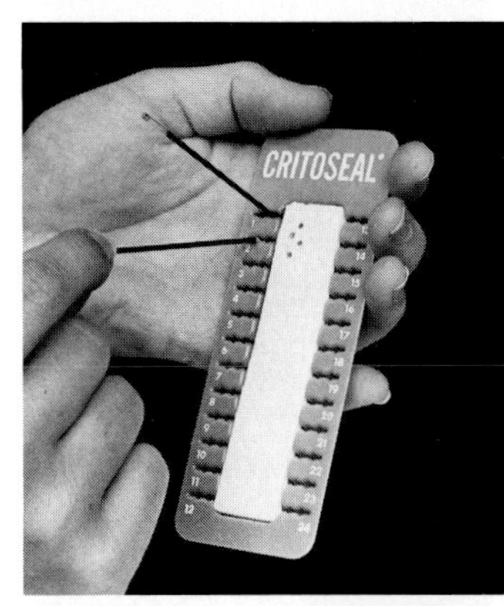

8 Next, place the tube in the sealing putty container. Repeat steps 6 and 7 until you've filled the required number of tubes.

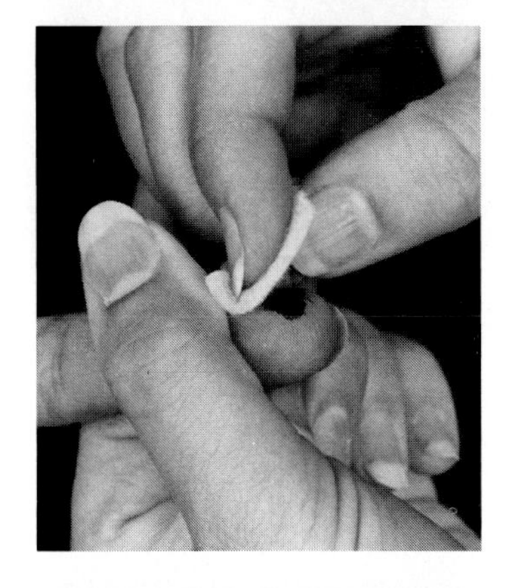

9 What if the blood flow decreases before you've collected the required amount of blood? Firmly squeeze the patient's fingertip several times, until more blood collects. Pause briefly between squeezes to allow the capillaries to refill. Or, try wiping your patient's finger with a clean alcohol swab, as shown.

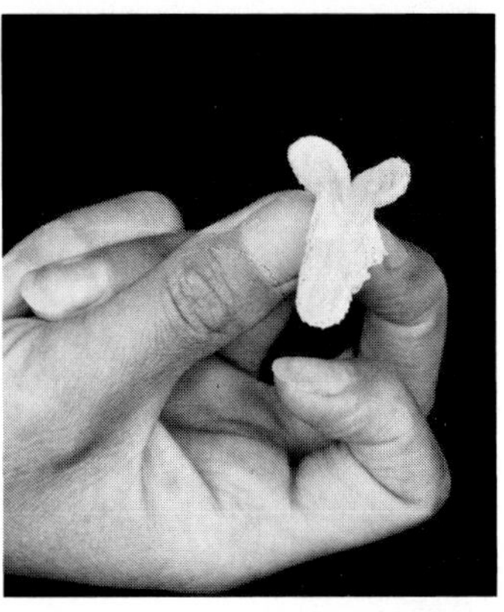

10 When the collection's complete, press a dry sterile gauze pad over the puncture site. When the bleeding's stopped, cover the site with an adhesive bandage strip.

Finally, document the procedure on the appropriate form.

Blood tests

Taking blood from the earlobe

Shortly after lunch, 22-year-old Barbara Batz comes into the blood bank where you work. She tells you she wants to donate a pint of blood. After documenting her patient history, you'll collect a blood specimen to determine hematocrit and blood group. This photostory shows you how.

To collect the blood specimen, prepare to perform an earstick on your patient. First, gather the following equipment: sterile lancet, capillary collection tubes, sealing putty, two sterile gauze pads or cotton balls, and alcohol swab. Thoroughly wash and dry your hands.

Then, explain the procedure to Ms. Batz. Assure her that it'll take only a few seconds to complete, but inform her she'll briefly feel a sting when you pierce her earlobe.

Next, unwrap an alcohol swab. Using a circular motion, cleanse the earlobe you'll be sticking.

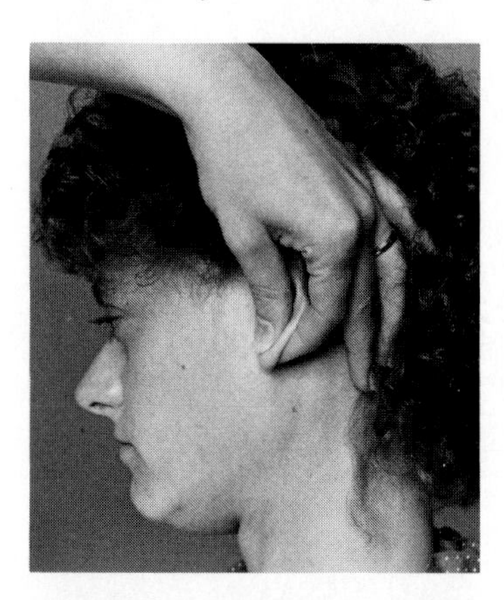

1 Now, grasp the earlobe just above the puncture site. If necessary, gently stroke toward the end of the lobe to increase blood flow; however, avoid contaminating the puncture site with your fingers.

Next, hold the lancet between the thumb and forefinger of your dominant hand. Position the lancet about 1" (2.5 cm) away from the side of the earlobe.

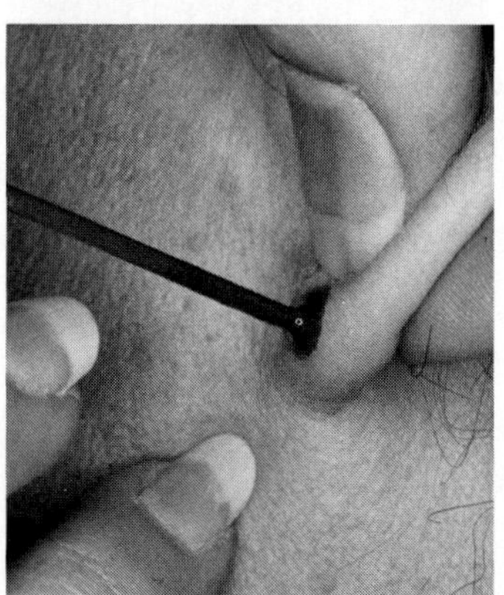

2 Then, with one quick, firm motion, move the lancet in a short arc so it penetrates the earlobe at a 90° angle. Immediately withdraw the lancet.

Use a gauze pad to clean away the first large blood drop. Then, squeeze out another drop of blood, and place the capillary tube's tip in the drop, as the nurse is doing here.

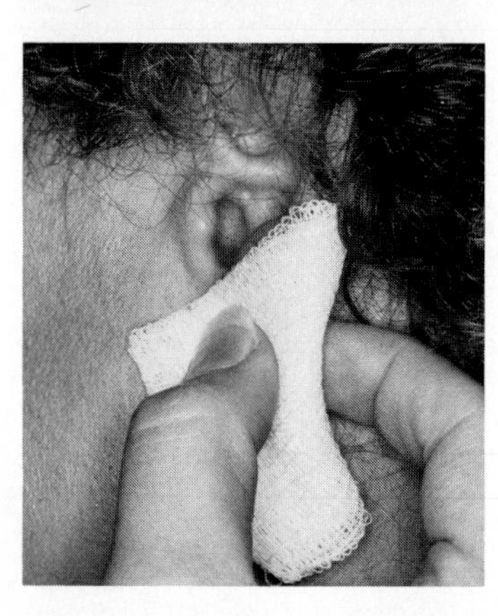

3 When the tube's full, seal the bottom with putty, as explained in the preceding photostory. Fill additional tubes until you've collected all the blood you need.

Then, apply a clean, dry gauze pad to the puncture site, and ask your patient to hold the pad firmly in place until bleeding stops.

Finally, document the procedure on the appropriate form.

Understanding hematocrit testing

As you know, hematocrit is the volume percentage of red blood cells in a blood specimen. What's a normal value? This depends on your patient's age, sex, and physical condition. As a rule, a male's hematocrit is between 40% and 50%. Consider a value between 37% and 47% normal for a female. For newborns, normal hematocrit is about 60%; for children, it's about 35%.

What can hematocrit tell you? A low value signifies a low red blood cell count, possibly caused by hemorrhage, anemia, or hemodilution (from fluid overload or congestive heart failure, for example). A high value may indicate polycythemia or hemoconcentration from fluid loss.

Collecting a specimen for testing

You may collect a blood specimen with either the micromethod or the macromethod. To use the micromethod, you'll perform a fingerstick and collect blood in capillary tubes. Although you can analyze the specimens yourself, test results may be 5% lower than the patient's actual hematocrit value.

When using the macromethod, you'll draw blood into a 7-ml lavender-top collection tube. Testing a specimen drawn this way provides more accurate results but is more time-consuming and requires laboratory analysis.

As a rule, a single hematocrit value has little diagnostic significance. By studying a *series* of values, however, you can identify trends. For example, although a patient with hidden gastrointestinal bleeding may appear stable, progressively decreasing hematocrit values indicate active bleeding.

Remember: Your clinical observations are important. Supplement the hematocrit test results with them.

How to determine hematocrit

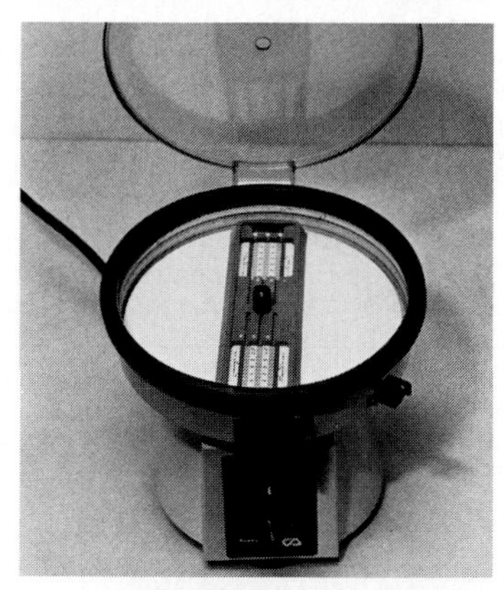

1 Determining your patient's hematocrit value with the micromethod? Use a centrifuge like this one. By spinning blood specimens at high speed, it separates red blood cells from plasma. To determine hematocrit, you'll measure the area occupied by red blood cells in relation to total blood volume. Here's how.

To begin, place the centrifuge on a flat, secure surface near a standard electrical outlet. Plug it in.

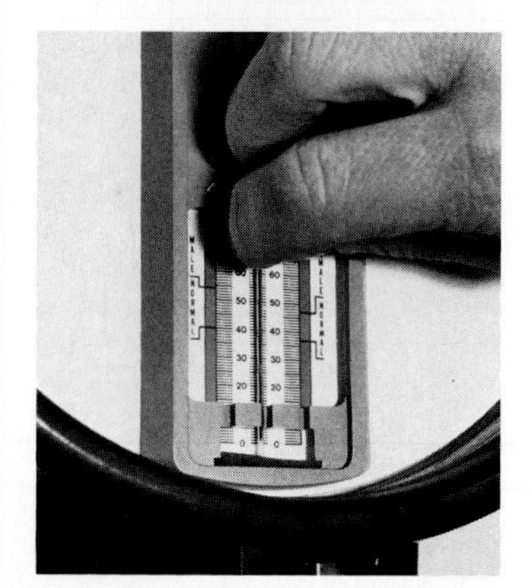

2 Next, place a capillary tube containing a blood specimen in one of the scale's grooves, as shown here. Make sure the sealed end faces outward. Repeat the procedure with the remaining tubes. *Note:* To ensure accurate results, make sure the tubes are filled correctly.

Understanding blood groups

Before a donor's blood is transfused, it undergoes laboratory testing to assure compatibility with the intended recipient's blood. But you can perform important preliminary testing. In the photostory at right, you'll see how. First, review this information on blood groups.

As a rule, red blood cells contain on their surfaces genetically determined antigens. The presence or absence of these antigens determines basic blood group classification: group A (A antigens only), group B (B antigens only), group AB (A and B antigens), and group O (neither A nor B antigens).

Between ages 2 and 8 months, an infant develops antibodies in his plasma designed to attack foreign blood antigens. He retains these antibodies for life. If he has group A blood, for instance, he has antibodies against B antigens found on group B red blood cells. For such a patient, transfusion of group B blood causes agglutination—and possibly death. (If he has group B blood, transfusion of group A blood is dangerous for the same reason.)

But what about group AB blood? Because it has both A and B antigens, it has no antibodies designed to attack either A or B antigens. As a result, a person with group AB blood can receive a transfusion of any of the four blood groups.

Finally, consider group O blood, which contains no A or B antigens. It won't trigger an antibody attack when mixed with another blood group. A person with group O blood is called a universal donor.

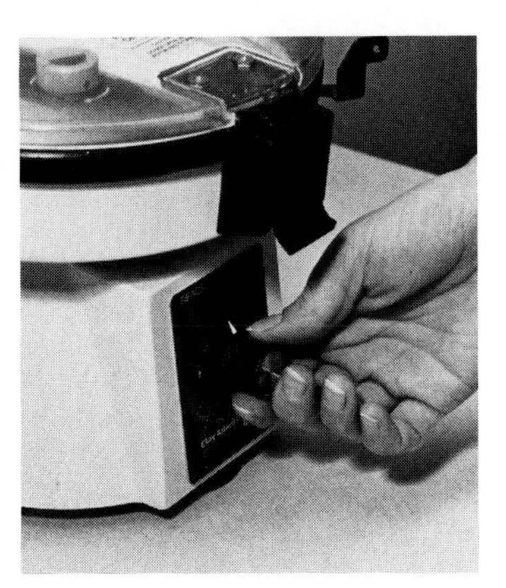

3 Lower the centrifuge's lid. Adjust the power dial to allow the blood to spin for 5 minutes.

Then, turn off the power and lift the lid. You'll see a column of packed red blood cells in each tube.

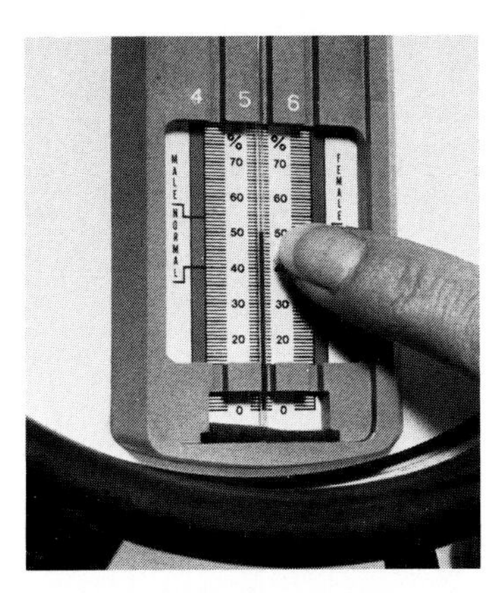

4 Align each tube so the base of the column parallels the 0 on the scale. To determine your patient's hematocrit, note the reading at the *top* of the packed red blood cells (as shown).

Finally, document the measurement on the appropriate form.

Assessing blood group and Rh factor

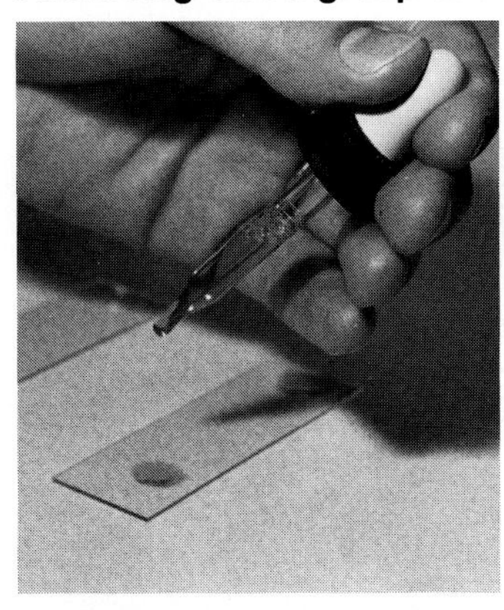

1 Now, you're ready to determine Barbara Batz's blood group and Rh factor. You'll need only a few drops of blood for this basic screening test.

In addition to the blood specimen, gather this equipment: two clean glass slides, two applicator sticks, and anti-A, anti-B, and anti-D typing serums. Then, place one drop of anti-A serum on one end of a slide and one drop of anti-B serum on the other end, as shown.

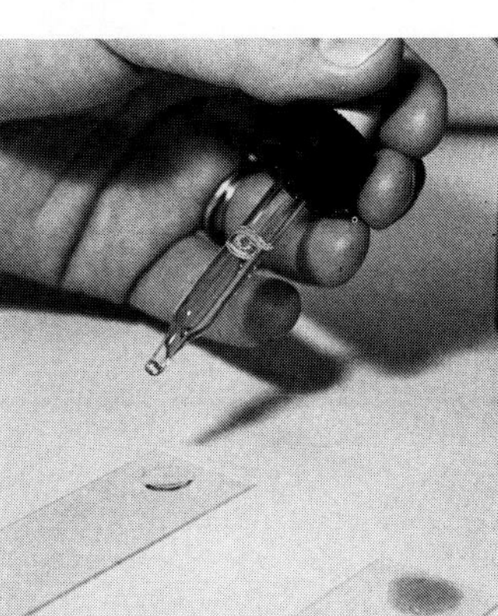

2 Now, place one drop of anti-D serum on the second slide, as shown here.

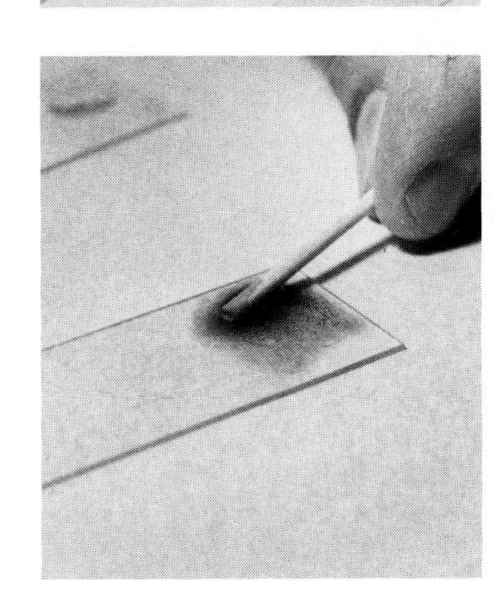

3 Place one drop of blood in the anti-A serum and another drop in the anti-B serum. Using separate ends of an applicator stick, thoroughly mix each specimen. As you do, watch for agglutination (clump formation). If agglutination occurs in the anti-A drop, Ms. Batz's blood group is A; if it occurs in the anti-B drop, her blood group is B. If agglutination occurs in both, her blood group is AB; if it occurs in neither, her blood group is O.

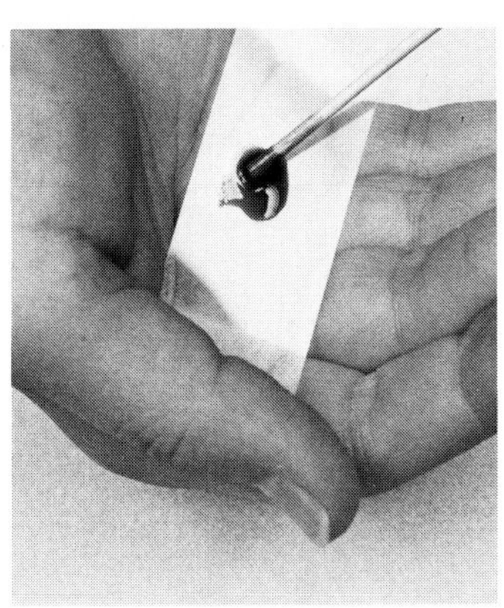

4 To determine your patient's Rh factor, add one drop of blood to the anti-D serum. Mix the specimen with a fresh applicator stick while you warm the slide in your hand. If agglutination occurs, your patient's blood is Rh positive. If agglutination doesn't occur, her blood's Rh negative.

Document all test results.

Blood tests

Learning about Dextrostix

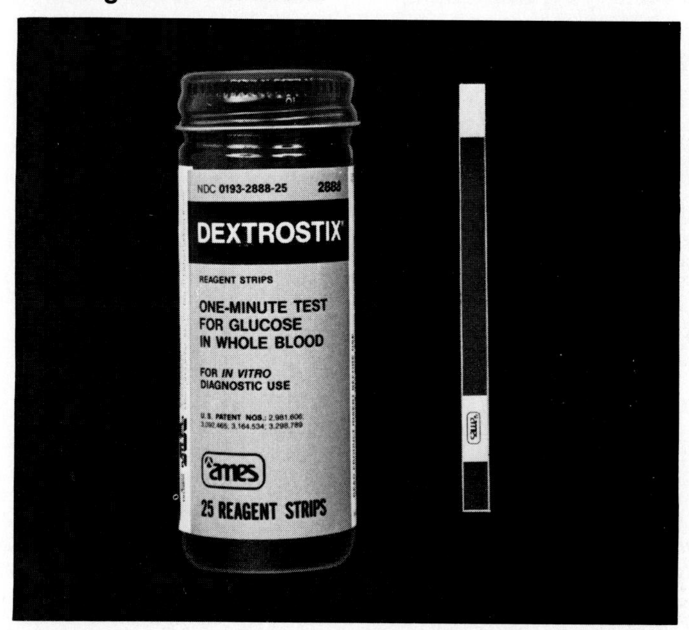

Dextrostix is a firm, plastic reagent strip that allows you to quickly and easily measure your patient's blood glucose level. It has a small, yellow test block at one end. When you place a drop of whole blood on the test block, the block turns gray, slate, blue, or violet, depending on blood glucose level. In the following photostory, you'll see how to use this reagent strip.

To ensure accurate test results, follow these guidelines:

- Document your patient's dietary intake of carbohydrates—especially sugar—over the previous 2 hours.
- Follow the procedure directions closely.
- Compare the test block with the chart at the specified time. Make the comparison in a well-lighted area, to ensure accurate color identification.

Note: To obtain more accurate results, read the strip in a reflectance photometer, an instrument designed especially to distinguish test block color. For details, see pages 27 through 29.

Ensuring freshness

To keep Dextrostix reactive, take the same precautions you'd use to preserve any reagent strip. For example:

- Don't store the Dextrostix bottle at a temperature higher than 86° F. (30° C.); however, don't refrigerate it.
- Keep the bottle away from light, moisture, and excessive heat.
- Check the bottle's expiration date. Dispose of the bottle and its contents if the expiration date has passed.
- When you open a new bottle, mark the date on the label. To ensure freshness, use the strips within 4 months following this date.
- When you need a test strip, remove the bottle cap and quickly take one out. Then, tightly recap the bottle.
- Before using a reagent strip, check the test block. If the block's discolored, don't use it.
- Avoid touching the test block.
- Store the reagent strips in their original bottle.

Measuring your patient's blood glucose level

Monitoring a diabetic patient's insulin therapy? Use Dextrostix to measure her blood glucose level. Here's why.

Insulin stimulates the body to convert carbohydrates and other sugars to a form of glucose that muscle and fat cells can easily use. So, as a rule, your patient's blood glucose level depends on the amount of insulin in her bloodstream. A high glucose level usually indicates an insulin deficiency; a low level may signify liver disease or an overabundance of insulin.

To proceed, you'll need this equipment: Dextrostix reagent strips with color chart, paper towel, wash bottle with water, alcohol swab, gauze pads, watch with a second hand, and lancet.

Before you start, explain the test to your patient and ask her to tell you what she's eaten during the past 2 hours. A high-carbohydrate meal before the test significantly increases her blood's glucose level.

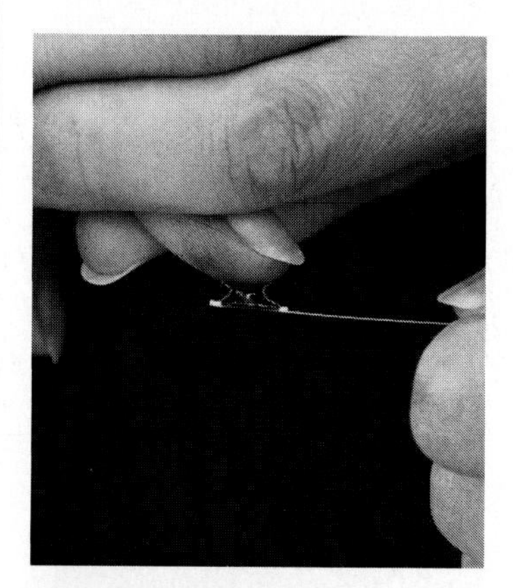

1 To begin, remove a reagent strip from the bottle, recap the bottle, and make sure the strip's test block isn't discolored. Cleanse the fingerstick site and puncture it with the lancet. Wipe away the first drop, position your patient's finger so the nail is facing upward, as shown here, and hold the strip under the site.

Squeeze enough blood onto the block to cover it; then apply a gauze pad to the puncture site. Wait 60 seconds.

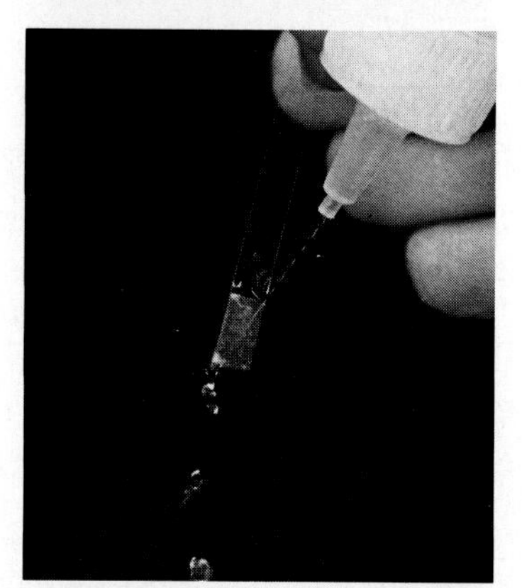

2 Grasp the strip at the corner, and hold it over a sink or other receptacle. Then, rinse the test block for 2 seconds with the water in the wash bottle, as the nurse is doing here. *Caution:* Rinse the block for *only* 2 seconds. Rinsing it for a longer period may affect test results.

Next, dry the reagent strip by blotting it on a paper towel.

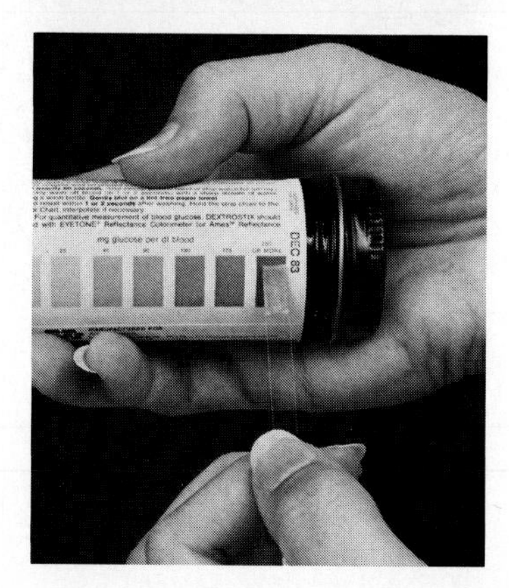

3 Immediately compare the test block color with the color chart, as shown here. Normal results range from 45 to 130 mg/dl. Report abnormal test results to the doctor.

Finally, document your results on the appropriate form.

Getting acquainted with the Glucometer

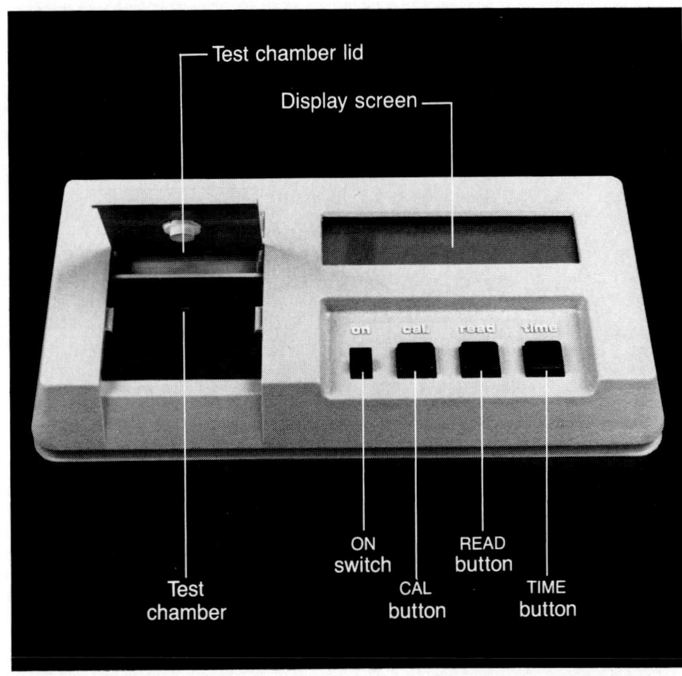

Now you know how to determine your patient's blood glucose level with a Dextrostix reagent strip. But, you can obtain more accurate results with a reflectance photometer, such as the Glucometer shown above.

Although you still use a Dextrostix reagent strip with this instrument, you don't compare the test block's color with a color chart. Instead, you insert the strip into the Glucometer, which reads the test block's color electronically and displays a digital value.

Because the Glucometer is portable and provides quick, accurate results, you'll find it useful no matter where you work. And a diabetic patient who routinely monitors his blood glucose levels may choose to use it at home.

How the Glucometer works

The Glucometer uses four AA alkaline batteries, which provide enough power for about 1,000 readings. These batteries fit in the back of the instrument.

Now, look at the Glucometer's front panel. You'll see an ON switch and three buttons below a display screen. The reagent strip test chamber, located on the Glucometer's left side, has a lid that flips up to reveal a molded groove designed to hold a reagent strip.

You'll use the CAL button (located to the right of the ON switch) to calibrate the instrument.

For accurate test results, routinely calibrate the Glucometer at least once daily. Also calibrate it under these circumstances:

- if it hasn't been used for a week or more
- after replacing the batteries
- when using a new bottle of Dextrostix
- when a different operator will perform the test.

For directions on calibrating and using the Glucometer, carefully read the following photostories.

Calibrating the Glucometer

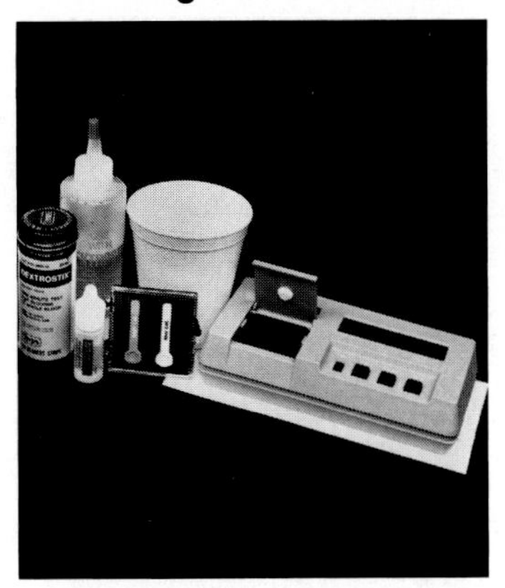

1 You've just placed fresh batteries in the Glucometer reflectance photometer. Now, you need to calibrate the instrument before using it. Here's what to do.

In addition to the Glucometer, gather this equipment: bottle of Dextrostix reagent strips, wash bottle with water, empty cup, paper towel, low and high calibration chips, and Dextro-Chek control solution.

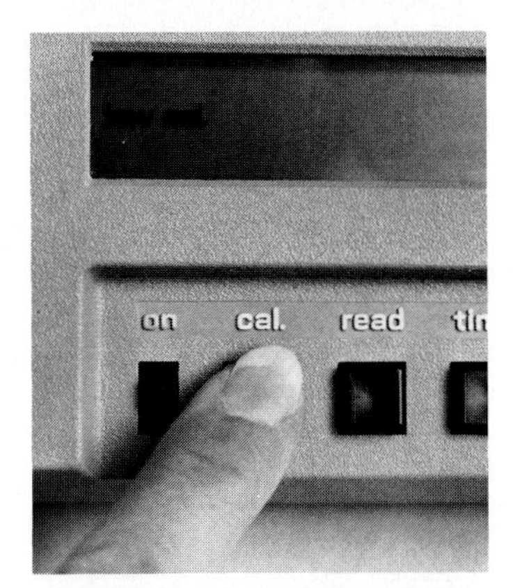

2 To start, slide the ON switch forward. Expect to see *mg/dl* appear on the display screen.

Next, press the CAL button. When you see *LOW CAL* on the left side of the screen, you've activated the calibration process.

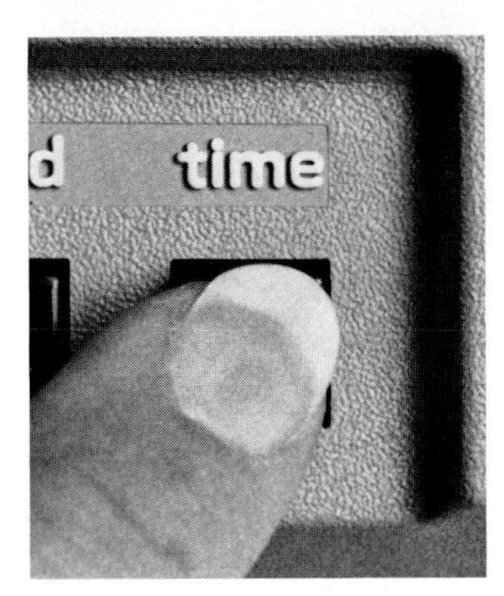

3 Now, press the TIME button. In the screen's bottom right-hand corner, expect to see three dashes and the word *SECONDS*. A few seconds later, the Glucometer buzzes briefly and the number *60* appears. Now, you'll see a countdown from 60 on the display screen. When the countdown concludes, the Glucometer buzzes again.

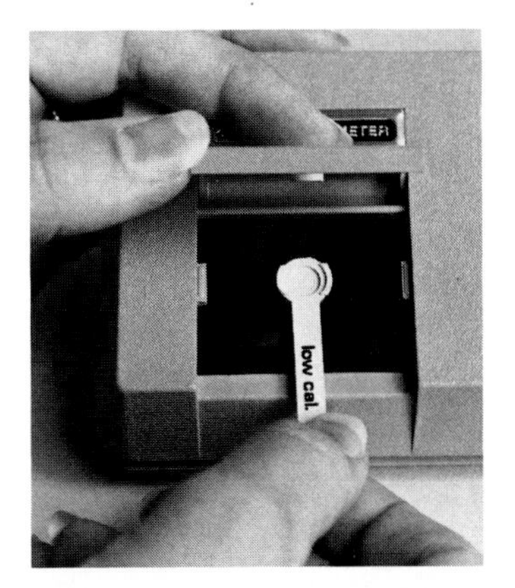

4 Immediately flip up the test chamber lid. Take the light gray chip (marked LOW CAL on the handle) and insert it into the test chamber with the marking up, as shown.

Then, gently lower the lid over the chip. *Caution:* Don't force the lid closed.

Blood tests

Calibrating the Glucometer continued

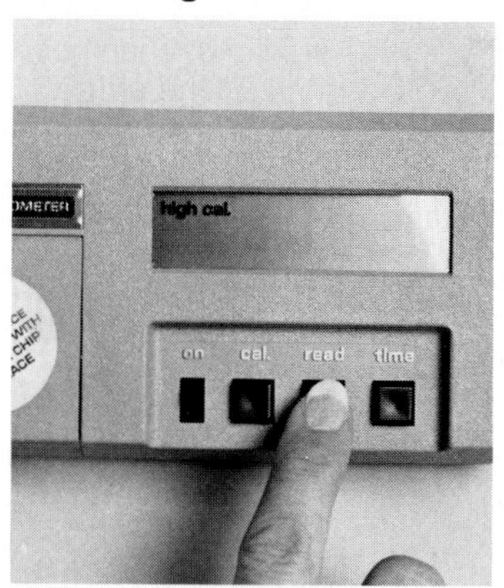

5 Next, press the READ button. When three dashes appear in the center of the display screen, the Glucometer is partially calibrated. Then, look for the words *HIGH CAL* to appear in the screen's left-hand corner, as shown here.

When this occurs, remove the LOW CAL chip from the test chamber. Repeat steps 3 through 5 with the darker chip marked HIGH CAL.

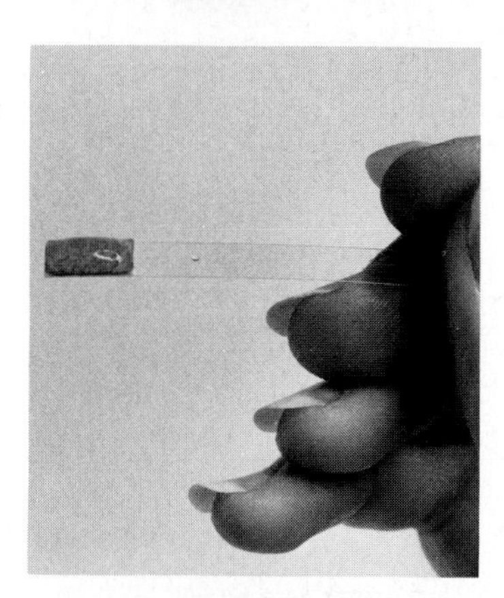

6 By completing the preceding steps, you've established low and high reference points for the Glucometer. Now, perform a control test to verify that the Glucometer is working properly.

First, remove a reagent strip from its bottle and replace the bottle cap. Next, remove the control solution cap and press the TIME button. When the buzzer sounds, gently squeeze a large drop of solution on the test block.

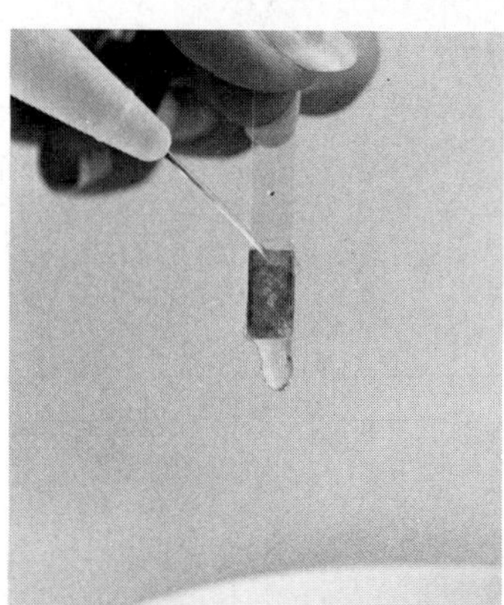

7 Position the strip over the cup. After 60 seconds, the buzzer sounds again. Rinse the excess control solution from the strip, using the wash bottle water. (Take care to rinse for only 2 seconds.) Then, gently blot the test block on the paper towel. *Note:* Always use a paper towel—not a cloth towel or tissue. Cloth and tissue attract lint that may interfere with results.

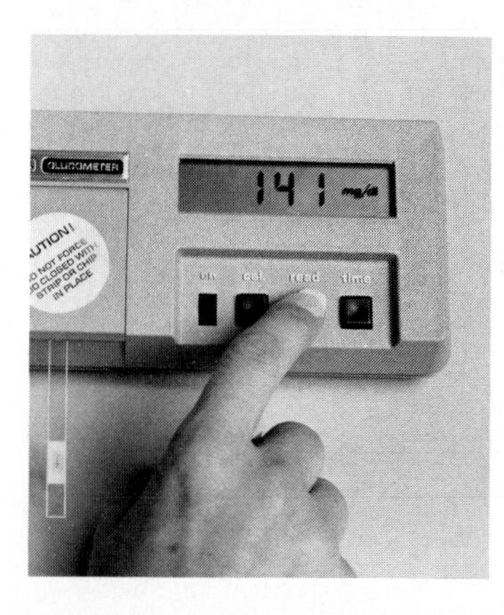

8 Now, insert the reagent strip into the test chamber, block side down. Gently close the lid and press the READ button. Observe the control test result on the screen.

If the result falls within the desired range (see the manufacturer's instructions), you're ready to begin testing. The next photostory shows you how.

Using the Glucometer

You're caring for 41-year-old storekeeper Sedgewick Durney. Mr. Durney's diabetes mellitus was diagnosed several years ago. For the past few days he's experienced symptoms of hyperglycemia. To help pinpoint the cause, the doctor's asked you to monitor Mr. Durney's blood glucose level four times daily, using a reflectance photometer. (Of course, he'll also ask you to monitor Mr. Durney's urine for glucose and ketones.) If you're using the Glucometer reflectance photometer, follow these steps.

In addition to the Glucometer, gather this equipment: bottle of Dextrostix reagent strips, wash bottle containing water, cup, alcohol swab, lancet, paper towel, and cotton ball (not shown).

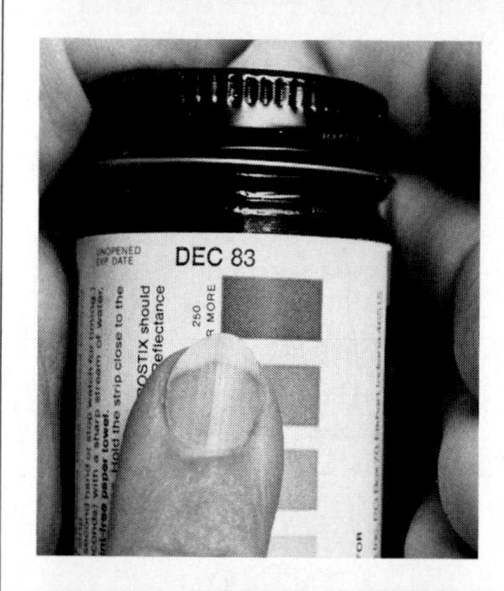

1 First, check the expiration date on the Dextrostix label to be sure the strips are fresh. Then, remove the cap and take a strip from the bottle. Immediately replace and tighten the cap.

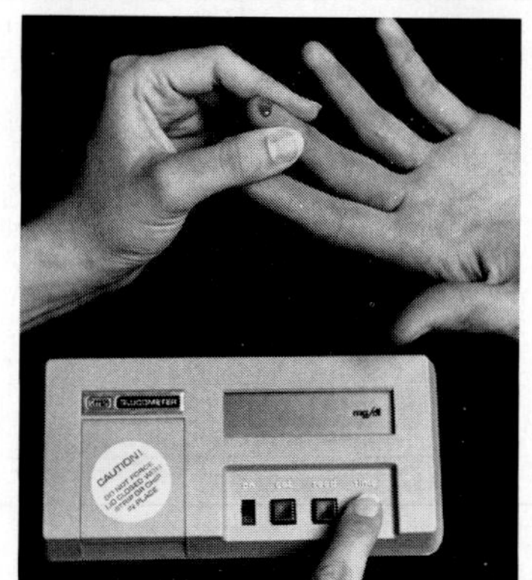

2 Next, use a lancet to collect a blood specimen. (For details on this procedure, see pages 22 and 23.)

Wipe the first drop of blood off your patient's finger with a clean, dry cotton ball. When a new drop of blood begins to form, press the TIME button on the Glucometer, as shown.

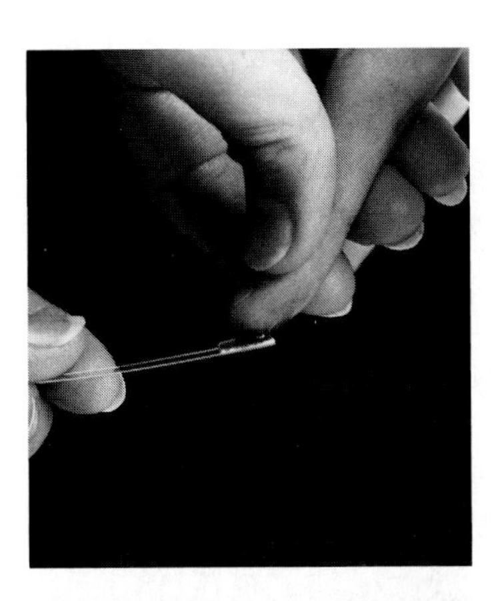

3 Now, reposition your patient's hand as shown. Hold the reagent strip under the blood drop and squeeze around the puncture site. When the Glucometer buzzes, let blood drop onto the reagent strip test block. Make sure you apply a generous amount of blood to the block. *Note:* To avoid spilling the blood, hold the reagent strip level.

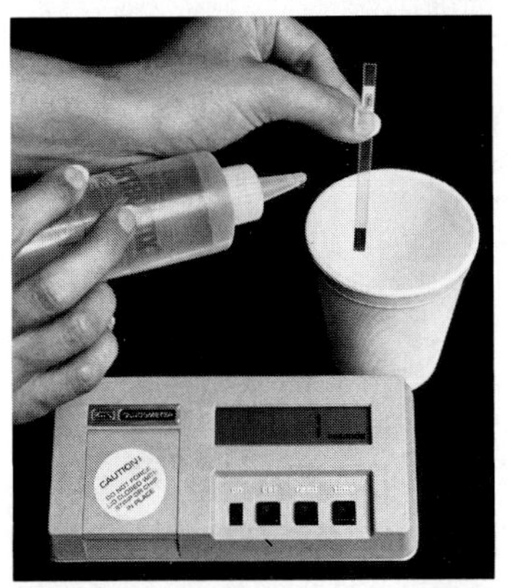

4 Now, watch the Glucometer's display screen. You'll see a countdown from 60 seconds to 0. When the digital display approaches 0, position the reagent strip over the cup.

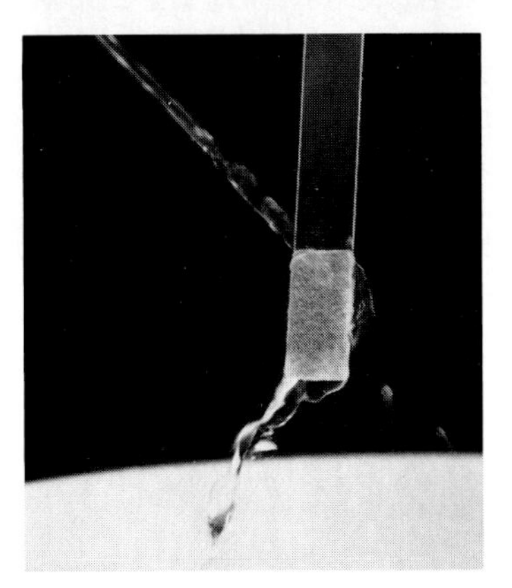

5 As soon as the buzzer sounds, remove excess blood by rinsing the reagent block for 2 seconds with the water in the wash bottle.

Caution: Avoid rinsing the block too long or with too much solution; this may produce false results.

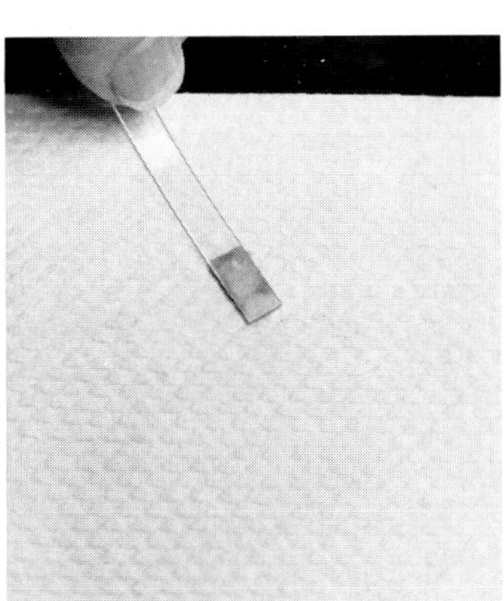

6 Now, gently blot the test block on a paper towel. *Remember:* Use a paper towel for this step because it's relatively lint-free.

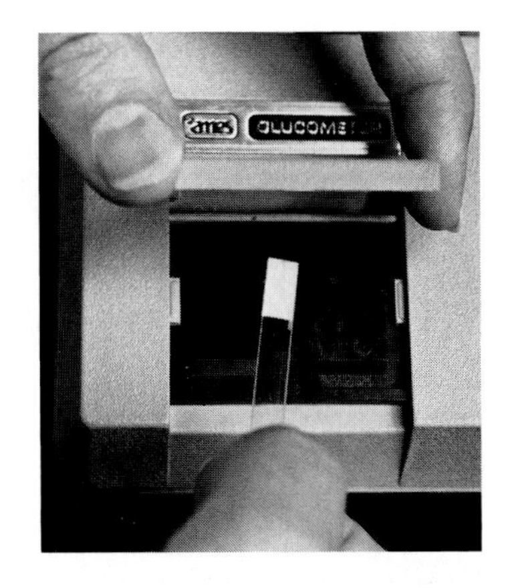

7 Next, lift the test chamber lid, and place the strip test-block side down in the chamber's molded groove.

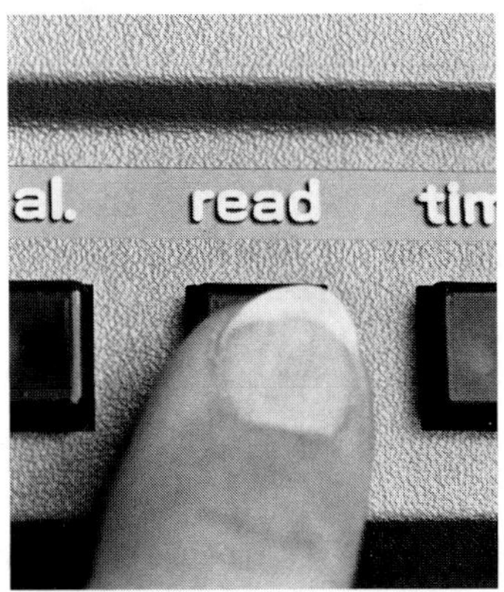

8 Then, press the READ button, as the nurse is doing in this photo.

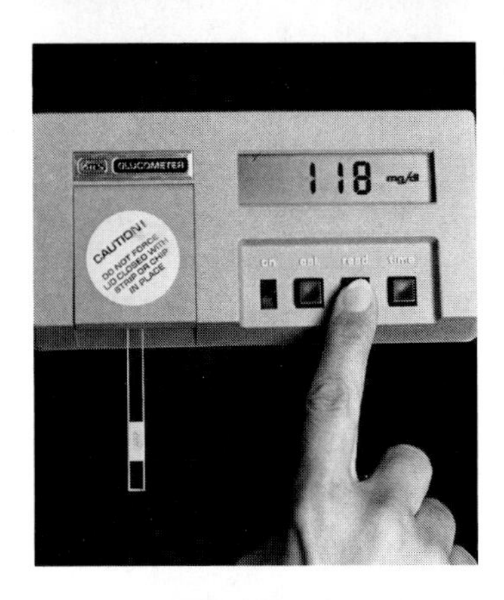

9 After several seconds, expect to see the glucose level reading appear on the display screen.

Document the reading in your nurses' notes.

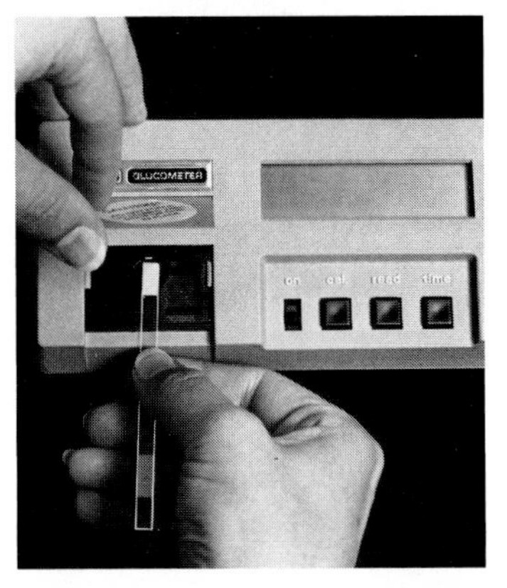

10 Now, remove the strip from the test chamber and dispose of it.

Lower the chamber's lid. Turn off the Glucometer unless you're planning to perform another blood glucose test immediately.

Blood tests

How blood clots

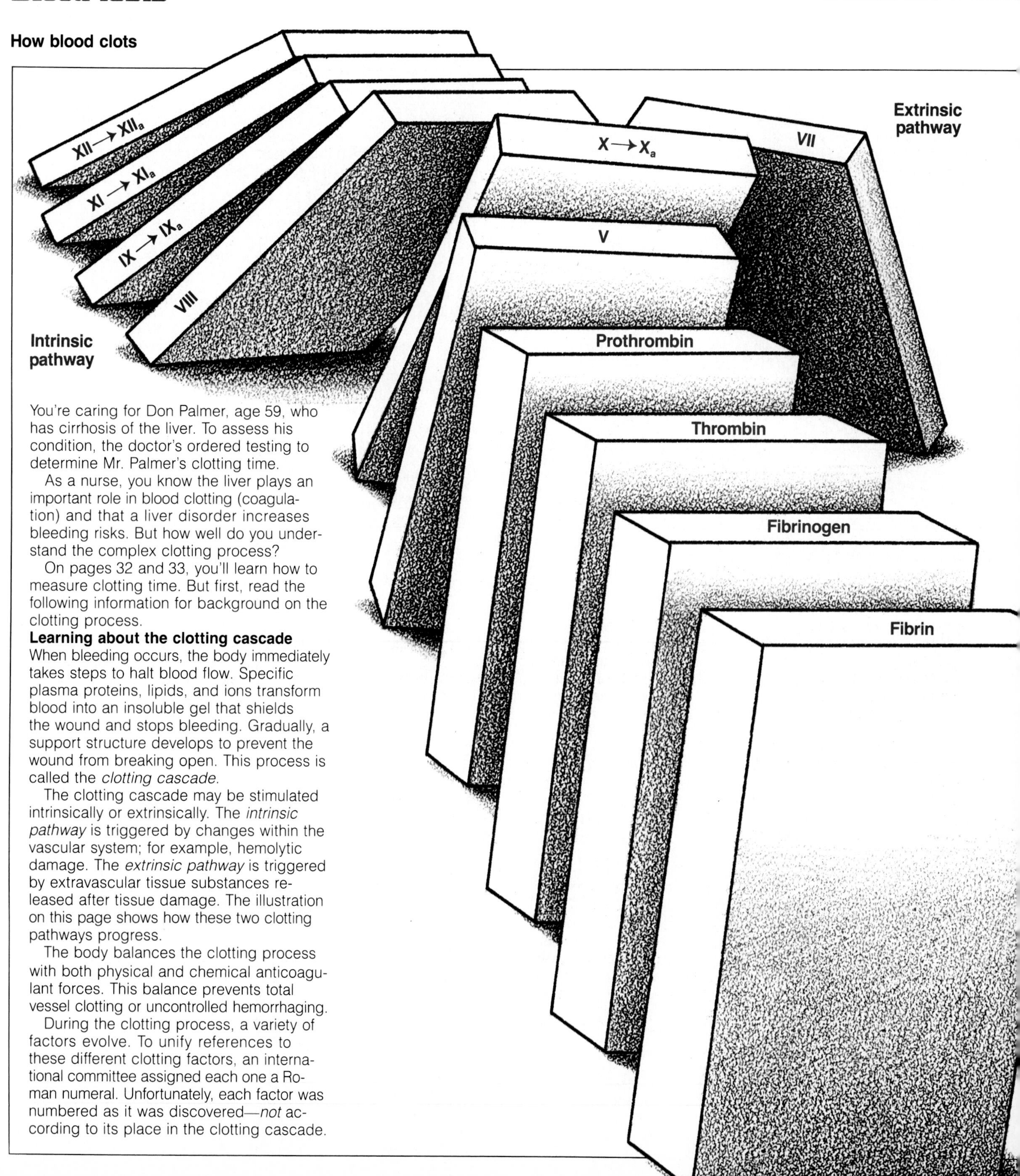

You're caring for Don Palmer, age 59, who has cirrhosis of the liver. To assess his condition, the doctor's ordered testing to determine Mr. Palmer's clotting time.

As a nurse, you know the liver plays an important role in blood clotting (coagulation) and that a liver disorder increases bleeding risks. But how well do you understand the complex clotting process?

On pages 32 and 33, you'll learn how to measure clotting time. But first, read the following information for background on the clotting process.

Learning about the clotting cascade
When bleeding occurs, the body immediately takes steps to halt blood flow. Specific plasma proteins, lipids, and ions transform blood into an insoluble gel that shields the wound and stops bleeding. Gradually, a support structure develops to prevent the wound from breaking open. This process is called the *clotting cascade.*

The clotting cascade may be stimulated intrinsically or extrinsically. The *intrinsic pathway* is triggered by changes within the vascular system; for example, hemolytic damage. The *extrinsic pathway* is triggered by extravascular tissue substances released after tissue damage. The illustration on this page shows how these two clotting pathways progress.

The body balances the clotting process with both physical and chemical anticoagulant forces. This balance prevents total vessel clotting or uncontrolled hemorrhaging.

During the clotting process, a variety of factors evolve. To unify references to these different clotting factors, an international committee assigned each one a Roman numeral. Unfortunately, each factor was numbered as it was discovered—*not* according to its place in the clotting cascade.

As a result, a factor's number doesn't indicate its place in the clotting sequence. *Note:* The subscript *a* after a factor number means that the factor is active.

To help you understand each factor's significance in the cascade, we identify and define each one and explain what causes its values to increase or decrease. To determine the cascade's proper sequence, study the illustration at left.

Factor I (fibrinogen)
- Part of common pathway (common to both intrinsic and extrinsic pathways)
- Relatively insoluble glycoprotein synthesized by the parenchymal cells in the liver
- Normally found in the bloodstream, the lymph system, and many tissues
- Converted into fibrin by action of thrombin
- Essential to normal platelet function and to wound healing
- Normal level increase associated with pregnancy and anovulatory drug administration
- Fibrinogen metabolism may be increased by such diseases as cirrhosis, multiple myeloma, and nephrosis. Any disorder associated with stress, inflammation, or tissue necrosis may produce fibrinogen excess.
- Depressed level associated with hypothyroidism

Factor II (prothrombin)
- Part of common pathway
- Active prothrombin is the most powerful clotting force in the body.
- Constantly present in blood in excess of clotting requirement. Even with 50% blood volume reduction, blood can clot normally.
- Dependent on vitamin K for synthesis. Vitamin K deficiency causes a marked decrease in levels. When intestinal flora (which produce vitamin K) are disturbed (for example, by certain antibiotics), levels decrease.
- Diseases that interfere with fat absorption, such as obstructive jaundice and steatorrhea, may impair vitamin K absorption, leading to decreased levels.
- Severe liver disease and use of oral anticoagulants (when given in therapeutic doses) may alter circulating levels.

Factor III (tissue thromboplastin)
- Part of extrinsic pathway; interacts with Factor VII
- Sources include brain, lung, prostate, and placental tissue.
- Tissue damage (or tissue disease that causes damage) may increase levels.

Factor IV (calcium)
- Part of intrinsic pathway
- Only small quantities are required to promote coagulation.
- Calcium deficiency may result from infusion of large quantity of banked, citrated blood after severe hemorrhage.
- Abnormal binding of calcium may result from hyperglobulinemia and dysglobulinemia, associated with sarcoidosis and myeloma. These conditions may produce a calcium deficiency even though test results indicate a normal calcium level or hypercalcemia.

Factor V (labile factor)
- Part of common pathway
- Also known as AcG or proaccelerin
- Essential in prothrombin formation in common pathway
- Synthesized in the liver
- A labile (unstable), water-soluble globulin
- Because factor is difficult to isolate and stabilize, biochemical role and actual contribution to coagulation process is unknown.
- Congenital deficiency results when an autosomal recessive trait is inherited from both parents.
- Characterized by excessive bleeding from vascular areas of body
- Acquired deficiency may occur in severe liver disease or from circulating anticoagulants.

Factor VI
- Activated Factor V. (Factor VI is an obsolete identification.)

Factor VII (stable factor, proconvertin)
- Part of extrinsic pathway
- Active only in presence of Factor III
- Related to prothrombin
- Can be converted to prothrombin by the liver
- Like prothrombin, dependent on vitamin K for synthesis
- Levels decrease during administration of oral anticoagulants.
- Levels increase after stored-serum administration.

Factor VIII (antihemophiliac factor)
- Part of intrinsic pathway
- Important in Factor IX evolution
- Primary source appears to be liver; may have other sources. The spleen is the major storing area.
- Circulating levels increase after vigorous exercise or epinephrine administration and in certain metabolic states.
- Inadequate levels cause classic hemophilia (hemophilia A).

Factor IX (plasma thromboplastin)
- Part of intrinsic pathway
- Also known as Christmas factor
- Present in serum and plasma; depressed in plasma by pharmacologic activity of oral anticoagulants
- Inherited abnormalities are associated with hemophilia B (Christmas disease).
- Associated with vitamin K deficiency, advanced liver disease, and prolonged anti–vitamin K therapy

Factor X (Stuart factor)
- Part of common pathway
- Activates Factor IV
- Glycoprotein found in plasma and serum
- Necessary for intrinsic thromboplastin formation and for prothrombin conversion
- Method of action and production unknown.
- Deficiency is a hereditary disorder (hemophilia C) that's produced by an incompletely recessive autosomal trait. Acquired deficiency seen in liver disease and vitamin K deficiency.

Factor XI (plasma thromboplastin antecedent)
- Reacts with Factor XII to form an active prothromboplastic substance, initiating the intrinsic pathway
- Deficiency is inherited, leading to a mild hemophilia-like state after trauma or surgery.

Factor XII (Hageman factor)
- Stimulated in intrinsic pathway by cell damage or release of platelets
- Deficiency causes prolonged venous clotting time and partial thromboplastin time, as well as an abnormal thromboplastin generation test. May also produce a hemorrhagic state.

Factor XIII (fibrin stabilizing factor)
- Part of common pathway; forms a stabilizing covalent bond within fibrin strands
- Glycoprotein; as much as 50% found in platelets
- Deficiency occurs with liver damage.
- Hereditary deficiency may be associated with abnormal scar formation, wound dehiscence (splitting), postcircumcision bleeding, and bleeding from the umbilical stump.

Blood tests

Assessing whole blood clotting

Normally, whole blood clots in 5 to 15 minutes. If your patient's blood clotting is incomplete or clotting time is prolonged—for any reason—he faces possible complications ranging from bruising to fatal hemorrhage.

For such a patient, your accurate assessment of whole blood clotting time may be crucial. In the following pages, you'll learn two ways to measure the interval required for a blood specimen to clot at body temperature.

Keep in mind that while a prolonged clotting time suggests a severe deficiency in clotting factors, it doesn't pinpoint the cause. To do this, the doctor will order additional testing, as indicated.

(Of course, if your patient's receiving anticoagulant therapy, you'll expect clotting time to be prolonged.)

Measuring clot retraction

You can use the same blood specimen to measure the time necessary for platelets and a fibrinogen network to form a firm clot (clot retraction time). Within an hour after it's collected, the specimen should have clotted and retracted from the tube's sides and its original volume should have been reduced by half. Abnormal results may indicate thrombocytopenia, hyperfibrinogenemia, anemia, DIC, or secondary fibrinolysis.

Measuring clotting time

You're caring for Anna Martz, a 35-year-old pianist admitted to your unit with deep vein thrombosis. To treat her condition and prevent complications, the doctor's begun anticoagulant therapy with heparin sodium.

To help the doctor evaluate the effects of therapy, you'll assess Ms. Martz's blood clotting time. To do so, you'll determine the time it takes for a fresh whole blood specimen to clot in vitro at 98.6° F. (37° C.). This photostory shows you how.

First, gather this equipment: tourniquet, alcohol swab, gauze pad, two 3-ml syringes, 21G needle, three 12x75-mm test tubes, water bath, and stopwatch. Wash and dry your hands.

Then, fill the bath with water and warm it to 98.6° F. Place the glass tubes upright in the water.

Explain the procedure to Ms. Martz. Prepare her to feel momentary discomfort from the venipuncture.

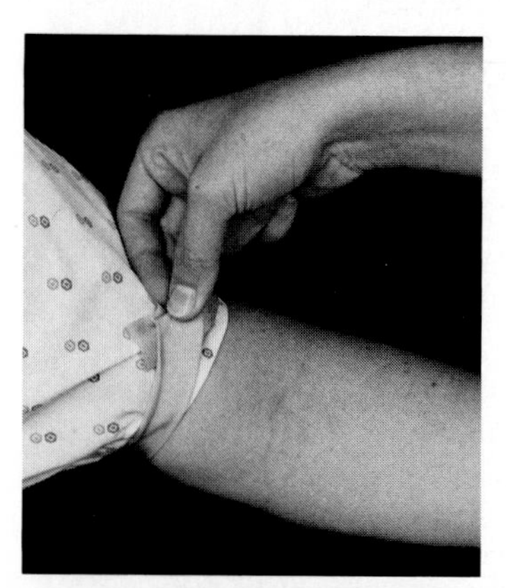

1 Dilate her vein by tying the tourniquet 2" to 6" (5 to 15 cm) above the venipuncture site you've selected. Apply enough pressure to impede venous flow without stopping arterial flow. To protect her skin from pinching, tuck part of her gown sleeve under the tourniquet, as shown.

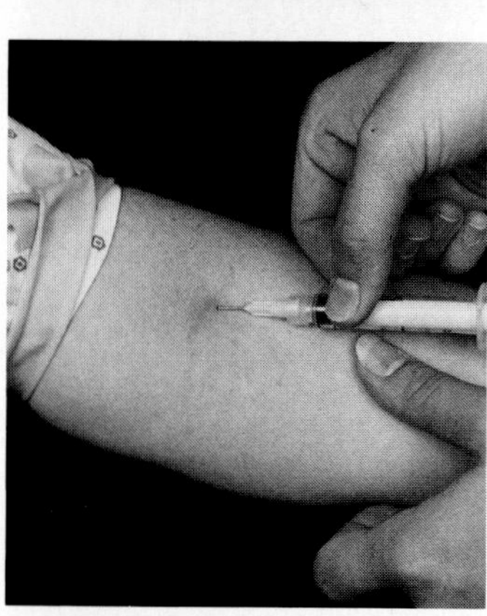

2 When Ms. Martz's vein is adequately dilated, prep the site. Then, insert the needle through the subcutaneous tissue and into the vein, as shown. As you guide the needle into the vein, exert a gentle, lifting pressure to avoid piercing the vein's opposite wall.

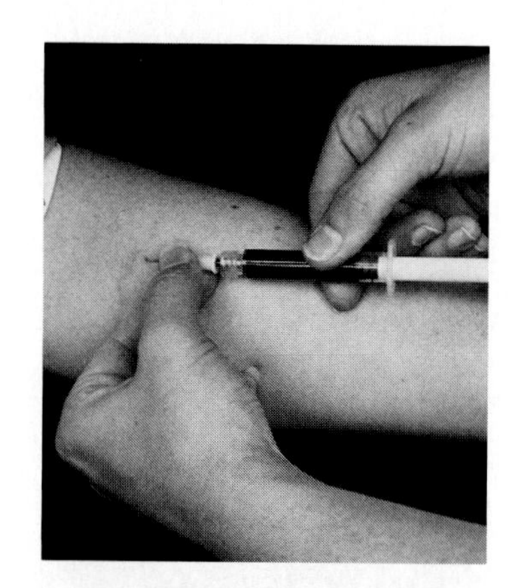

3 Draw 3 ml of blood into a syringe. Then, detach the syringe from the needle, as the nurse is doing here, and dispose of the syringe. This minimizes the risk of contaminating the blood specimen with tissue thromboplastin released when you punctured the vessel.

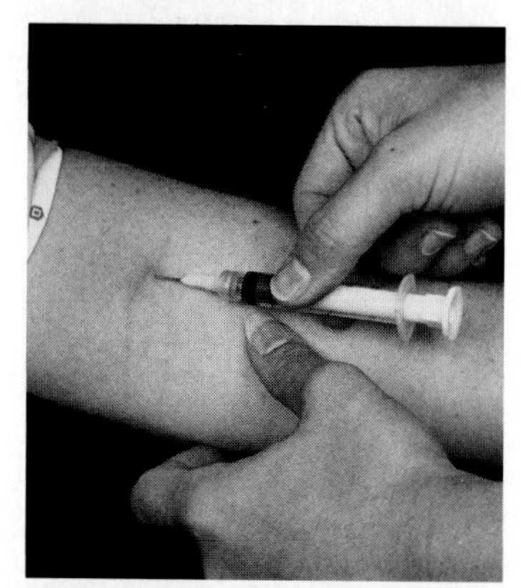

4 Now, attach a new syringe to the needle and begin drawing a blood specimen, as shown. Using the stopwatch, start timing as soon as blood enters the syringe.

When you've filled the second syringe, withdraw the needle and apply pressure to the puncture site with a gauze pad. Then, instruct Ms. Martz to maintain this pressure until the bleeding stops.

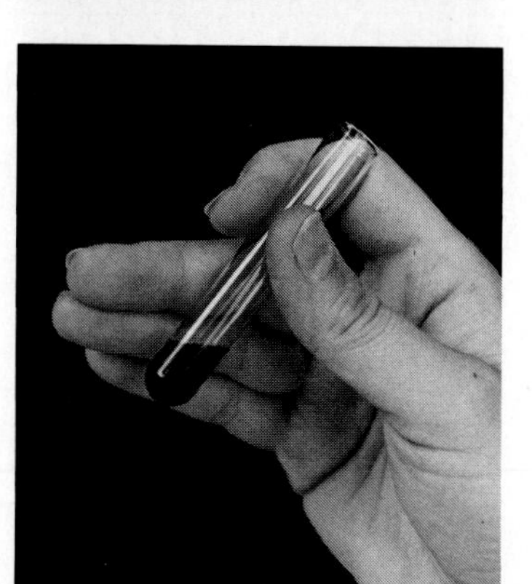

5 Remove the needle from the syringe. To minimize cell damage, *slowly* inject 1 ml of blood into each test tube.

Take the last tube you fill and tilt it gently once every 30 seconds until a clot forms. Return it to the water bath. Repeat the procedure with the second tube you fill and then with the first.

Stop timing when the blood's clotted in all three tubes. Document the results.

Using the Hemochron

Let's say your cardiac patient's receiving heparin therapy. To prevent complications (such as hemorrhage) from an extremely prolonged clotting time, you need a fast, precise way to monitor his whole blood clotting time. The Hemochron Portable Blood Coagulation Timing System, shown at right, usually provides you with clotting time measurements within 10 minutes of specimen collection.

Because the Hemochron doesn't have a water bath or heating block, it's easy to operate. And you can monitor your patient at his bedside, which eliminates laboratory delays and specimen mix-ups. The Hemochron runs on either battery or outlet power.

To use the Hemochron system, first perform venipuncture. Collect the specimen in a specially prepared test tube provided by the manufacturer. Then, place the tube in the Hemochron's incubated test well. When clotting has been detected, you'll hear a tone and see the results on the Hemochron's display screen.

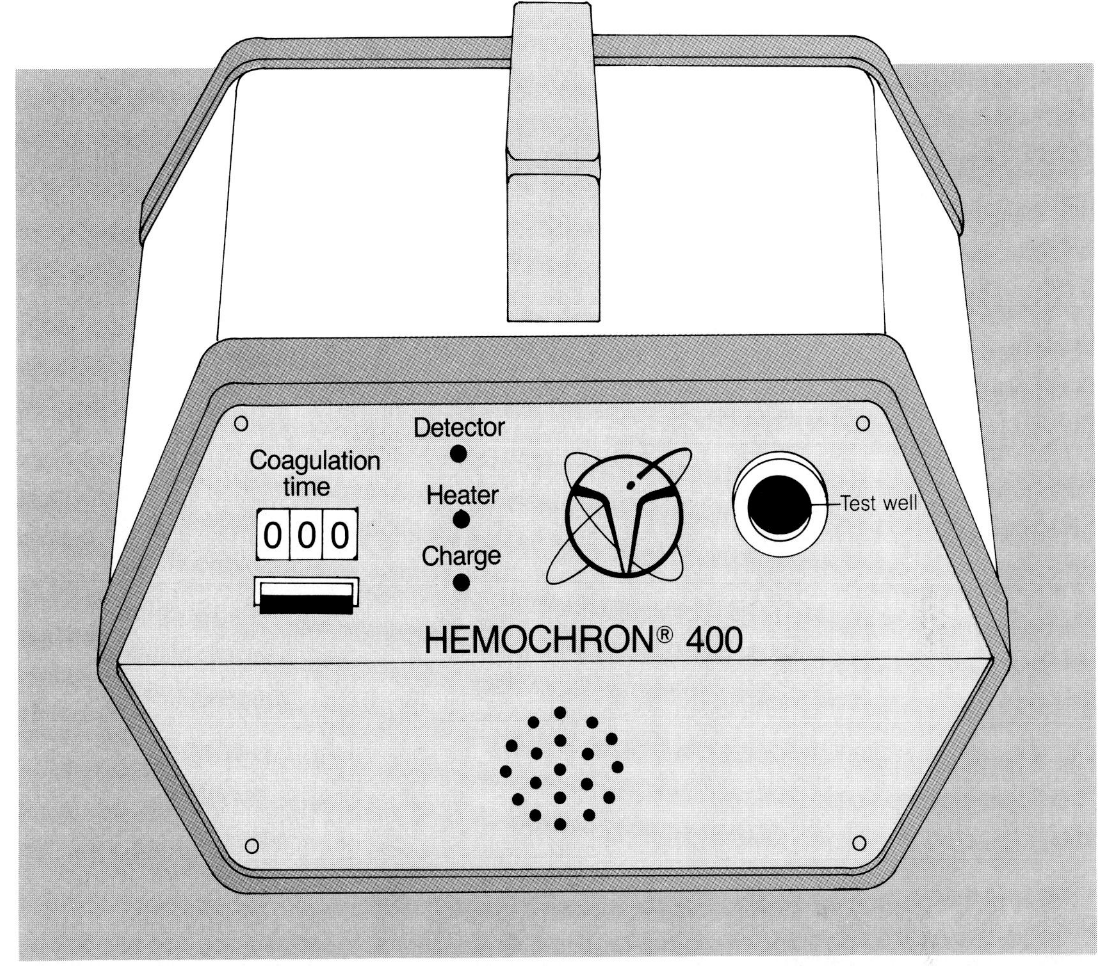

Because you use only one test tube, you needn't transfer the blood to different tubes (as when using the water bath method). In addition to simplifying the procedure, this feature makes possible more accurate test results.

When monitoring a patient receiving heparin therapy, use the Hemochron to:

- detect any initial sensitivity or resistance to the heparin.
- detect any variation in heparin potency.
- evaluate the rate of heparin consumption.
- assess for heparin rebound.

Note: Consider using the Hemochron to monitor a patient undergoing hemodialysis. By doing so, you protect him against overheparinization and still prevent clotting in the artificial kidney.

Understanding anticoagulant therapy

The doctor has ordered anticoagulant therapy for your patient for one of these reasons:

- to prevent thromboembolism
- to reduce the risk of complications from a thromboembolus
- to prevent clotting during extracorporeal circulation, such as in hemodialysis.

Although the doctor is responsible for initiating and adjusting therapy, you're likely to be asked to monitor your patient's response.

Let's assume the doctor's ordered anticoagulant therapy to prolong clotting time. How familiar are you with the two principal types of anticoagulant he may order? Do you know how quickly they work and how to reverse their effects? If you're unsure, read the following chart.

heparin sodium

Action
Interferes with conversion of fibrinogen to fibrin

Administration
Subcutaneous or I.V. (isn't absorbed from the gastrointestinal tract)

Onset and duration
- Acts immediately; peaks in a few minutes
- Clotting time returns to normal in 2 to 6 hours.

Therapeutic level
Clotting time one and a half to two times above normal

Specific test to determine activity
Partial thromboplastin time (PTT)

Treatment of overdose
- If bleeding's minimal and can be controlled through local measures (for example, by applying pressure over the bleeding site), discontinue therapy, as ordered.
- If bleeding's severe, give protamine sulfate (1 mg per 95 units of heparin given), as ordered, to counteract heparin's effects.

warfarin sodium (Coumadin*), phenprocoumon (Liquamar)

Action
Inhibits vitamin K–dependent activation of clotting factors II, VII, IX, and X

Administration
P.O.

Onset and duration
- Starts acting in 1 hour and peaks in 12 hours
- Requires 1 to 3 days to produce therapeutic levels
- Duration is from 1 to 14 days, depending on the patient and the drug used.

Therapeutic level
Generally one and a half to two times above normal

Specific test to determine activity
Prothrombin time (PT)

Treatment of overdose
- Administer vitamin K I.M. or I.V., as ordered.

*Available in both the United States and Canada

Blood tests

Learning about the Autoclix lancet

Jack Talbot has diabetes. "I stick myself at least twice a day to test my blood glucose level, but I've never gotten used to it," he tells you. "I sure wish I knew an easier way to collect a blood specimen."

Consider teaching a patient like Jack how to use an automatic lancet, such as the Autoclix featured below. This device makes the self-sticking procedure quick, easy, and almost painless.

The Autoclix plastic case is wide at the base and tapered at the top. A plunger extends from the base, and a spring's located inside the top. A pressure platform snaps into place over the spring to regulate puncture depth.

Your patient may choose one of three color-coded platforms supplied by the manufacturer. The yellow platform usually provides sufficient puncture depth to obtain a blood specimen. The white platform decreases puncture depth, and the orange platform increases the depth.

Instruct your patient to practice with this automatic lancet on a soft object, such as a plastic cup, until he can use the device confidently. Then, he can use it to puncture his finger, heel, or earlobe. But advise him to take a few specimens from his finger before attempting to stick his heel or earlobe.

If your patient has poor circulation or the area he's puncturing is cold, he may have a problem collecting enough blood. To stimulate blood flow in the puncture area, suggest that he first wash the area in warm water and then massage it.

Teaching your patient to use the Autoclix

You're teaching Jack Talbot how to use the Autoclix lancet to collect a blood specimen from his fingertip. After briefly explaining how he'll collect the specimen, tell him to gather the following equipment: Autoclix case, yellow pressure platform, lancet, gauze pad or cotton ball, and alcohol swab.

Then, show your patient the equipment and explain how it works. Don't forget to tell him how the three color-coded platforms differ and to explain why he should use the yellow platform for his first puncture attempt.

Have him wash his finger in warm water and massage it to promote blood flow. Next, tell him to hold the case vertically and to gently snap the platform on the tapered end of the case. Then, have him place his thumb on the plunger located at the case's base. Tell him to press the plunger as close to the base as possible and hold it there.

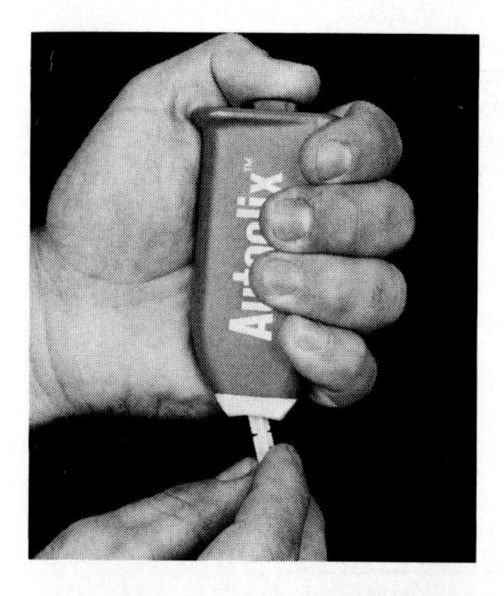

1 Next, instruct him to take a lancet and insert the flat end through the hole in the platform's middle. He should twist the lancet slightly as he pushes it into place.

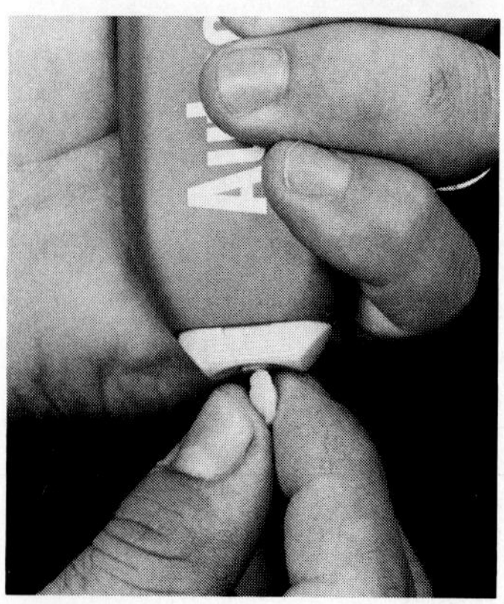

2 While your patient's still depressing the plunger, have him slowly twist off the lancet's round protective cap. Instruct him to put the cap aside.

Then, tell him to release the plunger, so the lancet withdraws into the case. Make sure he understands that the case is now cocked and can be activated by pressing on the platform.

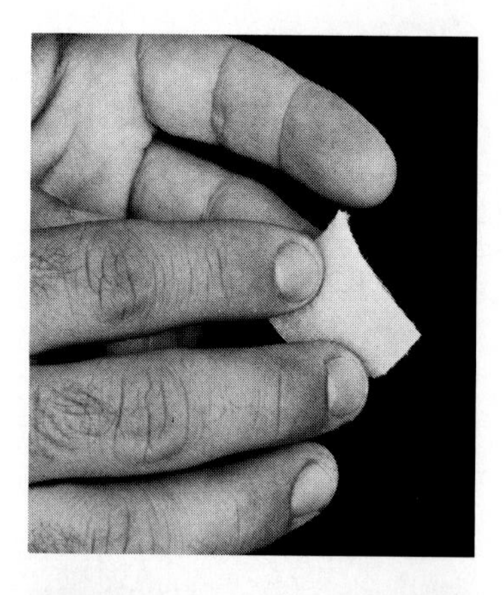

3 Now, tell him to take the alcohol swab and thoroughly cleanse his fingertip. Remind him to allow his skin to air-dry before proceeding.

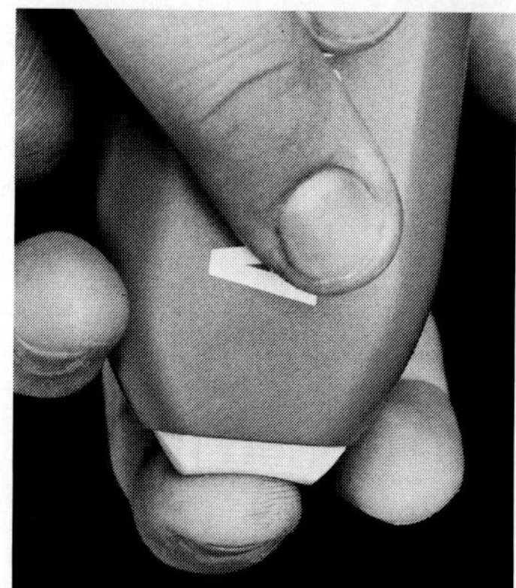

4 Instruct him to firmly hold the Autoclix case in his free hand, without touching the plunger.

Now, have him *gently* press his cleansed fingertip over the platform hole, as shown here. The pressure releases the lancet, which then punctures the skin.

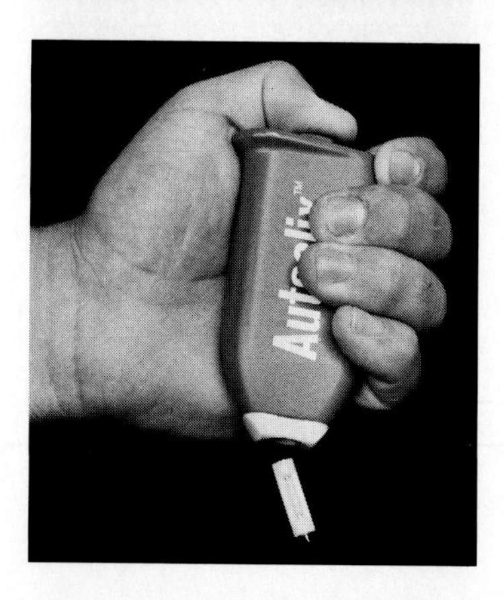

5 Now, tell him to put the case down and squeeze just below the fingertip. Remind him to wipe away the first drop with a clean gauze pad or cotton ball. After he's collected an acceptable blood specimen and tested it, have him hold the case as shown and press the plunger to eject the lancet. Then, instruct him to recap the lancet and discard it.

Finally, document your teaching in your nurses' notes.

Nutritional tests

Maintaining your patient's nutritional status is an integral part of his care. By keeping him sufficiently nourished, you can prevent complications, speed his recovery, and promote a positive attitude.

In this section, we describe the important role you play in sustaining your patient's nourishment. You'll learn how to:

- take a nutritional history.
- perform a visual assessment to detect signs and symptoms of malnutrition.
- weigh your nonambulatory patient.
- take skin-fold measurements to determine fat and protein reserves.
- perform a skin test to detect anergy, which usually indicates malnutrition.
- provide total parenteral nutrition, if ordered.

What's your role in maintaining your patient's nutritional status? Find out on the following pages.

Becoming aware of nutritional needs

With all the other patient needs you satisfy, nutrition often takes a backseat. After all, the doctor decides the diet and the dietitian plans the meals. Where do you fit in? How important is your role in responding to your patient's nutritional needs?

Actually, you play the biggest part. When your patient is admitted to the hospital, you take a complete history (see box at right) that alerts you to possible nutritional problems. By providing care during his hospitalization, you observe and document changes in his condition and daily eating habits. All these factors enable you to assess your patient's needs and recommend diet changes; for example, a change from full liquids to solid foods.

You can also recognize and solve problems before they become serious. For example, suppose you notice that your patient hasn't eaten a meal. Try to pinpoint the reason. Is he nauseated or depressed? Do his dentures hurt him? Does he dislike the food being served? Once you know the reason, you can try to solve the problem before he becomes malnourished.

Malnutrition's consequences

As you know, malnutrition may lengthen a patient's recovery time by making him susceptible to infections. But that's not all. A malnourished patient is also at risk of developing marasmas or kwashiorkor, two disorders resulting from dietary deficiencies. At one time, these disorders were thought to afflict children in third world countries only. Now, we know they can afflict hospitalized patients as well.

Marasmas results from an inadequate calorie-protein intake. The condition usually causes weight loss (which may be excessive), skin dryness, frequent diarrhea, weakness, and muscle wasting. Patients who can't maintain adequate oral nutrition are most susceptible.

Kwashiorkor is a protein malnutrition disorder affecting patients who consume many more carbohydrates than proteins. This leads to a well-nourished (even obese) appearance, as the excess calories are stored in body fat. The appearance is deceiving, however, because a patient with kwashiorkor is severely protein-deficient and a high mortality risk.

Kwashiorkor-marasmus mix (marasmic kwashiorkor), a combination of the two disorders, has signs and symptoms of both.

DOCUMENTING

Taking a nutritional history

Don't assume your patient's well nourished just because he *looks* well nourished. Remember, appearances can be deceiving. To properly assess his nutritional status, first take a complete history. Knowing his background will help you anticipate problems that may interfere with proper nutrition and enable you to suggest dietary modifications to the doctor.

Remember to explain to your patient why you're asking these questions and how his answers will benefit him. *Important:* Watch for nonverbal and visual clues to your patient's condition. For example, a patient whose clothing fits loosely may have lost weight recently.

For an overview of your patient's nutritional history and condition, ask him these questions:

- What is your height? Your weight? Your age?
- Have you gained or lost weight over the past few days or weeks? How much? Are you trying to lose weight; for example, by dieting?
- Do you maintain a special diet at home?
- How frequently do you eat at home? Do you live alone? Who cooks for you?
- Are your teeth in good condition? Do you have any problems chewing your food? Do you wear dentures? If so, do they fit well?
- Do you frequently have mouth sores or episodes of gum bleeding?
- What's the condition of your skin? Your hair?
- Have you noticed any swelling of your legs or feet recently? Have you noticed any general weakness or diminished strength recently?
- Are your bowel movements regular?
- Do you have problems with diarrhea or constipation?
- Do you ever feel nauseated or have heartburn or a lot of gas?
- Have you ever lost your appetite for any length of time?
- Does anyone in your family have diabetes? Are any family members obese?

After taking the history, supplement the information with the results of your patient's admission screening tests; for instance, his total serum protein level, including the albumin fraction. Then, perform a physical assessment. The chart on the following page will help you interpret your assessment findings.

Nutritional tests

Interpreting assessment findings

Suppose, while performing a physical assessment and taking a history, you discover that your patient has chronically sore, swollen gums. Do you automatically attribute the problem to poor dental hygiene? If so, you may be overlooking an important clue to his nutritional status.

Your patient's general condition can tell you a lot about how well nourished he is. Read this chart for details.

Hair

Finding	Possible deficiency
• Appears dry, fine, and brittle; pulls out of scalp easily; brown or black hair lightens	• Protein

Eyes

Finding	Possible deficiency
• Frothy, irregular white or yellow spots on conjunctivae; dry, rough conjunctivae; lids red and swollen; loss of light reflex; corneal ulceration	• Vitamin A
• Conjunctivitis; arteriole penetration into corneas; moist, red lesion formation at outer edges of eyelids	• Riboflavin (vitamin B_2)
• Ocular hemorrhage	• Vitamin C, vitamin K

Mouth

Finding	Possible deficiency
• Bleeding or swollen gums, loose teeth	• Vitamin A, niacin, riboflavin (vitamin B_2), or vitamin C
• Thick, red, beefy mouth and lips; red tongue; atrophied papillae	• Niacin
• Purple tongue (magenta tongue)	• Riboflavin (vitamin B_2)

Neck

Finding	Possible deficiency
• Large, palpable thyroid gland (goiter)	• Iodine

Skin

Finding	Possible deficiency
• Oiliness, dermatitis, fissuring, and exfoliation; especially along nasolabial folds, scrotum, or vulva	• Riboflavin (vitamin B_2)
• Dry, scaly, and red (gooseflesh appearance, especially on outer arms and thighs)	• Vitamin A
• Dry, rough, and brown	• Vitamin C
• Petechiae or bleeding	• Vitamin K
• Marked pitting edema of legs, arms, and thighs	• Protein
• Pallor	• Folic acid, thiamine, vitamin B_{12}, or iron

Cardiovascular system

Finding	Possible deficiency
• Cardiomegaly or tachycardia	• Thiamine

Gastrointestinal system

Finding	Possible deficiency
• Diarrhea	• Calorie, niacin, folic acid, or vitamin B_{12}
• Anorexia, nausea, or vomiting	• Thiamine, niacin, vitamin B_{12}, or iron
• Constipation	• Iron or thiamine
• Gastrointestinal bleeding	• Vitamin K

Identifying body frames

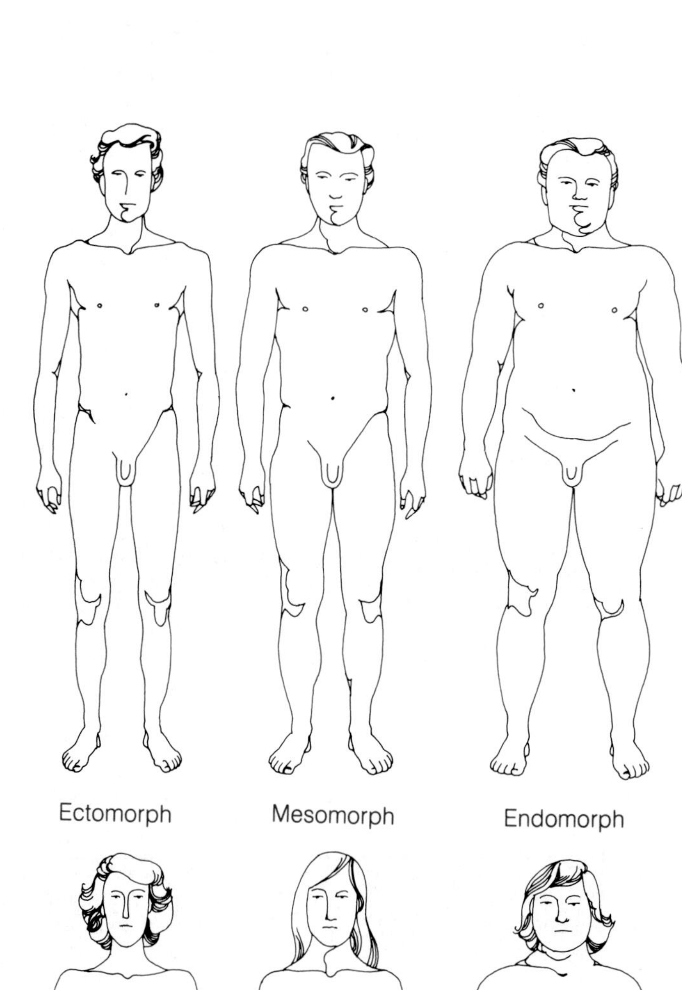

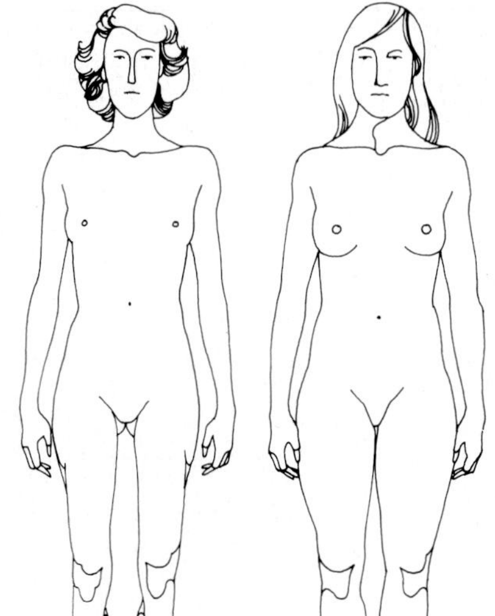

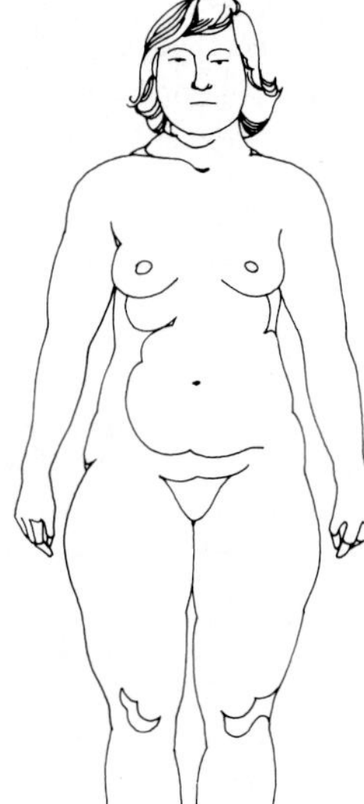

Imagine that you have two patients, each weighing 165 lb (74.8 kg). Despite their equal weight, one could be overweight and one could be underweight. Wondering how to tell the difference? As a rule, by considering each patient's body frame type, which relates directly to weight.

Depending on your patient's body frame, you may classify him as an ectomorph, a mesomorph, or an endomorph. Read the chart below to learn the characteristics of each classification.

Note: These classifications apply to both males and females.

Ectomorph
- Small, slender body that appears weak
- High proportion of skin and bones
- Long arms and legs
- Slender, delicate bone structure
- Stringy muscles
- Thin subcutaneous tissue
- Slightly developed abdominal viscera

Mesomorph
- Athletic appearance
- Well-developed muscles
- High proportion of muscle
- Prominent body joints, particularly at the shoulders and hips
- Massive, muscular chest (in males); chest more prominent than abdomen
- Flat stomach
- General hardness and ruggedness in all regions (especially in males)

Endomorph
- Large body type with short arms and legs
- High proportion of fat
- Arms and legs appear to taper from proximal to distal.
- Abdominal mass dominates body section in males (females may be proportioned somewhat differently).
- Large abdominal viscera overhangs pelvis
- General roundness, with soft contours in all regions

Determining body frame type

Aside from observation, how can you determine your patient's body frame type? Try this technique. First, measure his wrist at the narrowest circumference (between the wrist joints and the hand). Then, measure his height without shoes.

On the chart at right, find the wrist measurement on the horizontal axis and the height measurement on the vertical axis. The block corresponding to both measurements tells you the patient's body frame type.

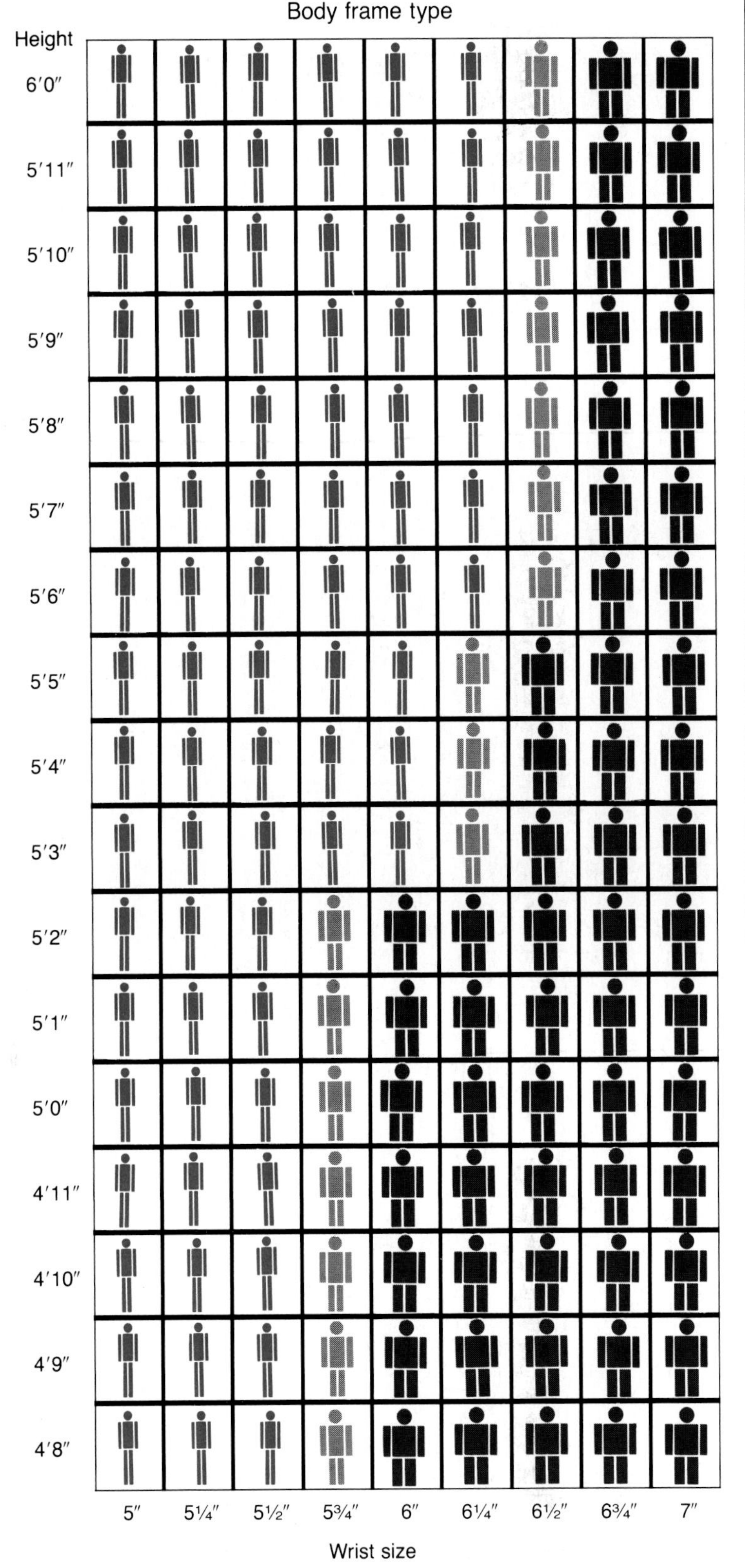

Small frame

Medium frame

Large frame

Nutritional tests

Weighing your patient: Some guidelines

Like most nurses, you probably overlook the value of weighing your patient daily. Yet it's an easy way to assess his nutritional status. Scales are available on all nursing units, and usually you can weigh your patient without a doctor's order.

By weighing your patient daily, you can observe any changes that occur over time and note any trends. For an accurate daily assessment, observe these guidelines:

- Weigh him at the same time each day.
- Use the same scale.
- Make sure your patient's wearing the same (or similar) clothing each day.
- Support all equipment (for instance, an indwelling catheter, ventilator tubing, or I.V. lines) during the procedure so it doesn't add to the patient's weight.
- Make sure the scale's set at 0 before placing your patient on it.

In addition to weighing your patient, monitor his daily intake and output. Be aware that rapid daily weight gain or loss (0.6 to 1 kg) occurs from a fluid shift. Protein changes occur over a longer period.

How much should your patient weigh? Of course, this depends on his dietary intake and his body type. To estimate his ideal weight, use the following guidelines.

A male should weigh 106 lb (48 kg) for the first 5′ (1.5 m) of height and another 6 lb (2.7 kg) for each inch (2.5 cm) of height beyond 5′ (for example, a 5′8″ male should weigh approximately 153 lb). A female should weigh 105 lb (47.6 kg) for 5′ of height and another 5 lb (2.2 kg) for each additional inch of height.

Now, read the next few pages to learn how to weigh a nonambulatory patient.

Understanding the Scale-Tronix bed scale

To monitor a nonambulatory patient's nutritional status, use a bed scale, such as the Scale-Tronix 2001 model shown at right.

This battery-powered scale, which can weigh up to 450 lb (204 kg), provides a measurement that's accurate within 0.1 lb (50 g). Four swivel casters under the base make the scale easy to transport, and two handles located midway up the vertical post enable you to grasp the scale securely while maneuvering it into place. *Caution:* Because the scale contains sensitive electronic transducers within the arms of its frame, be especially careful when moving or repositioning it.

The legs of the scale spread, providing additional support during the weighing procedure. The base even fits under very low beds. In addition, the scale's hydraulic system and flexible sling make it possible for you to weigh your patient without assistance. *Important:* Plug the scale into a wall outlet when it's not in use. Doing so keeps the battery charged. An uncharged battery takes 14 hours to fully recharge.

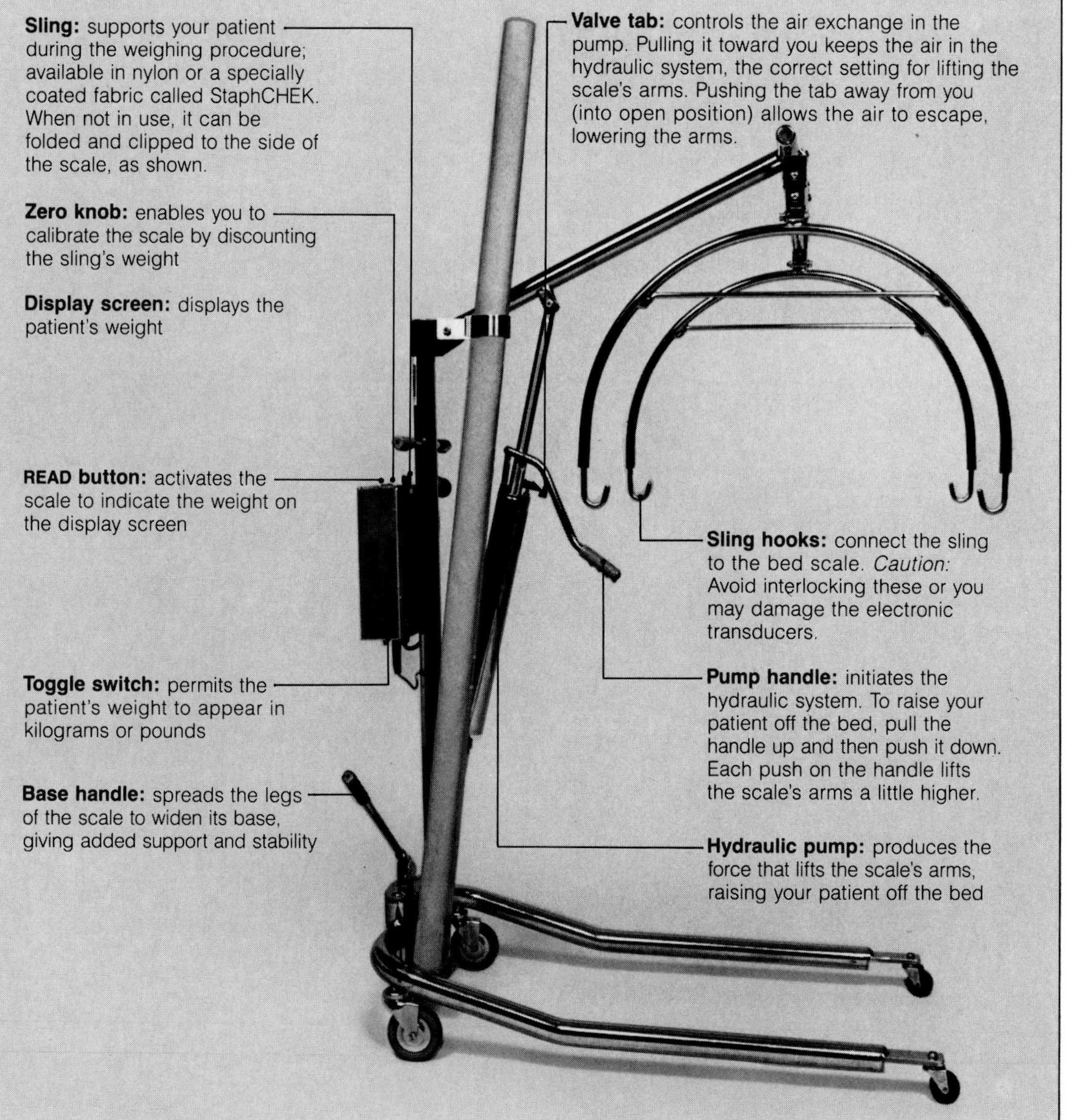

Calibrating a bed scale

Grace Myers, a 40-year-old lab technician, has been admitted to your unit with congestive heart failure. The doctor has asked you to weigh Ms. Myers daily to determine if she's retaining fluids. Because she's been instructed to remain in bed, you'll weigh her with the Scale-Tronix 2001 bed scale.

Before you use this bed scale, calibrate it by weighing the empty sling. This automatically deducts the sling's weight from the final measurement. As a rule, you'll calibrate the scale only once daily. Perform this procedure again, however, when you change slings, jar the equipment, or switch the measurement from pounds to kilograms (or vice versa). For convenience, perform the calibration procedure in your patient's room, just before weighing her. Because the scale is battery-powered, unplug it before beginning. A safety lock system prevents the scale from being operated when the power cord is plugged in.

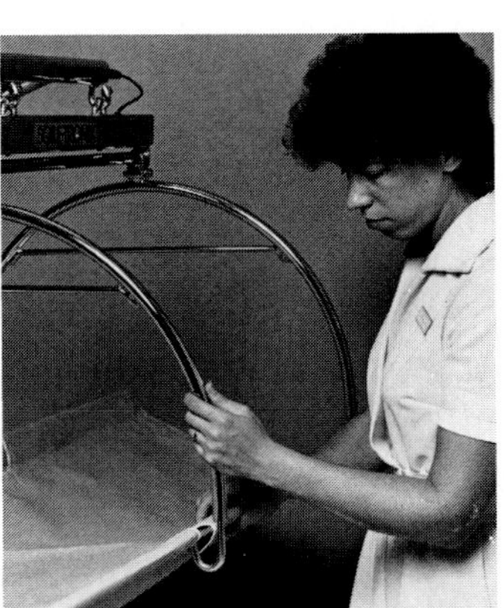
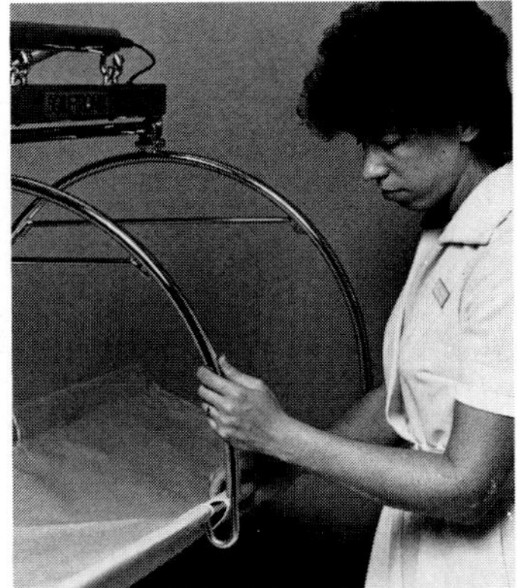

1 To begin, remove the sling from its safety clip and unroll it. Then, attach the sling to the hooks, as shown here.

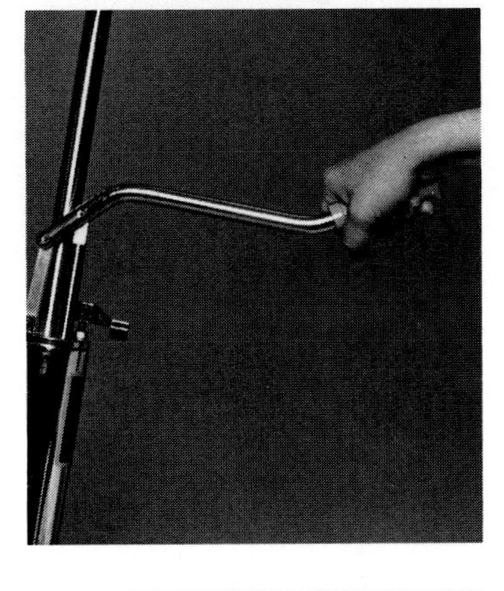

2 Make sure the sling is hanging freely. Then, pump the hydraulic pump handle to raise the sling, if necessary.

3 Now, decide whether you want to record your patient's weight in kilograms or pounds. Make your selection by adjusting the toggle switch located under the display screen. (In this photostory, we'll record measurements in pounds.)

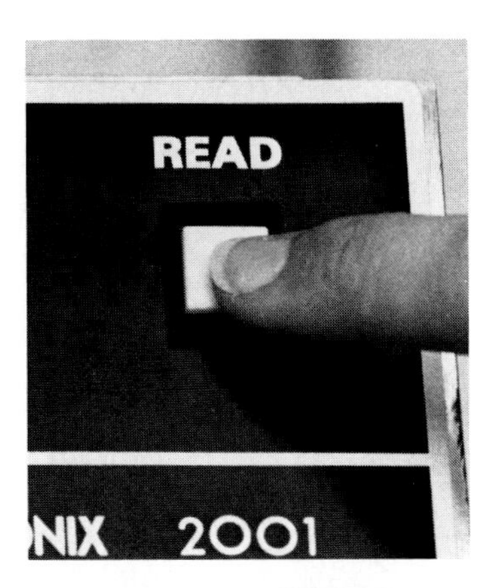

4 Next, press the READ button, as shown in this photo.

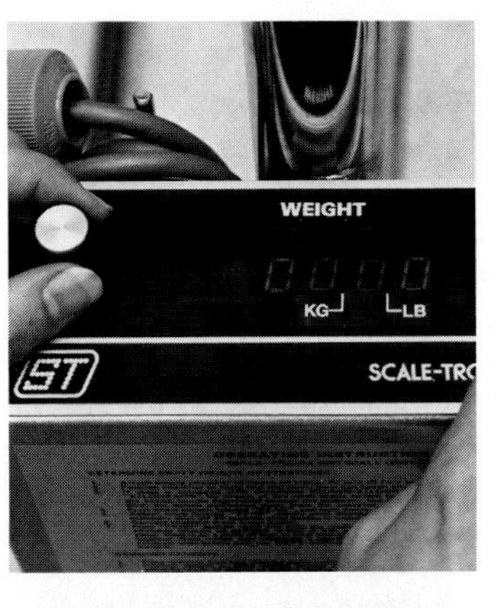

5 Then, twist the ZERO knob until you see 0.00 on the display screen.

Note: The scale shuts off automatically 20 seconds after the READ button is released.

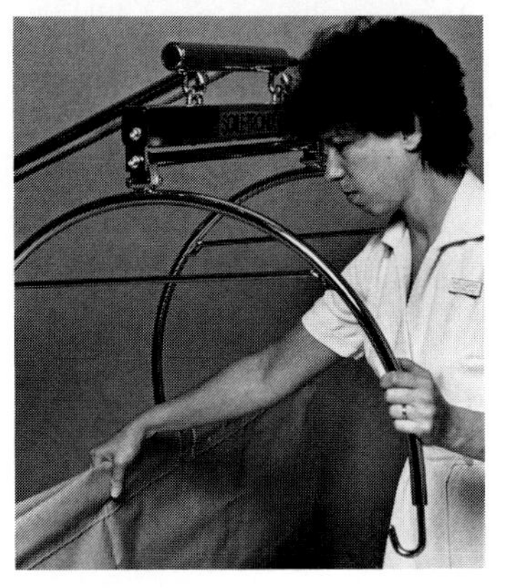

6 Now, remove the sling from the hooks.

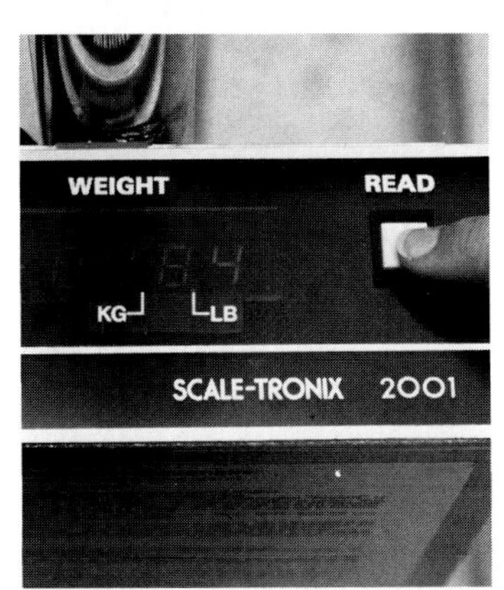

7 Press the READ button again. Wait 3 seconds, and then observe the display screen for the sling's weight measurement. The screen will show the sling weight as a negative value; for example −8.4. (This reading's in pounds because of the toggle switch adjustment you made in step 3.) Most slings weigh between 6 and 9 lb. Record this figure on a piece of tape and attach it to the scale. You'll use this figure when you weigh the patient.

Nutritional tests

Using a bed scale to weigh your patient

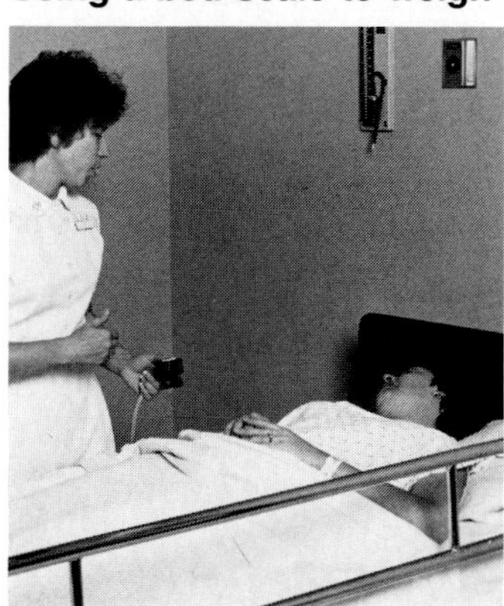

1 You've calibrated the Scale-Tronix 2001 bed scale, as shown on the preceding page. Now you're ready to weigh your patient. Here's how.

First, make sure your patient's bed is flat and that she's lying in a comfortable position. Explain the procedure to Ms. Myers and reassure her.

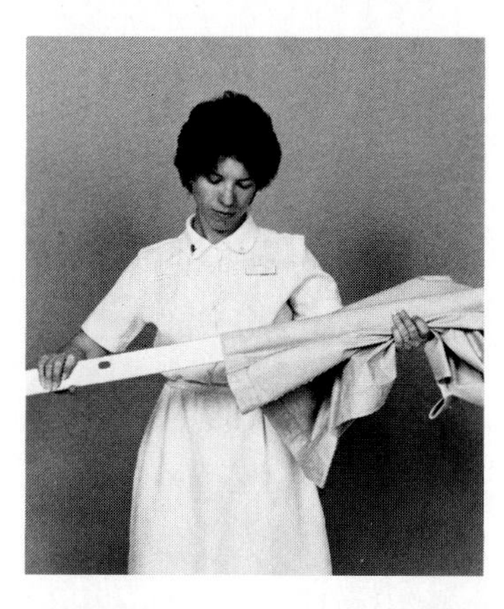

2 Now, remove the metal bars from both sides of the sling.

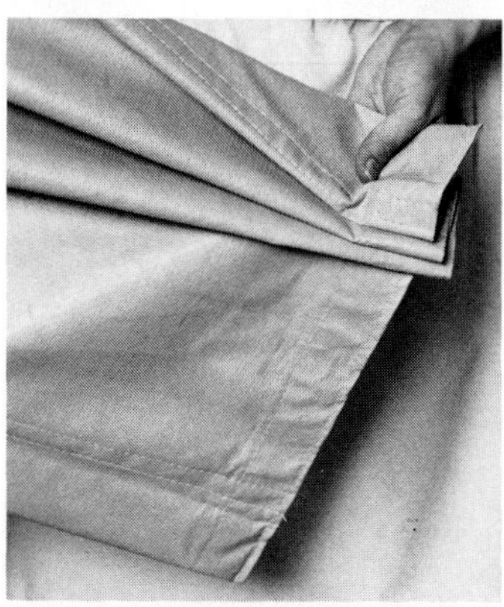

3 Next, fanfold the sling, as the nurse is doing in this photo.

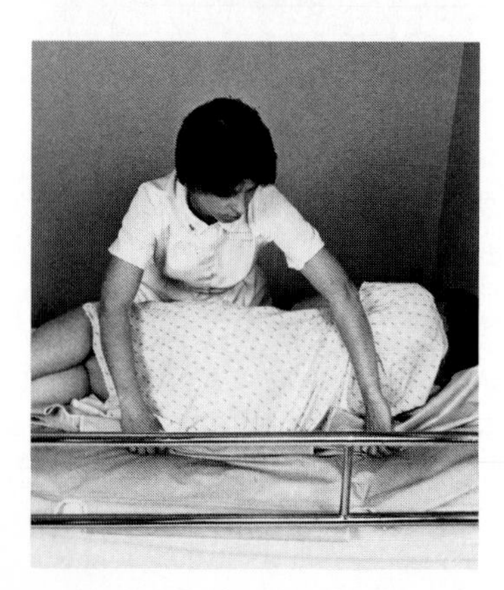

4 Gently roll Ms. Myers toward you. Then, place the fan-folded sling behind her, as shown here. Make sure the hem's open ends face toward the foot of the bed, so you can easily insert the metal bars.

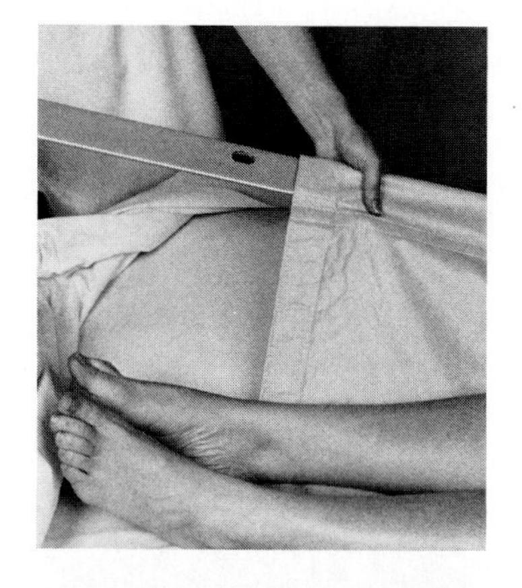

5 Then, roll Ms. Myers onto her other side, and unfold the sling. Remove the pillow.

Now, place her in a supine position in the center of the sling and align her body. Position her heels over the sling's edge. *Note:* The Scale-Tronix 2001 model accurately weighs your patient in any position.

Next, insert a metal bar in each hem's open end, as shown.

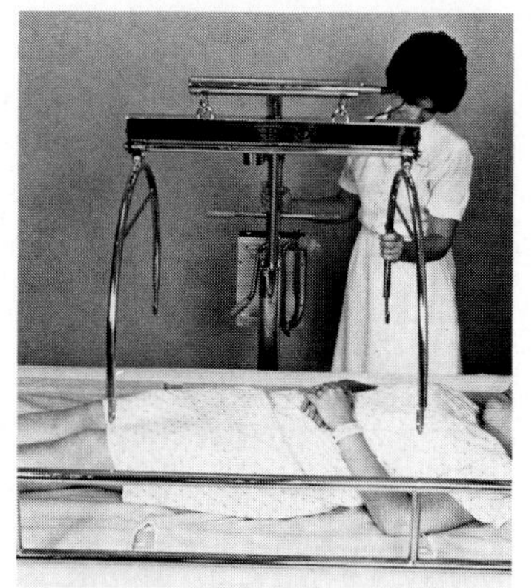

6 Now, move the scale to bedside. Press its READ button and adjust the ZERO knob until the display screen registers the empty sling weight that you previously determined (see the preceding page). *Important:* Make sure the sling weight is displayed as a negative value.

Next, pump the hydraulic pump handle to raise the scale's top portion. Then, position the arms over your patient, as shown.

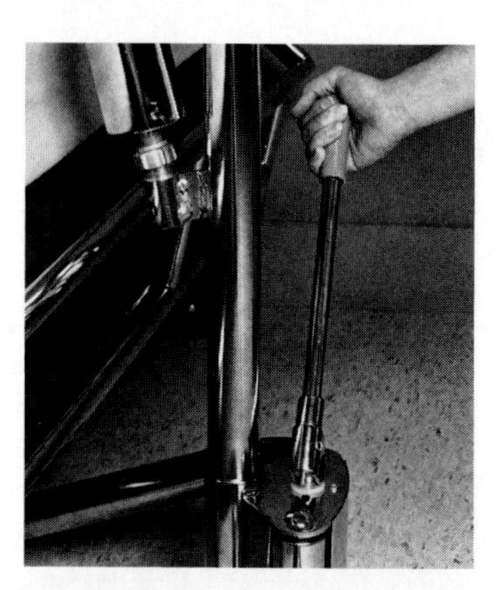

7 Now, firmly turn the base handle counterclockwise until the scale's legs are far enough apart to properly stabilize the scale.

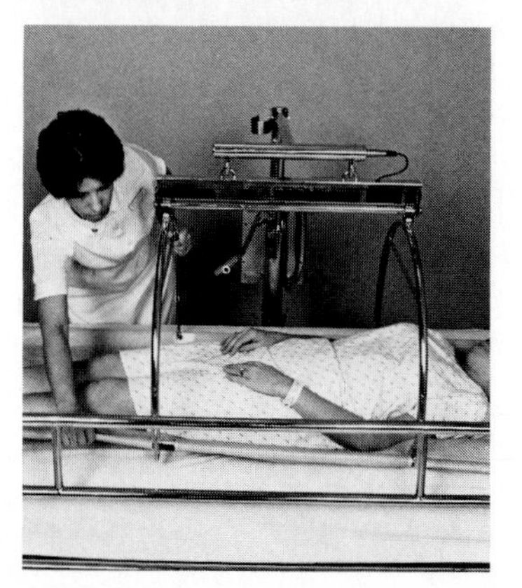

8 Push the valve tab to the open position. As you do, expect the scale's arms to lower toward the bed.

When the hooks are within 1″ (2.5 cm) of the bed, pull the tab back to the closed position. Then, attach the sling, as the nurse is doing here.

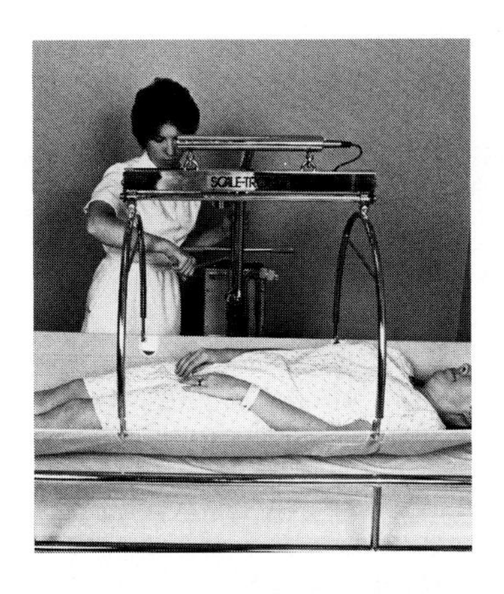

9 Next, pump the hydraulic pump handle to raise the bottom of the sling about 1″ (2.5 cm) off the bed. *Caution:* Don't move the scale or transport your patient away from the bed.

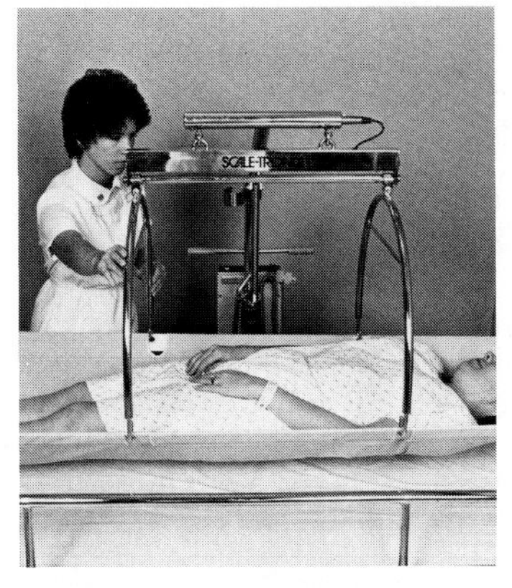

10 Wait for the sling to stabilize. If the sling continues to sway, steady it with your hands.

Note: Before recording your patient's weight, make sure any tubes that are connected to her are supported away from the scale.

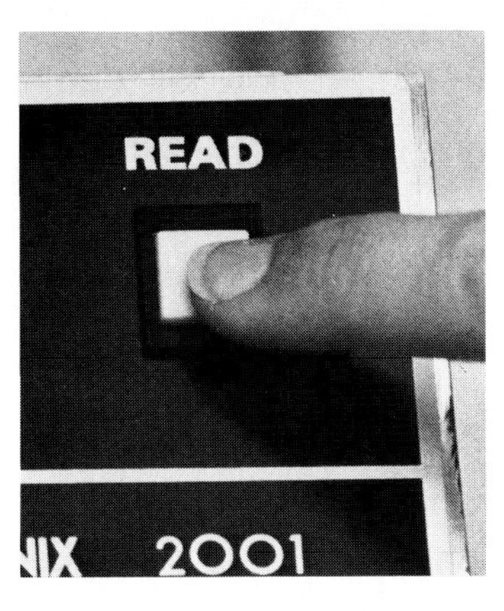

11 Now, press the READ button. The display screen will show your patient's weight. Record the figure. After 20 seconds, the screen automatically becomes blank.

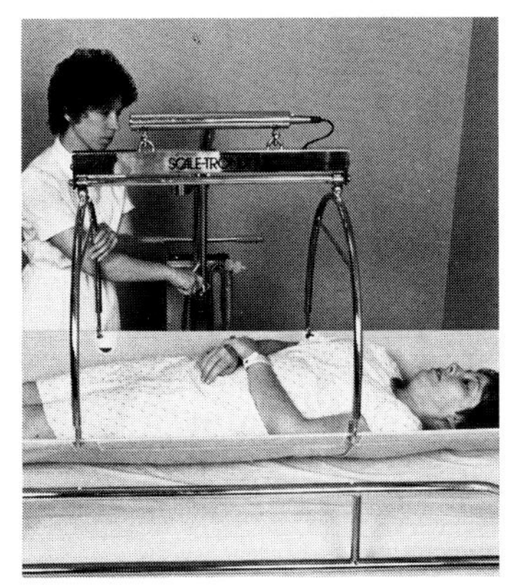

12 Push the hydraulic pump's valve tab to the open position to lower the sling and your patient to the bed.

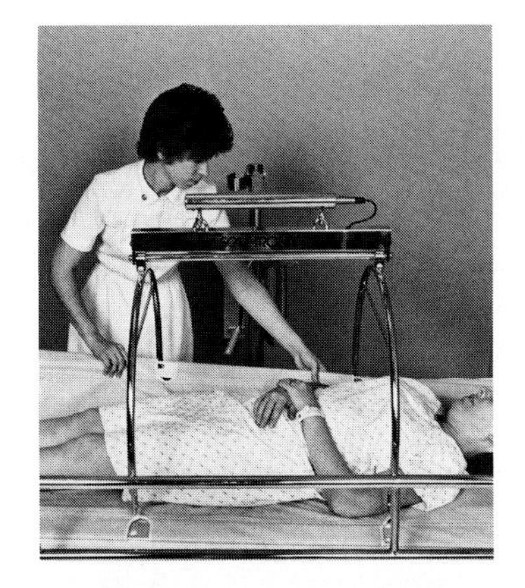

13 When the sling settles on the bed, pull the valve tab back into the closed position. Then, disconnect the hooks from the sling, as the nurse is doing here.

Now, pump the hydraulic pump handle to raise the scale's arms until they clear your patient.

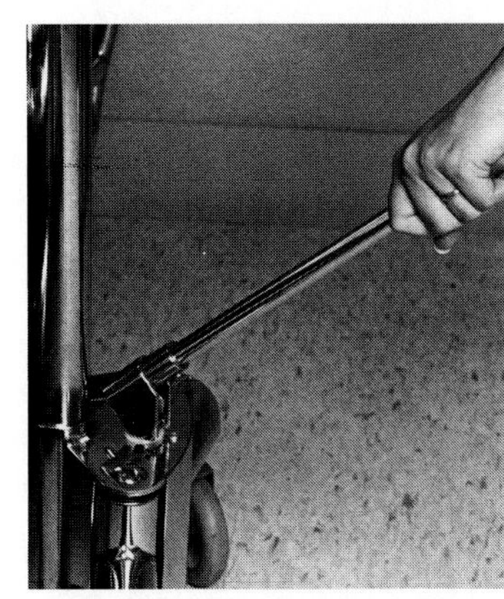

14 Next, return the scale's legs to their original position by turning the base handle clockwise. Then, return the base handle to a vertical position.

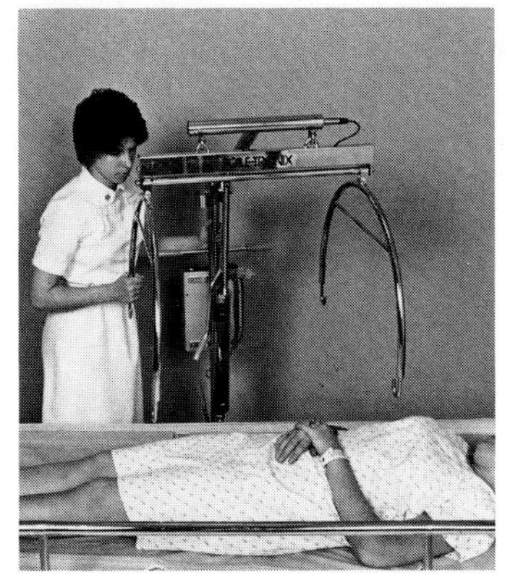

15 Move the scale away from the bed, as shown.

Then, pull the metal bars from both sides of the sling. Roll Ms. Myers onto her side and remove the sling. Make her comfortable and raise the side rail.

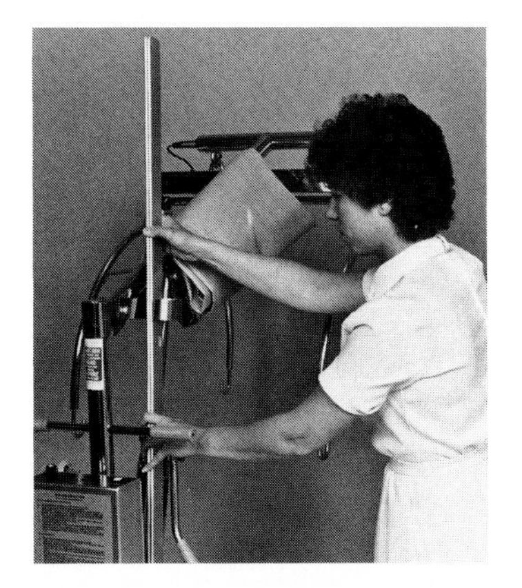

16 Fold the sling and place it over the scale, as shown. Position one end of each metal bar in the scale's base, and rest the bars in the spring clip located at the top of the scale's mast.

Finally, document the patient's weight and how she tolerated the procedure.

Nutritional tests

Learning about skin-fold measurements

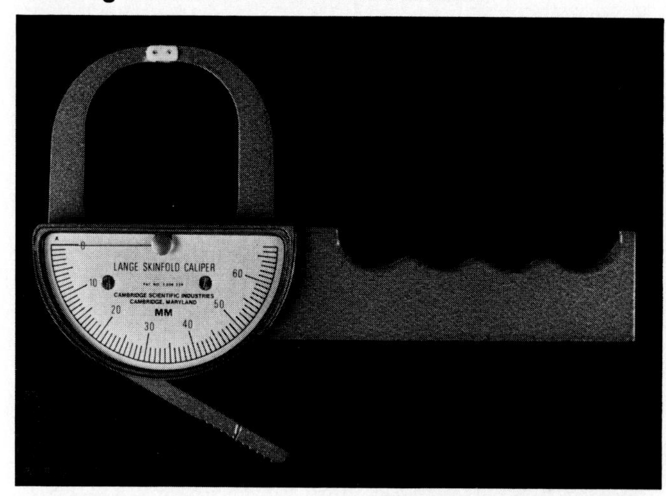

Now you know your patient's weight. But this tells you only part of what you need to know about his nutritional status. Next, you'll perform a skin-fold measurement to estimate the amount of body fat that's stored in subcutaneous tissue. This measurement will help you assess your patient's energy reserves.

In many parts of the body, subcutaneous fat is only loosely attached to underlying tissue, allowing you to easily grasp it between your thumb and forefinger. After doing so, you'll apply skin-fold calipers to take a skin-fold measurement.

Look at the Lange calipers, shown above. This instrument consists of two jaws that grip either side of the skin fold, a lever that opens the jaws, and a gauge to measure skin-fold width.

You can take a measurement wherever the skin's loose enough to grasp. But for accurate test results, some sites are preferable to others. Consider the following points.

Choosing a site

As a rule, the triceps site is best, because it's easily accessible in both men and women. The following photostory shows you how to measure a skin fold at this site.

If the triceps site isn't usable, however, you can obtain a reliable measurement at one of these sites:

- below the tip of the scapula
- over the biceps
- above the iliac crest
- under the costal (rib) margin.

Assessing fat and protein reserves

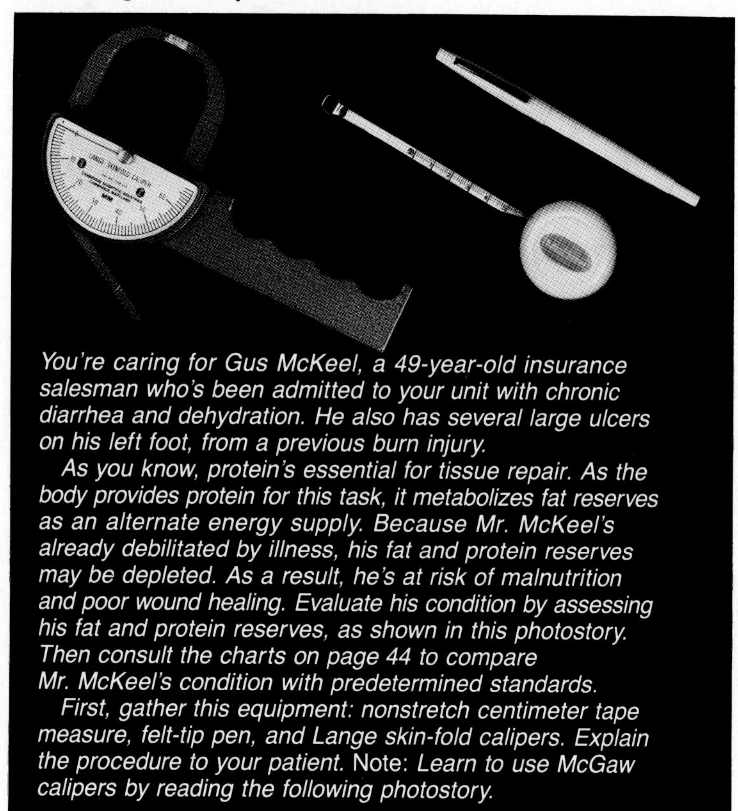

You're caring for Gus McKeel, a 49-year-old insurance salesman who's been admitted to your unit with chronic diarrhea and dehydration. He also has several large ulcers on his left foot, from a previous burn injury.

As you know, protein's essential for tissue repair. As the body provides protein for this task, it metabolizes fat reserves as an alternate energy supply. Because Mr. McKeel's already debilitated by illness, his fat and protein reserves may be depleted. As a result, he's at risk of malnutrition and poor wound healing. Evaluate his condition by assessing his fat and protein reserves, as shown in this photostory. Then consult the charts on page 44 to compare Mr. McKeel's condition with predetermined standards.

First, gather this equipment: nonstretch centimeter tape measure, felt-tip pen, and Lange skin-fold calipers. Explain the procedure to your patient. Note: *Learn to use McGaw calipers by reading the following photostory.*

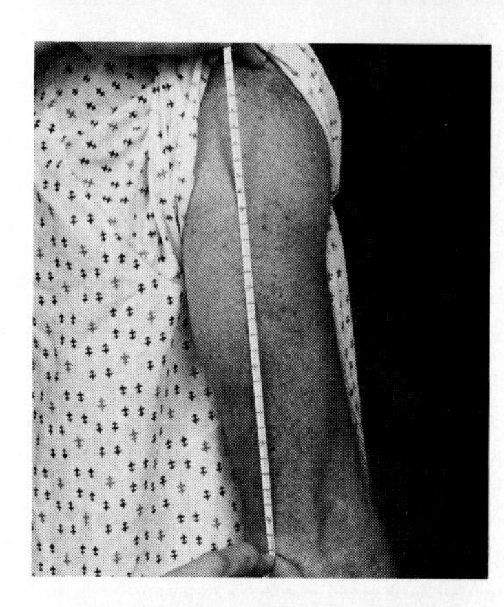

1 Now, have your patient align his nondominant upper arm with his side. Measure the distance between the tip of the scapula's acromial process and the tip of the ulna's olecranon process, as shown.

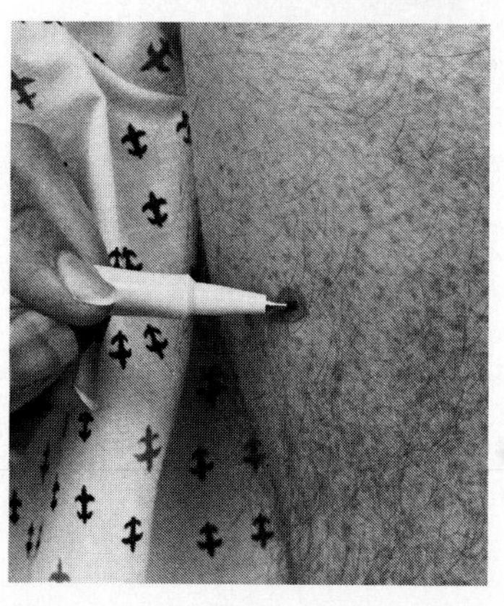

2 Locate the midpoint and mark it with a felt-tip pen.

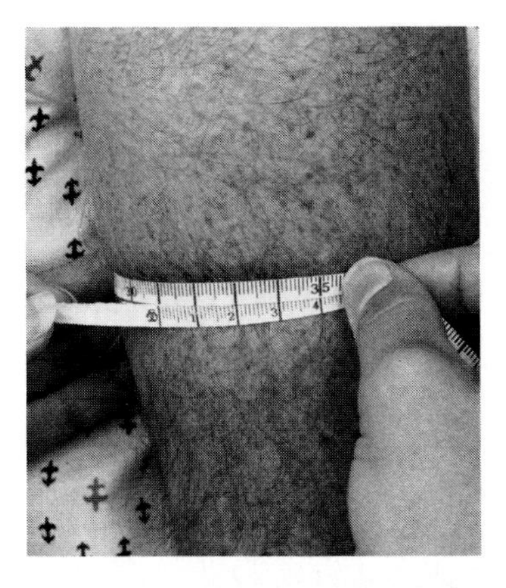

3 Then, measure the circumference at the midpoint. Document the results in centimeters.

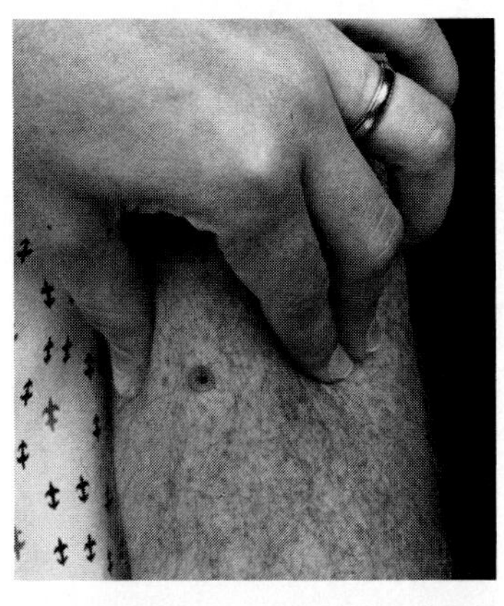

4 Now, measure the triceps skin fold. To do so, firmly grasp a skin fold at the back of his upper arm, about 1 cm above the midpoint dot. Pull the skin fold away from the arm so it's parallel to the arm's long axis.

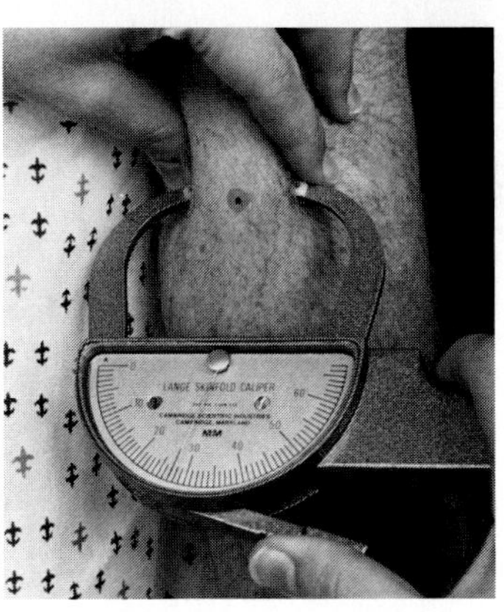

5 Then, open the calipers' jaws by pressing the lever. To measure skin-fold thickness, release the lever and let the jaws close beside the midpoint dot. Wait 2 or 3 seconds for the calipers to settle around the skin fold before taking a reading.

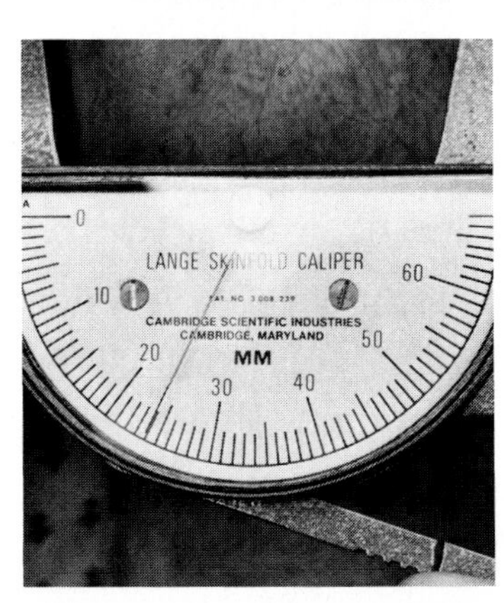

6 Round off the measurement registered on the gauge to the nearest 0.5 mm. Then, take two more readings (releasing the skin fold between readings) at the same site. Record the average reading.

To calculate midarm *muscle* circumference (which indicates protein reserve), multiply the triceps skin-fold measurement (in millimeters) by 0.314, and then subtract your answer from the midarm circumference measurement (in centimeters).

Using McGaw calipers

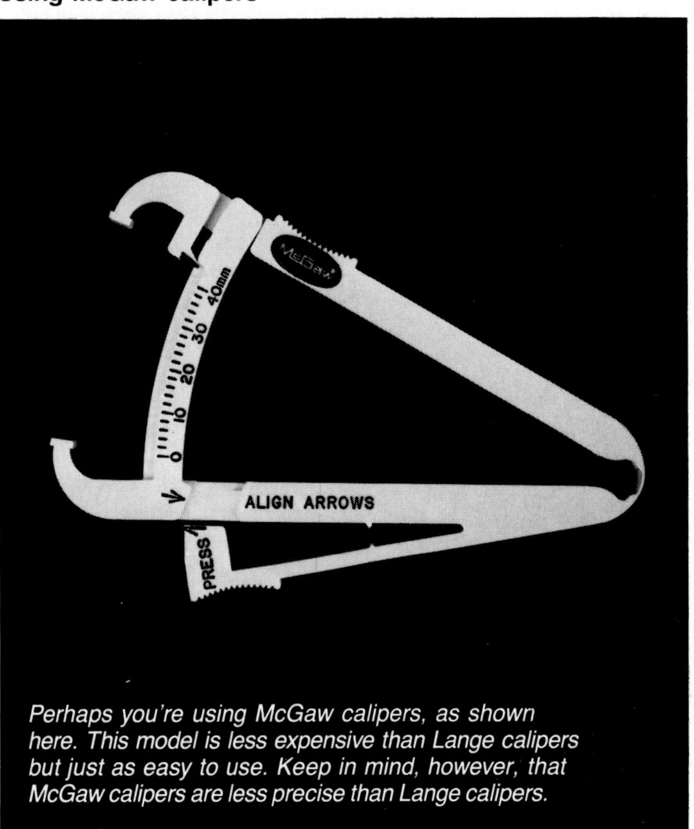

Perhaps you're using McGaw calipers, as shown here. This model is less expensive than Lange calipers but just as easy to use. Keep in mind, however, that McGaw calipers are less precise than Lange calipers.

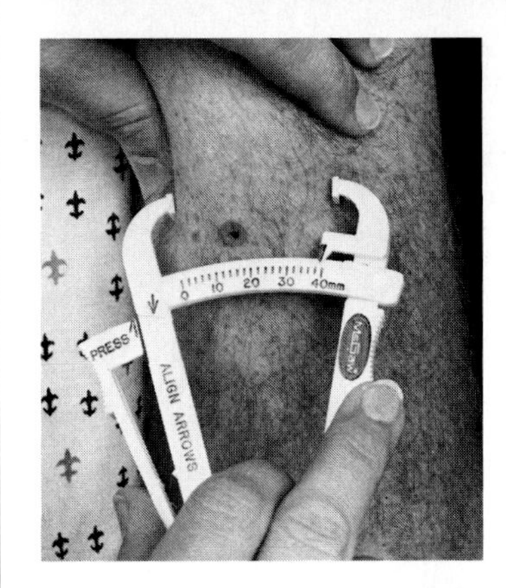

1 To proceed, find the upper arm's midpoint and gently pinch the skin fold, using your thumb and forefinger. Then, apply the calipers over the skin fold, as shown.

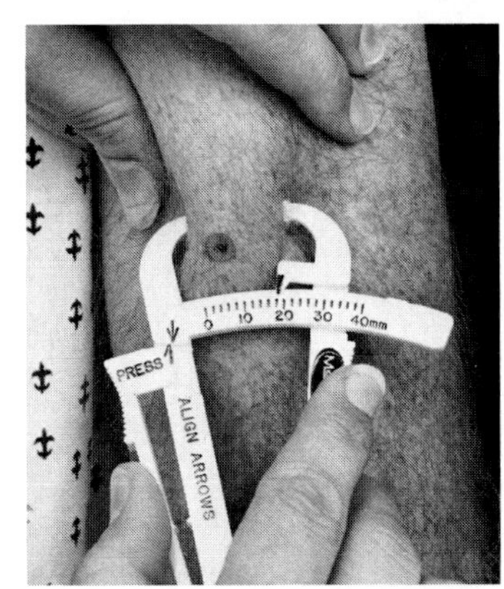

2 Now, use your thumb to align the calipers' two arrows, as shown. Wait 2 or 3 seconds for the calipers to settle against the skin before taking a reading. Then, record your results to the nearest 1 mm. Take two additional readings and average the results.

Finally, document the results in your nurses' notes.

Nutritional tests

Protein and fat reserves: Making an assessment

You've just finished measuring your patient's mid–upper-arm circumference and triceps skin-fold thickness. Can you interpret the results? For guidance, consult the charts shown below.

You'll recall that upper-arm *muscle* circumference is calculated by multiplying the triceps skin-fold measurement (in millimeters) by 0.314 and then subtracting that value from the upper-arm circumference (in centimeters). By comparing the result to the chart at right, you can assess your patient's protein reserves. Likewise, by comparing his triceps skin-fold measurement to the chart at left, you can assess his fat reserves.

The 100% values you see are standard for a patient of ideal weight for his height. If your patient's values are standard according to the charts, he suffers no fat or protein depletion. A value that's 80% to 90% of standard indicates mild depletion; 60% to 80% of standard, moderate depletion; and less than 60%, severe depletion.

Triceps skin-fold measurement

	100% (standard)	90%	80%	70%	60%
Male	12.5 mm	11.3 mm	10 mm	8.8 mm	7.5 mm
Female	16.5 mm	14.9 mm	13.2 mm	11.6 mm	9.9 mm

Mid–upper-arm muscle circumference

	100% (standard)	90%	80%	70%	60%
Male	25.3 cm	22.8 cm	20.2 cm	17.7 cm	15.2 cm
Female	23.2 cm	20.9 cm	18.6 cm	16.2 cm	13.9 cm

Skin testing for nutritional deficiencies

If your surgical patient's nutritionally deficient, he's more susceptible to infection and other postop complications. Why? Because nutritional deficiency causes *anergy*, a failure of the body's defense mechanisms to activate.

If surgery can be delayed, the doctor may want you to test your patient for anergy by performing a series of skin tests. If the tests indicate anergy, the doctor will postpone surgery while the patient receives nutritional supplements.

To test your patient for anergy, administer a series of intradermal antigen injections. If he's nutritionally fit (and if he's been previously exposed to the antigen-producing organism), red, hardened wheals will appear at the injection sites. If your patient fails to respond positively to at least one of the injections, his defense mechanisms may be compromised by a nutritional deficiency.

To ensure reliable test results, inject three to five common antigens; for example, those caused by exposure to mumps, *Trichophyton*, or a *Candida* fungus. Chances are, your patient's been exposed to at least one—and probably all—of these organisms. So, expect to see at least one positive reaction if he's nutritionally fit.

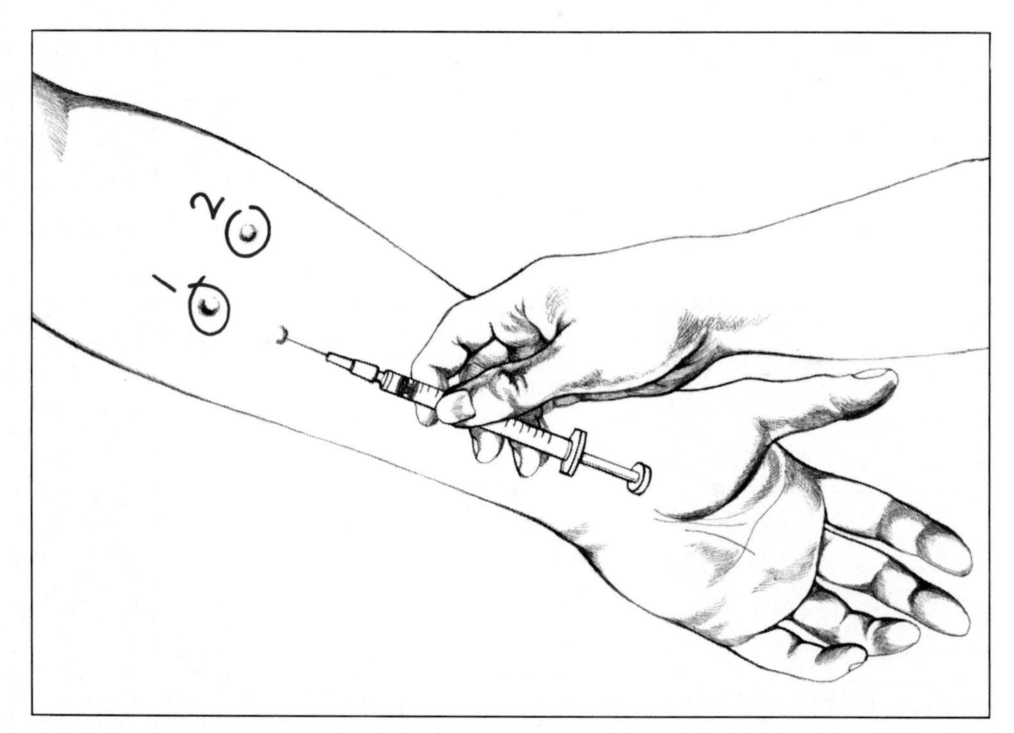

Performing a skin test

Carefully read the antigen manufacturer's instructions before beginning. Some antigens are ready for use; others require dilution.

Caution: Keep epinephrine hydrochloride (Adrenalin Chloride, Sus-Phrine*) handy in case of anaphylaxis.

After injecting the antigens, circle and number each injection site, as shown above. Then, record each site and what you injected there in your nurses' notes. By documenting each site's location, you'll know which antigen your patient reacts to.

Observe the skin sites for a red, hardened wheal. Measure the diameter of each wheal at 24-hour intervals for 3 days. Be sure to record your results.

A hardened wheal signifies a positive response to the antigen. Your patient's anergic only if *none* of the antigens causes a skin reaction.

Before performing the test, make sure your patient understands the procedure and the expected outcome. Reassure him that if no reaction develops, you can improve his condition with nutritional supplements.

Be aware that several other factors may affect your patient's skin reaction to antigens. For example, lack of previous exposure to the antigen will cause false results. Steroid therapy and immunosuppressives may suppress reactivity; chemotherapeutics can produce a false-negative response. Accidentally injecting the antigen subcutaneously also causes a false-negative response, but it won't harm your patient.

*Available in both the United States and Canada

Providing total parenteral nutrition (TPN)

Let's say your patient's skin test reveals that he's anergic. To avoid postop complications from a nutritional deficit, the doctor has postponed surgery.

In the meantime, try to improve your patient's condition by giving him feedings high in protein and calories. If he can't tolerate oral or nasogastric tube feedings, or if his gastrointestinal tract isn't functional (for example, because of inflammatory bowel disease), the doctor will probably order TPN. The sooner the patient begins receiving TPN therapy, the more effective it's likely to be.

Learning about TPN

As you may know, a TPN solution is a mixture of 50% dextrose in water, amino acids, and other special components (see chart at right). Dextrose and amino acids serve as the major calorie sources, generally providing about 1,000 calories per liter. In addition to these basic substances, the doctor prescribes a combination of additives in appropriate amounts to meet your patient's specific needs.

After receiving the doctor's order, the pharmacist prepares the TPN solution under a laminar flow hood to ensure sterility. When the solution's delivered to your unit, refrigerate it until therapy begins.

Beginning TPN therapy

To assure adequate dilution and quick distribution, you'll administer TPN through a central I.V. line resting in the patient's superior vena cava. The doctor may insert the line through the subclavian vein (direct line) or advance it through the jugular vein or a large peripheral vein.

TPN is administered into the superior vena cava to allow adequate dilution of the solution with blood. Otherwise, the solution's high osmolarity could cause thrombosis at the I.V. catheter tip.

Of course, like any invasive procedure, a central line insertion risks complications. During the insertion procedure, be alert for signs and symptoms of air embolism, cardiac arrhythmias, hemothorax, pneumothorax, and thromboembolis. (For details on assisting with central line insertion, see the NURSING PHOTOBOOK MANAGING I.V. THERAPY.)

When beginning TPN therapy, your patient's body needs time to adjust to the TPN solution's high osmolarity. So, begin feedings slowly, according to the doctor's order and hospital policy. By doing so, you'll give the pancreas a chance to secrete enough insulin to handle the increasing carbohydrate loads.

Important: Discontinue TPN therapy gradually, too. Otherwise, the patient may experience rebound insulin shock.

Nursing considerations

To enhance the success of TPN therapy and reduce its risks, observe the following guidelines:

- Before beginning therapy, make sure the doctor's confirmed correct catheter placement with a chest X-ray.
- Use an infusion pump to administer TPN solution. Doing so helps maintain an accurate flow rate and minimizes the risk of clotting in the catheter.
- Maintain a constant flow rate, as ordered. If the infusion falls behind, increase the rate slowly, to give the pancreas time to adjust to the increased carbohydrate load. *Caution:* Don't try to catch up if therapy's 10% or more behind schedule.
- Maintain meticulous fluid intake and output records.
- Weigh your patient daily. He may gain up to ¾ lb (0.35 kg) through protein synthesis; attribute a greater weight gain to the fluids he's receiving.
- Measure his urine glucose, ketones, and specific gravity every 4 to 6 hours. For details, review the information beginning on page 13.
- Monitor his vital signs at least once every 4 hours. *Note:* A patient with kidney or liver disease may have problems associated with fluid imbalance and protein metabolism. Take care to monitor his vital signs more frequently.
- Maintain a regular schedule for blood studies, according to hospital policy. Watch for signs of these possible complications: hyperglycemia, hypernatremia, hyperkalemia, and fluid imbalance.
- Control infection by maintaining strict aseptic technique during dressing and I.V. tubing changes. Be alert for early signs of local or systemic infection.
- Keep your patient lying in bed during all tubing and dressing changes.
- Provide emotional support for your patient and his family. Explain each procedure to them, and keep the family informed of the patient's progress.
- Balance your patient's activity with rest.
- Routinely reevaluate your patient's condition by maintaining communication with the doctor, dietitian, nursing staff, and nutrition support team.
- If TPN administration's interrupted for any reason, maintain catheter patency and prevent insulin shock with an infusion of 10% dextrose in water. *Note:* In this book's second section, we provide details on intermittent TPN therapy through a Hickman catheter.

Understanding TPN solutions

After determining your patient's nutritional deficiencies, the doctor prescribes a combination of total parenteral nutrition (TPN) components to best meet your patient's needs. To understand the functions of each, review this chart.

Note: Fat emulsions are special TPN solutions. For details about them, see the NURSING PHOTOBOOK MANAGING I.V. THERAPY.

TPN component	Purpose
50% dextrose in water	Provides calories needed for metabolism
Amino acids	Supply protein needed for tissue repair
Potassium	Functions in cellular activity and tissue synthesis
Folic acid	Functions in deoxyribonucleic acid (DNA) formation
Vitamin D	Maintains serum calcium levels and functions in bone metabolism
Vitamin B complex	Aids final absorption of carbohydrates and protein
Vitamin K	Helps prevent bleeding disorders
Vitamin C	Promotes wound healing
Sodium	Helps control water distribution to maintain fluid balance
Chloride	Helps regulate acid-base equilibrium and maintain osmotic pressure
Calcium	Promotes blood clotting; aids teeth and bone development
Phosphate	Minimizes threat of peripheral paresthesia
Magnesium	Helps absorb carbohydrates and protein
Acetate	Prevents metabolic acidosis
Trace elements (zinc, cobalt, manganese)	Promote wound healing and red blood cell synthesis

Special tests

So far, you've learned basic tests that enable you to quickly assess your patient's condition. Now, we show you how to perform several specialized tests to detect some common problems.

For example, we familiarize you with glaucoma's signs and symptoms and show you how to use indentation and applanation tonometers to measure intraocular pressure.

Does your patient suffer from edema? We show you, step by step, how to perform an evaluation. In addition, we provide you with a chart that'll help you to quickly assess your findings.

And that's not all we cover. We also show you how to measure gastric pH and how to detect and absorb cerebrospinal fluid drainage.

Although the tests on the following pages have different purposes, they have a common quality: They help you provide expert nursing care.

MINI-ASSESSMENT

Assessing gastric pH

You've been feeding 82-year-old Marvin Hill with a nasogastric tube for the past week. You know prolonged intubation may stimulate his stomach to produce too much hydrochloric acid, possibly causing an ulcer.

To prevent ulcer formation in a patient with a gastric or nasogastric tube in place, monitor the pH of his stomach contents, as ordered. By doing so, you can detect abnormal gastric acidity before it causes a problem. Then, the doctor can order appropriate treatment; for example, with antacids.

For easy, accurate, and inexpensive monitoring, use pH tape (as shown in the following photostory). Like other types of reagent strip, pH tape changes color when it contacts the substance for which you're testing; in this case, gastric acid. By comparing the tape color to a corresponding color chart, you can accurately assess gastric pH.

If possible, use a brand of pH tape that detects pH values ranging from 1 to 14. Keep in mind that some brands can't detect values lower than 4.5. If you use one of these brands, a 4.5 reading may not accurately reflect your patient's gastric pH.

Performing gastric pH measurements

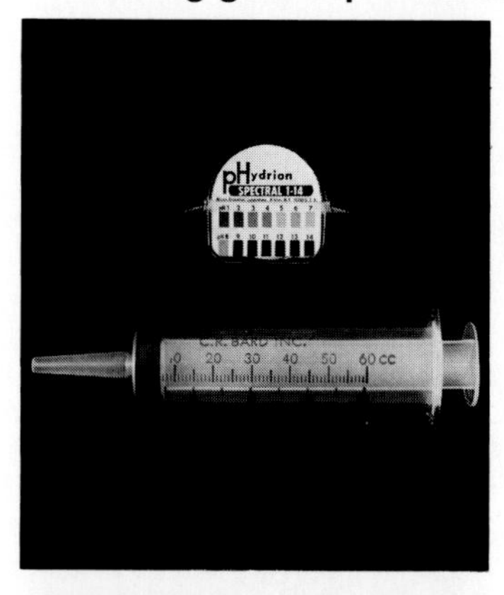

1 To determine how prolonged nasogastric (NG) intubation has affected Mr. Hill's gastric pH, test the acidity of his secretions with pH tape. To begin, gather a pH tape dispenser and an irrigating syringe.

After assuring Mr. Hill that the test won't hurt, confirm NG tube placement. (For information on checking NG tube placement, see the NURSING PHOTOBOOK PERFORMING GI PROCEDURES.)

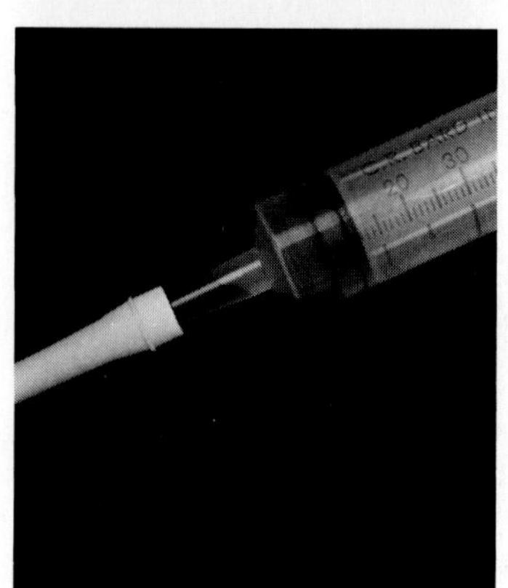

2 When you're sure the tube's correctly positioned in the stomach, withdraw at least 3 ml of gastric secretions, using the irrigating syringe.

Note: If your patient's undergoing continuous intermittent suctioning, you may need to stop the suction machine and clamp the NG tube to permit buildup of enough secretions for testing. After collecting a specimen, don't forget to unclamp the tube and resume suctioning.

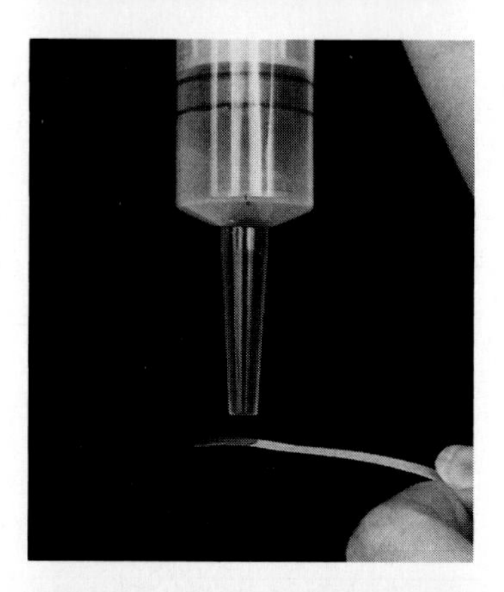

3 Now, remove a strip of pH test paper from the dispenser. Place a specimen drop on the strip, as shown.

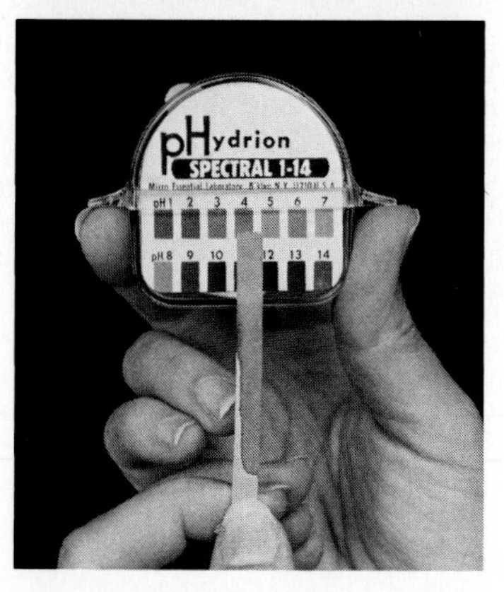

4 Then, compare the test strip color to the dispenser's color chart.

Document the results on the appropriate form. If gastric secretions are highly acidic (below 4.0), follow the doctor's order for antacid treatment. Then, repeat the test every 2 to 4 hours.

If secretions remain highly acidic despite antacid treatment, notify the doctor.

Testing for cerebrospinal fluid drainage

Has your patient suffered a head injury? If so, he may be prone to cerebrospinal fluid (CSF) drainage from his nose or ears, especially if the injury's in the basilar area of his skull. You should suspect CSF drainage if you notice clear or blood-tinged fluid coming from his ear or nose.

As you know, coughing, straining, and head position changes increase intracranial pressure (ICP). Elevated ICP, in turn, may increase the amount of CSF drainage.

To distinguish CSF drainage from mucous discharge, perform a quick preliminary test with a Dextrostix reagent strip. The Dextrostix will react to the glucose that's normally present in CSF. But be aware that the results aren't necessarily conclusive, because mucus and lacrimal fluid may also contain glucose. For example, drainage from a sinus infection may contain glucose.

To perform the test, obtain a bottle of Dextrostix with color chart and a watch with a second hand.

Before you start, tell your patient what you'll be doing. Also, make sure the Dextrostix bottle is still fresh. Then, follow these guidelines:

- Remove a reagent strip from the bottle, and recap the bottle.
- Place the test block directly in the drainage flowing from your patient's nose or ear.
- Allow drainage to completely cover the block.
- Wait 60 seconds from the time the drainage saturates the block.
- Compare the block's color with the bottle label's color chart.
- Document the results.

Note: For more details on using and preserving reagent strips, review pages 15 to 17 and 26.

Testing with filter paper

If your patient's drainage is blood-tinged, you may use filter paper or gauze to test for CSF, instead of a Dextrostix. To perform this test, place the filter paper in the drainage flow and allow the paper to absorb a few drops. Then, hold the paper under a bright light. If the drainage contains CSF, you'll see a colorless stain encircling a blood or serum spot (see photo below). Document your observation on the appropriate form.

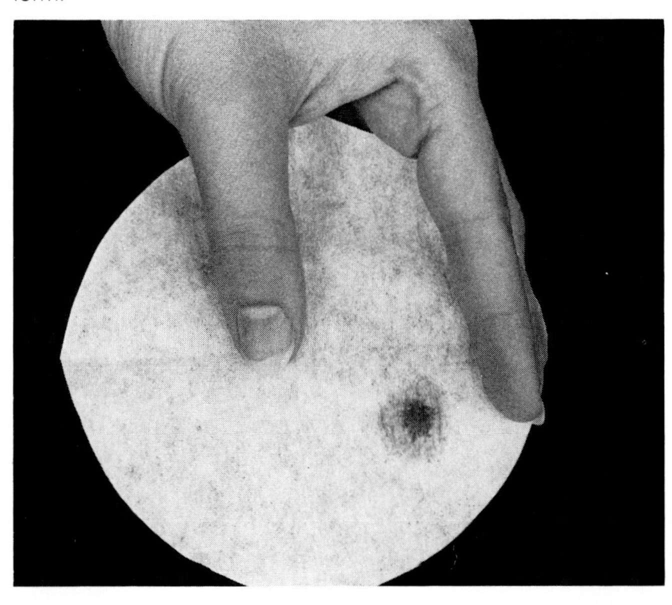

Absorbing CSF drainage

You've determined that cerebrospinal fluid (CSF) is draining out of your patient's nose and right ear. As you know, CSF is an excellent growth medium for bacteria. From CSF, bacterial infection can quickly spread to the brain or spinal column, causing a serious complication; for example, meningitis or encephalitis. To prevent such a complication, take steps to absorb CSF drainage. The following photostory shows you what to do.

First, elevate the head of your patient's bed 30° (if his condition permits). Caution him to avoid sniffing, blowing his nose, or picking at his ears or nose. Explain why these precautions are so important. Then, tell him how you plan to absorb the drainage, and answer his questions.

Now, gather two 4"x4" gauze pads and a roll of nonallergenic tape. Tear off two 3" (7.6-cm) strips of tape and place them within your reach.

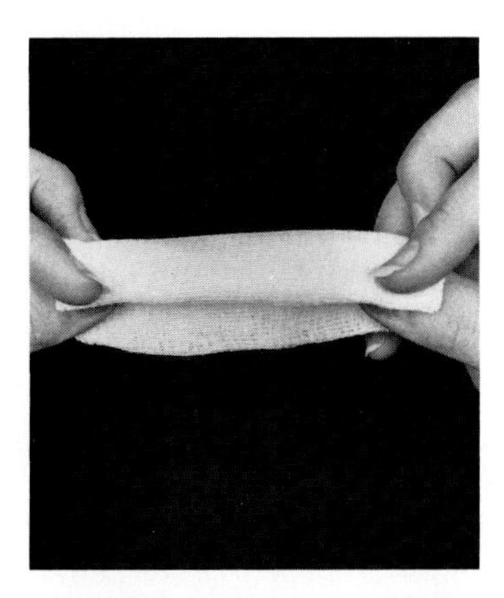

1 Now, fold a gauze pad lengthwise several times, as shown, or roll it up. Then, loosely position the pad on the patient's upper lip.

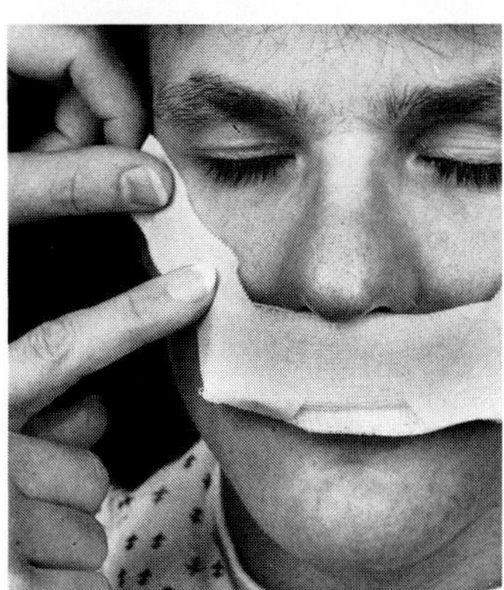

2 Next, apply a tape strip diagonally over one side of the pad and across your patient's cheek.

Then, apply the other tape strip on the opposite side in the same way, as the nurse is doing here. Or, secure the pad with one long tape strip that extends from cheek to cheek.

Replace the pad when it becomes saturated.

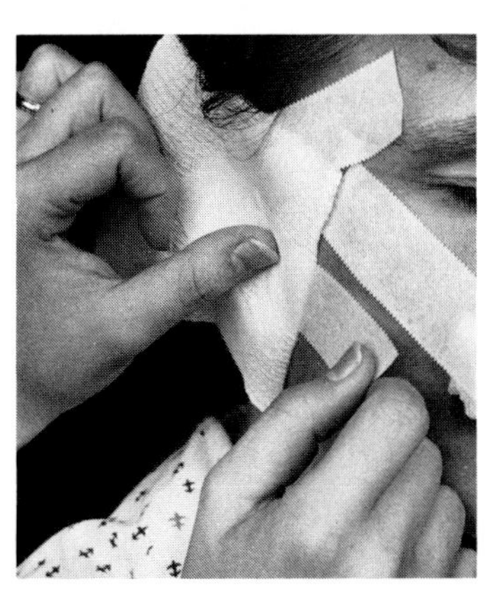

3 To absorb ear drainage, cover your patient's right ear with a gauze pad. Secure it with three 4" (10-cm) tape strips. *Note:* If your patient has a beard, anchor the pad with one 6" (15-cm) tape strip. Apply the strip diagonally from his neck to his forehead.

Replace the pad when it becomes saturated.

Document the procedure and the drainage type, amount, and color.

Special tests

Learning about glaucoma

What comes to mind when someone mentions glaucoma? If you're like most nurses, you know glaucoma is an eye disorder caused by increased intraocular pressure (IOP) and that it most commonly affects the elderly. But unless you specialize in eye care, these may be the only facts you know. That's why we highlight the disorder's characteristics here.

The normal eye

To understand what causes glaucoma, take a moment to review basic eye anatomy (see the first illustration at right). Three tissue layers (the sclera, choroid, and retina) form a covering around the eye's interior. These layers, along with the clear cornea, enclose the lens, the anterior and posterior chambers, and the vitreous cavity.

Aqueous humor—a clear, watery fluid—occupies the area within both chambers. Its specific gravity ranges from 1.002 to 1.004 and its pH ranges from 7.1 to 7.3. This protein-free fluid is produced by the ciliary bodies located in the posterior chamber. From the ciliary bodies the fluid circulates into the anterior chamber, passing through the outflow pathway (which includes the pupil, the trabecular meshwork, and a channel called Schlemm's canal). Finally, the fluid is absorbed into the venous system.

Normally, the rate of aqueous humor production balances aqueous humor outflow, maintaining stable IOP. Depending on the individual, IOP measurements range from 12 to 21 mm Hg.

Understanding glaucoma types

Elevated IOP, the hallmark of glaucoma, usually results from aqueous humor accumulation from an outflow pathway blockage. (A less common reason for IOP elevation is overproduction of aqueous humor.) When untreated, elevated IOP leads to optic nerve damage and blindness.

In general, glaucoma's classified as one of the following three types.

- *Chronic open-angle,* the most common type, results from overproduction of aqueous humor or obstruction of its outflow through the trabecular meshwork, Schlemm's canal, or aqueous veins.
- *Acute closed-angle* (narrow angle) may result from obstruction of aqueous humor outflow by anatomically narrow angles between the anterior iris and the posterior corneal surface; shallow anterior chambers; a thickened iris that causes angle closure on pupil dilation; or a bulging iris that presses on the trabeculae, closing the angle (see the second illustration above).
- *Chronic closed-angle* follows an untreated attack of acute closed-angle glaucoma or several mild, recurring, acute attacks that produce trabecular adhesions.

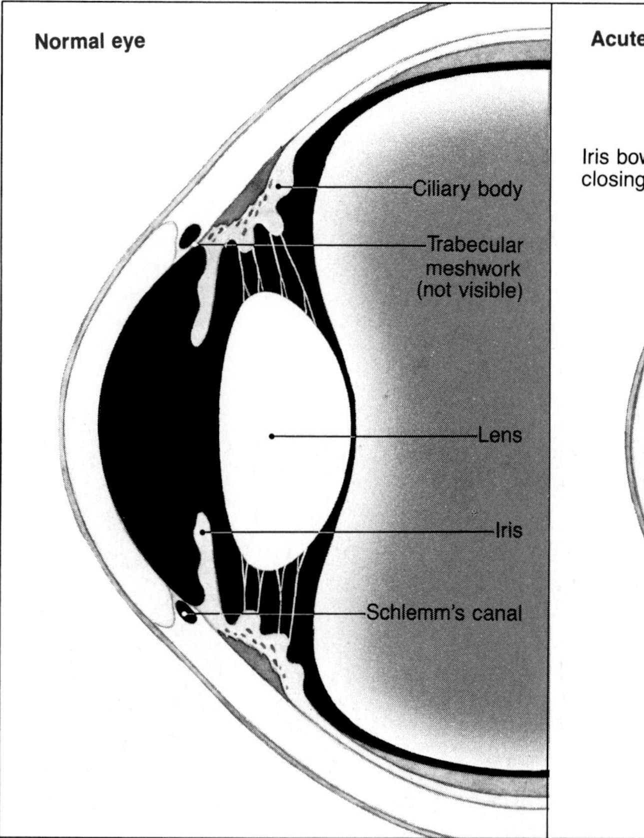

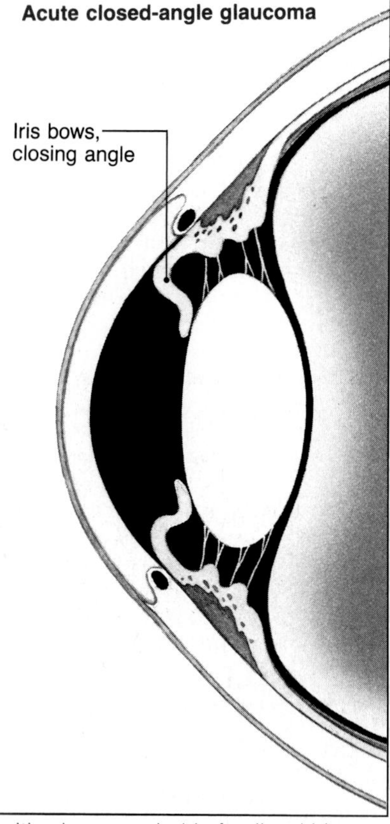

Glaucoma may be primary or secondary in origin. Primary glaucoma results from an anatomic abnormality. Most types of primary glaucoma develop after age 40; however, developmental (congenital) glaucoma may be present at birth. In contrast, secondary glaucoma results from a specific precipitating factor (for example, trauma, inflammatory eye disease, enlarged cataract, intraocular tumor, or corticosteroids).

Recognizing high-risk patients

Glaucoma isn't easy to identify. In its early stages, the disease causes little discomfort and no observable signs. By the time the patient notices symptoms, he's already suffered some irreversible damage.

The most reliable way to detect glaucoma is by measuring IOP with an instrument called a tonometer. (You'll learn more about tonometry beginning on the following page.) By using tonometry to screen all patients over age 40 (when they're more likely to develop chronic open-angle glaucoma), you can detect the disease before it causes damage. But many patients are unwilling to undergo tonometry—especially if they feel fine. This is why your ability to recognize high-risk patients and inform them of the danger is so important.

A family history of glaucoma, for example, is a significant risk factor. Regularly test a patient with glaucoma in his family within two generations. As a rule, regular testing should begin at age 25 and continue yearly. But if your patient's a child with a family history of *developmental* glaucoma, begin regular testing immediately.

Other high-risk patients include:

- those with diabetes or hypertension
- those who've suffered traumatic eye injuries; for instance, from a tennis ball or other blunt object
- blacks
- anyone over age 55.

Treating glaucoma

Let's say the doctor's diagnosed glaucoma in your patient. What's next? Chances are, the doctor will immediately begin drug therapy. Depending on your patient's condition, he may order a cholinergic to improve aqueous humor drainage or an adrenergic to reduce aqueous humor production. For more on glaucoma medications, see page 54.

The doctor may also recommend surgery; for example, a trabeculectomy or a peripheral iridectomy. Like any surgery, these procedures expose your patient to infection and other risks. On pages 54 and 55 you'll learn more about these surgical procedures.

Consider glaucoma screening one of your most important responsibilities. After all, your patient's eyesight may be at stake.

Identifying glaucoma's signs and symptoms

Can you recognize glaucoma's signs and symptoms? Carefully review this chart to make sure you know its warning signals.

Open-angle glaucoma
- Ocular discomfort
- Tired eyes
- As the condition progresses, an extensive vision field loss in one or both eyes

Closed-angle glaucoma
- Unilateral ocular and facial pain
- Nausea and possibly vomiting
- Decreased visual acuity
- Blurred vision
- Halo or rainbow vision
- Mottled diffuse light
- Pupil fixed in middilation
- Clouded cornea from edema
- Red and swollen conjunctiva

Developmental glaucoma
- Irritability
- Poor eating habits
- Tendency to rub eyes
- Developmental or learning problems from chronic discomfort

Understanding the Schiøtz tonometer

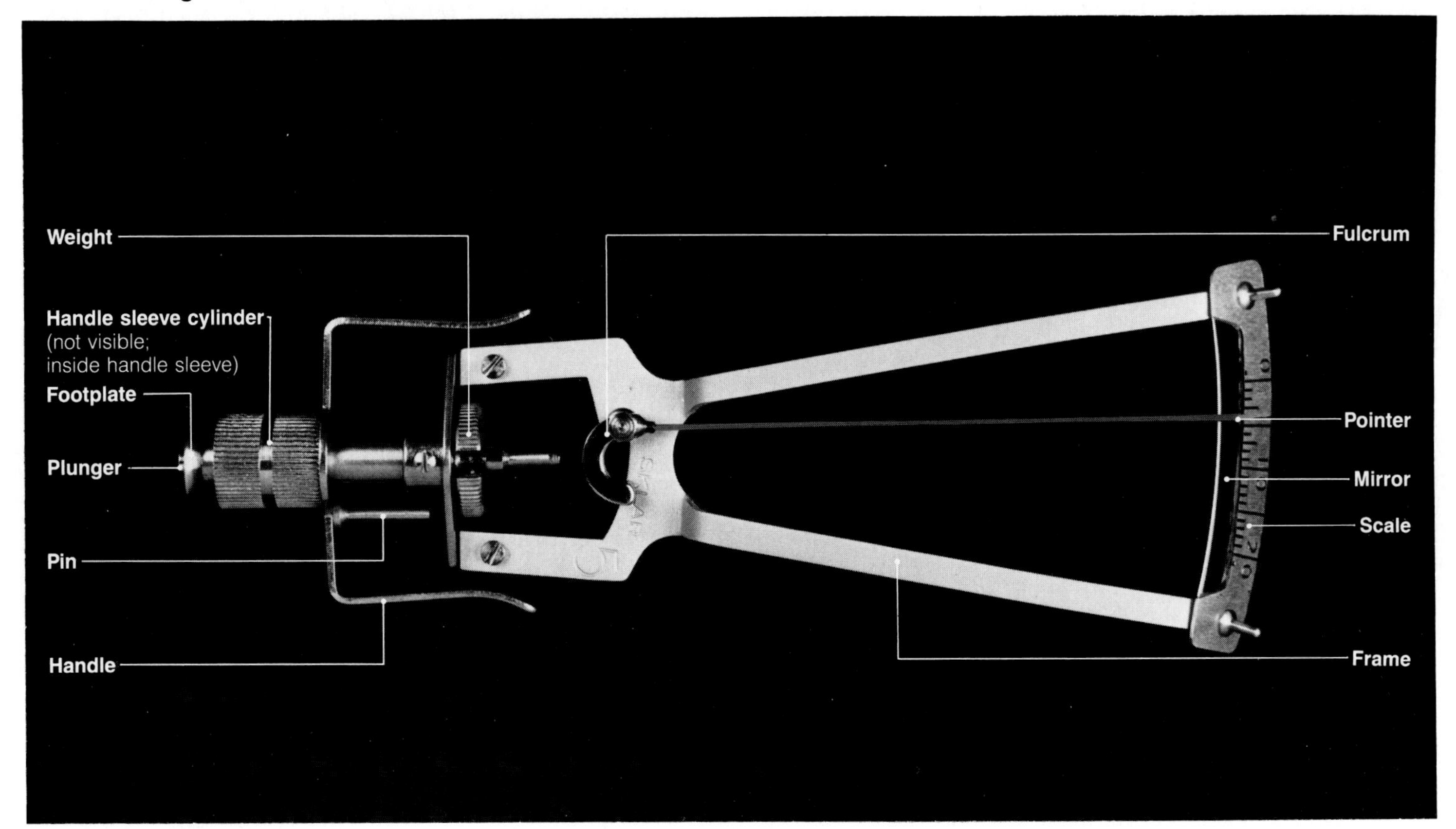

Testing your patient's eyes for glaucoma? Chances are, you'll use a Schiøtz tonometer like the one shown here. This lightweight, easy-to-use instrument is about 5″ (12.7 cm) long. With a little practice, you can use it to accurately assess your patient's intraocular pressure (IOP). In the following photostory, we show you how. But first, familiarize yourself with the Schiøtz tonometer by studying this photo.

Take a look at the tonometer's plunger. As you see, a metal weight fits around it. The manufacturer supplies four such weights: 5.5 g, 7.5 g, 10 g, and 15 g. As a rule, you'll use the lightest weight for IOP testing. But if your patient's IOP is unusually high, you'll need a heavier weight to obtain a reading.

How does the tonometer work? First, you rest its footplate on your patient's cornea (after anesthetizing his eye, of course). The cornea then forces the plunger (which protrudes slightly from the footplate's center) against the fulcrum. The fulcrum, in turn, moves the pointer across the scale. To determine IOP, you'll take this measurement and the plunger's weight and refer to a precalculated table.

Note: Because the plunger leaves a slight indentation in the cornea, this procedure is also called *indentation tonometry*.

These factors may prevent the Schiøtz tonometer from providing accurate results:
- the patient's refusal or inability to tolerate the procedure.
- a significant difference between the footplate's curvature and the cornea's curvature, preventing the plunger from resting properly on the cornea.

Also, indentation tonometry may be contraindicated; for example, if the patient's eye is infected.

Noncontact tonometry avoids these problems. Learn more about it on pages 52 and 53.

Special tests

Preparing the Schiøtz tonometer

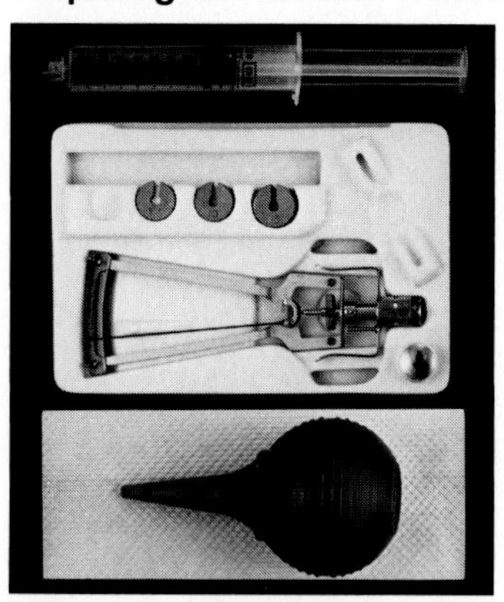

1 If you use a Schiøtz tonometer for glaucoma screening, periodically take it apart and clean it. By doing so, you remove contaminants that may have accumulated. In addition, routinely check the tonometer's calibration. As a rule, perform both procedures daily.

Gather this equipment: tonometer and test block, paper towel or gauze pad, medication syringe with water, and ear syringe.

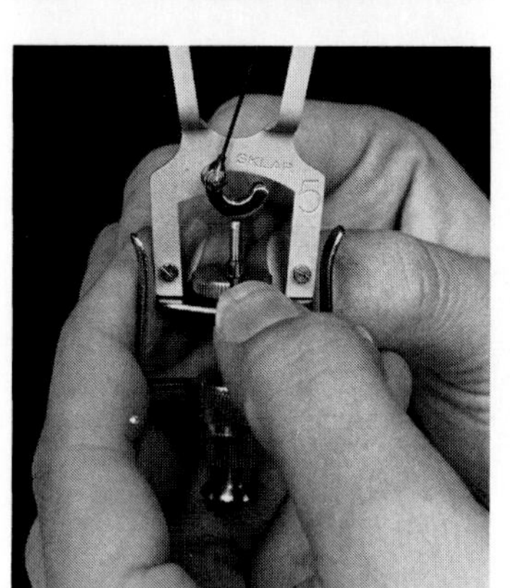

2 Take apart the tonometer by removing its weight and plunger, as the nurse is doing here. Clean the plunger by rinsing it in warm water.

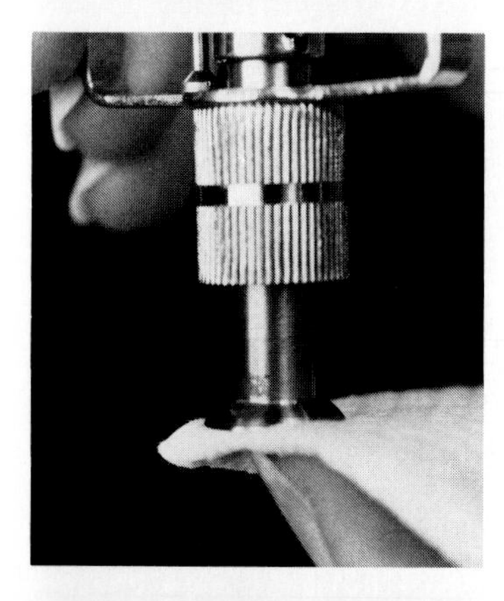

3 Use the water in the medication syringe to flush the handle sleeve cylinder's inside. Then, wipe dry the plunger and footplate with a paper towel or gauze pad.

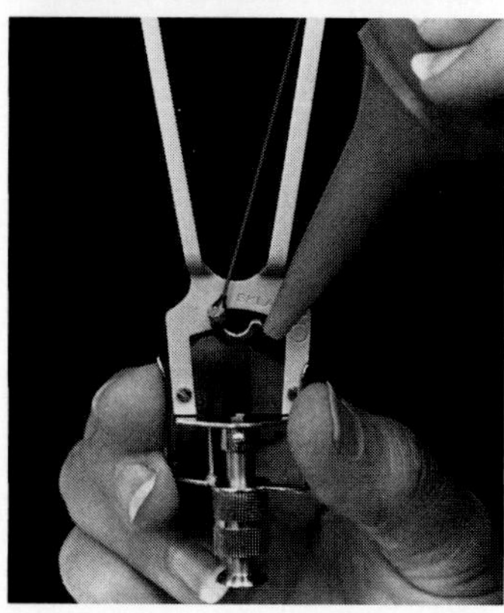

4 To dry the handle sleeve cylinder, use the ear syringe to blow air through it, as the nurse is doing here. (Or, pour alcohol through the cylinder. The cylinder dries as the alcohol evaporates. But take care to wipe the alcohol from the footplate with a paper towel or gauze pad.)

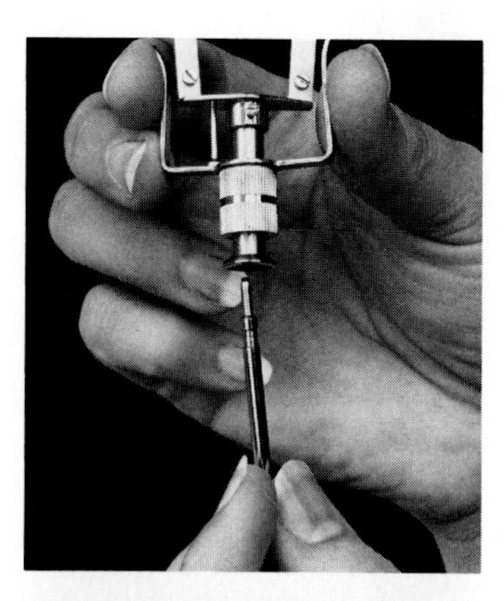

5 Now, reassemble the tonometer. First, insert the plunger, tapered side up, through the handle sleeve cylinder. *Note:* Continue to hold the plunger after insertion, because it isn't secure until you replace the weight.

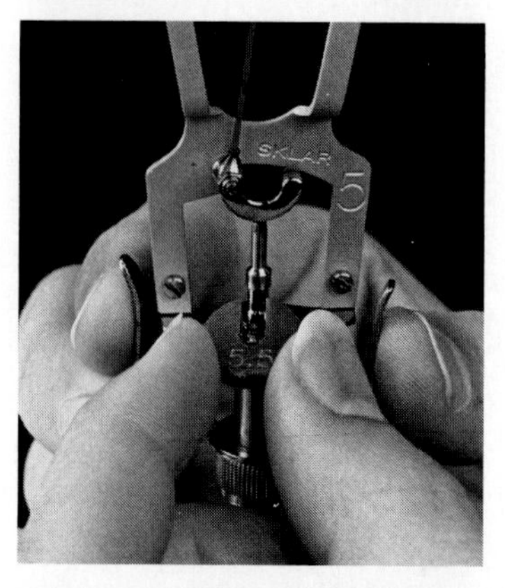

6 You'll check calibration with the standard 5.5 g weight. To attach it, press the plunger's tapered portion into the weight's slot, until the weight snaps securely in place.

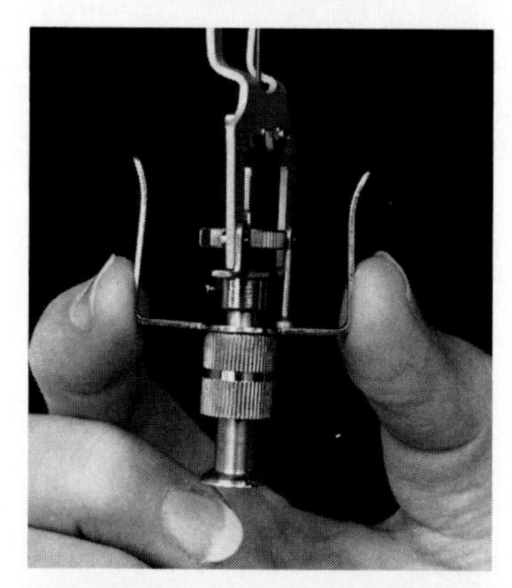

7 Next, turn the handle until the pin rests against the weight, as shown.

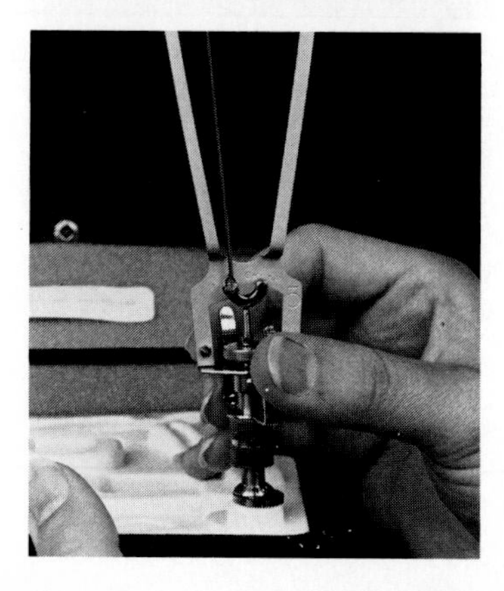

8 Now you're ready to check the tonometer's calibration. Gently set its footplate on the test block. Use the handle to steady the tonometer, as the nurse is doing here. Expect to see a 0 reading on the tonometer scale; this indicates that the tonometer's calibrated. If you don't see this reading, doublecheck the tonometer for dirt. If you can't confirm calibration, return the tonometer to the manufacturer and obtain a new one.

Your patient, 29-year-old Sheila Arnold, has come to your clinic for a routine eye examination. Because she has a family history of glaucoma, you'll test her intraocular pressure (IOP) with a Schiøtz tonometer.

Important: *Perform this test as the last part of your patient's eye exam. The tonometer may cause corneal indentations that'll interfere with corneal assessment.*

Have your patient sit in an exam chair that has a movable headrest. Or, ask her to lie on an examination table. Explain the procedure and assure her that it's painless.

Before beginning, wash your hands. Then, clean the tonometer's footplate by wiping it with an alcohol swab, as shown here. Caution: *Alcohol can cause severe corneal burns. To eliminate this risk, use a moist—not soaking wet—alcohol swab, and wipe it* lightly *across the footplate once or twice. Don't apply so much pressure that alcohol's forced up the plunger's sides. Allow the footplate to dry before proceeding.*

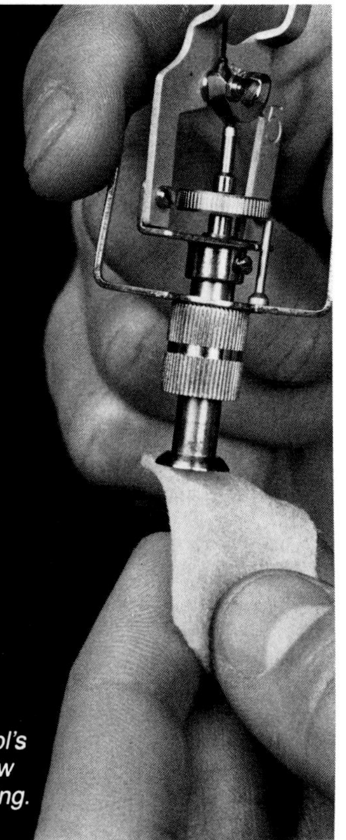

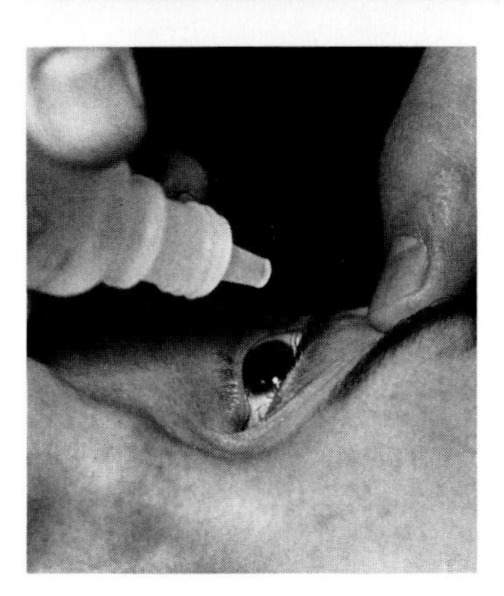

1 Now, inspect your patient's eyes. If you see signs of infection, postpone the test. If she's wearing contact lenses, ask her to remove them.

Place her in a supine position by tilting the chair backward.

Then, apply the prescribed ophthalmic anesthetic. Instill one drop in each eye, as ordered.

Instruct your patient to gently blot her eyes with a tissue to absorb excess medication. But caution her *not* to rub her eyes.

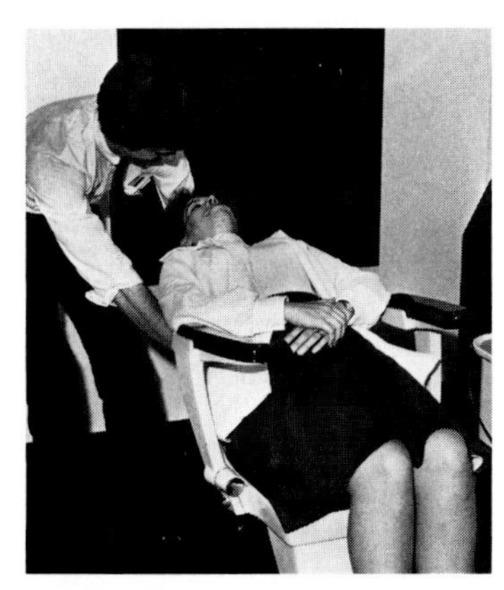

2 Wait about 30 seconds for the anesthetic to take effect. (Expect its effects to last 10 to 15 minutes.) Then, ask her to stare straight up.

Nursing tip: To help your patient maintain her gaze, have her make a fist directly above her nose and stick out her thumb. Then, instruct her to stare at her thumb.

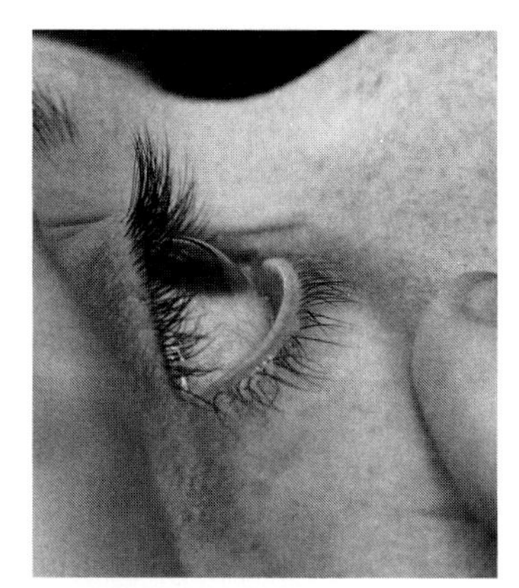

3 Next, use the thumb and forefinger of your nondominant hand to hold her right eyelids open. Gently press your fingers on her superior and inferior orbital rims, as shown here. *Caution:* Avoid pressing down on the eyeball, or you may cause false IOP elevation.

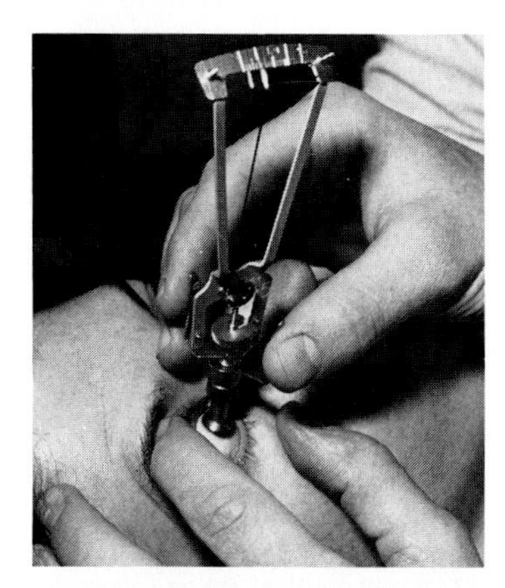

4 Using your dominant hand, hold the tonometer by its handle. To avoid breaking your patient's gaze, approach her cornea from the outer canthus. Gently place the footplate on the cornea's center. *Caution:* Avoid pressing down on the footplate; you may damage the eye or cause false IOP elevation.

Steady your hand by resting it on your patient's nose, cheek, or forehead.

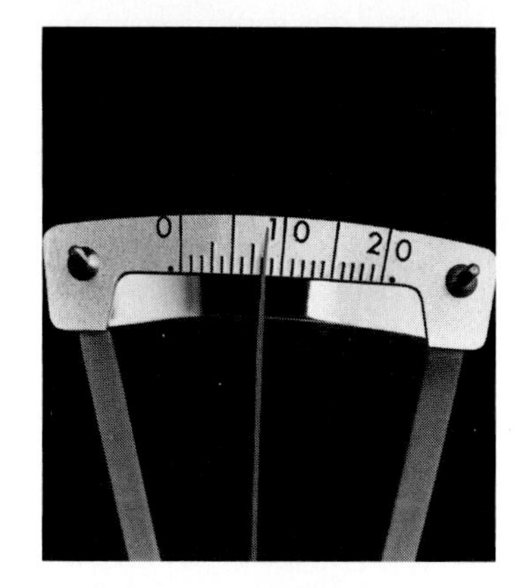

5 Make sure the plunger's perpendicular to the cornea. If you must reposition the plunger, *lift* rather than slide it. Instruct your patient to breathe normally.

Now, observe the pointer's tip in the tonometer's mirror, located below the scale. If the pointer oscillates or falls between two measuring rules, take the reading at the higher rule. Use the chart that accompanies the tonometer to calculate IOP in mm Hg.

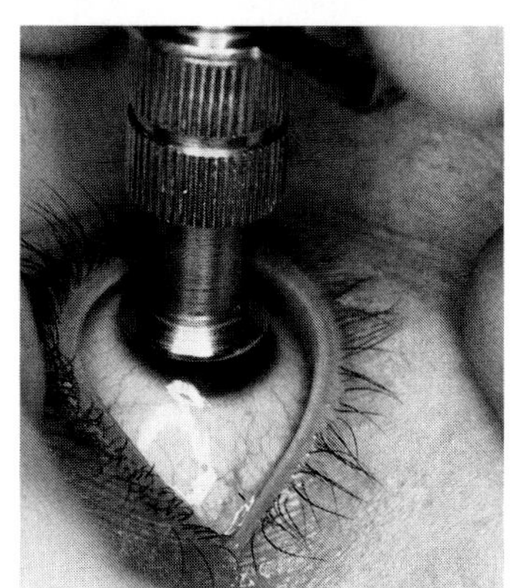

6 Next, perform the test on the other eye.

Document the results on the appropriate form. If the reading for either eye is abnormally high (for example, above 18 mm Hg, according to hospital or clinic guidelines) or if the pressure in both eyes is abnormally low, refer your patient to an eye-care specialist.

Special tests

Getting acquainted with noncontact tonometry

If you frequently screen for glaucoma with a Schiøtz tonometer, you've probably encountered patients like Betty Faulkner, age 59. Despite your efforts to reassure her, she can't remain motionless for indentation tonometry. You're reluctant to insist for fear of injuring her eye, but you know the importance of assessing her intraocular pressure (IOP). What's the answer?

For a patient like Ms. Faulkner, noncontact tonometry may be the solution. Because this procedure doesn't necessitate contact between the eye and the tonometer, it's also suitable for a patient with an eye infection. And because the procedure's painless, the patient doesn't need an ophthalmic anesthetic.

On these pages, we acquaint you with one type of noncontact tonometer: the AO (American Optical) Non-Contact II.

How the Non-Contact II tonometer works

When operated correctly (see following photostory), this tonometer directs a light beam against the patient's cornea. Then, it releases a short burst of air (air puff) that hits the cornea with increasing force. As the cornea flattens, it redirects the light until a predetermined amount of light is reflected directly toward a light detector. By analyzing the time necessary to receive this reflection, the tonometer calculates IOP and then shows a digital IOP reading (in mm Hg) on its display screen. *Note:* Because this type of test flattens the cornea, it's also called *applanation tonometry.*

When performed correctly on a relaxed, cooperative patient, noncontact tonometry is highly accurate. But keep in mind that anxiety may temporarily increase IOP, making initial readings falsely high. To compensate, test each eye at least three times and average the results.

Examining the instrument

Before using the Non-Contact II tonometer, take a moment to become familiar with its parts by studying the two photos at right. As you see, the tonometer has two override controls: the headrest override knob and the override button. Ordinarily, the tonometer won't function unless the patient's positioned correctly and his cornea is in focus. The override controls permit testing even when these criteria haven't been met. This feature is especially helpful if your patient's a frightened or uncooperative child, or if his cornea's highly irregular (from astigmatism or edema, for example), making focusing impossible. Of course, an IOP measurement obtained with override controls is only approximate.

Now, for details on checking calibration and using the tonometer, read the following photostory.

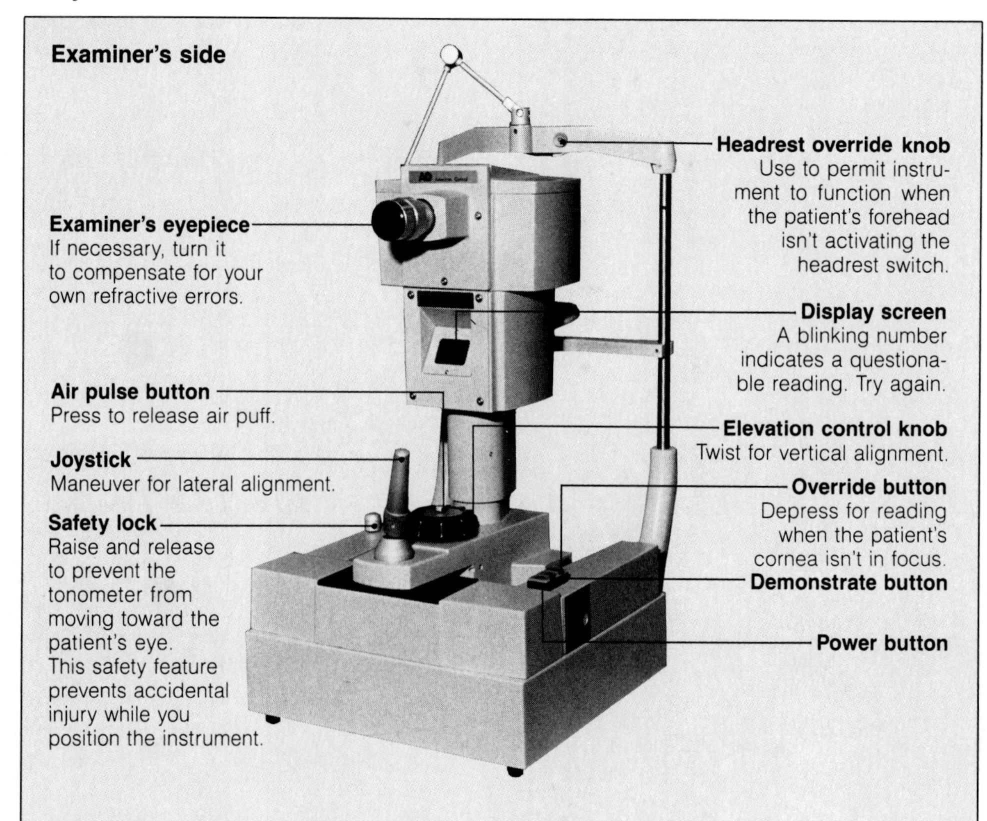

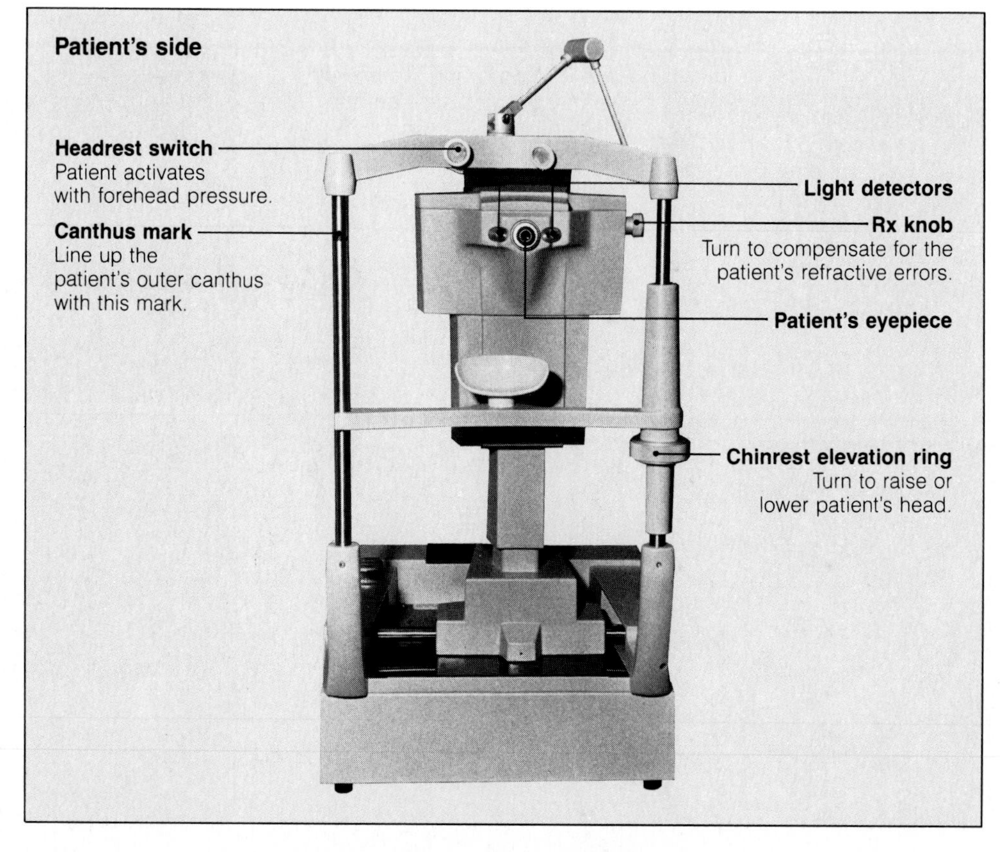

Using the Non-Contact II tonometer

Susan Grey, a 29-year-old cytologist, has a family history of glaucoma. Today, she's in your clinic for routine glaucoma screening. If you're using the AO Non-Contact II tonometer, follow the steps shown below.

First, explain the procedure to Ms. Grey, and assure her that it's painless. If she's wearing contact lenses, ask her to remove them. Warn her that she may be momentarily startled to feel the air puff against her eye. Tell her you'll help her become accustomed to the feeling by demonstrating the air puff on her hand. You'll test the tonometer's calibration at the same time.

Now, seat her on the tonometer's patient side, and adjust her chair (or the table) so her eyes are level with the patient's eyepiece when she's sitting straight.

Turn on the tonometer by depressing the power button. Wait 30 seconds for the instrument to warm up.

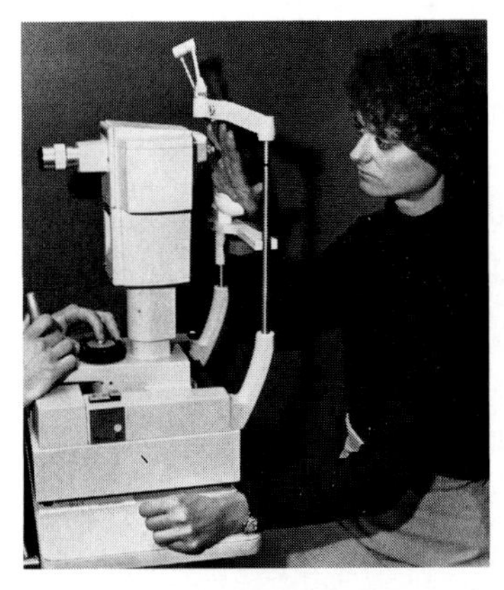

1 To accustom your patient to the air puff, ask her to place her hand an inch (2.5 cm) away from the patient's eyepiece, as shown. Next, depress the demonstrate button. Then, to release an air puff, depress the air pulse button. Ms. Grey will feel the air puff against her hand. *Note:* The manufacturer recommends that you always release an air puff before testing, to reduce the risk of blowing dust into the patient's eye.

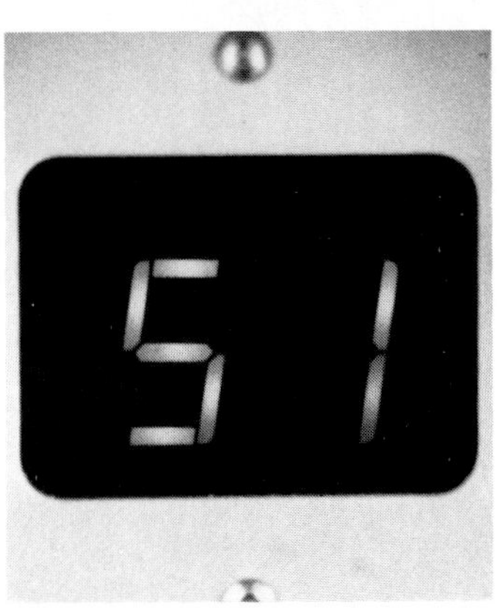

2 Now, look for the calibration number on the display screen. Expect to see a number from 49 to 51, as shown here. If the number you see is incorrect, contact the manufacturer for recalibration.

Release the demonstrate button by depressing it again.

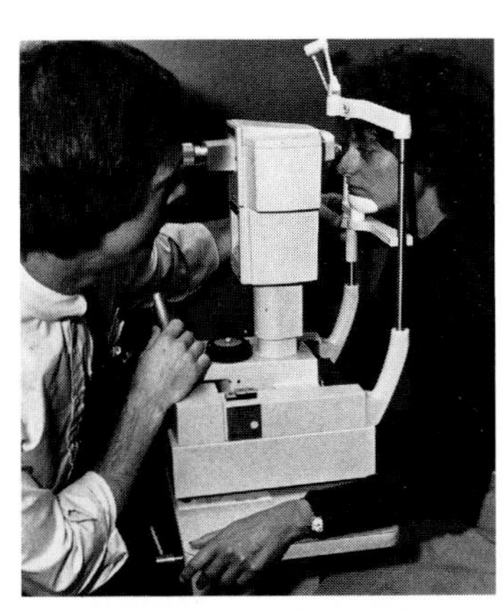

3 To position Ms. Grey, ask her to place her chin on the chinrest and to press her forehead against the headrest. *Remember:* She must press against the headrest to activate the headrest switch.

Using the chinrest elevation ring, position her head so her left eye is level with the eyepiece and her outer left canthus is aligned with the canthus mark.

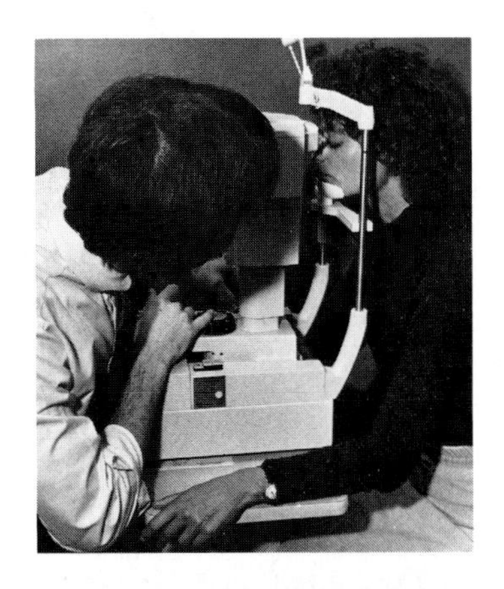

4 Now, instruct her to close her eyes. Pull up the safety lock knob. Using the joystick, slowly move the tonometer toward her. Stop when the eyepiece is no more than ¼" (6 mm) from her eye. Release the knob to lock the tonometer. Now, you can't accidentally move the instrument closer to the patient's eye.

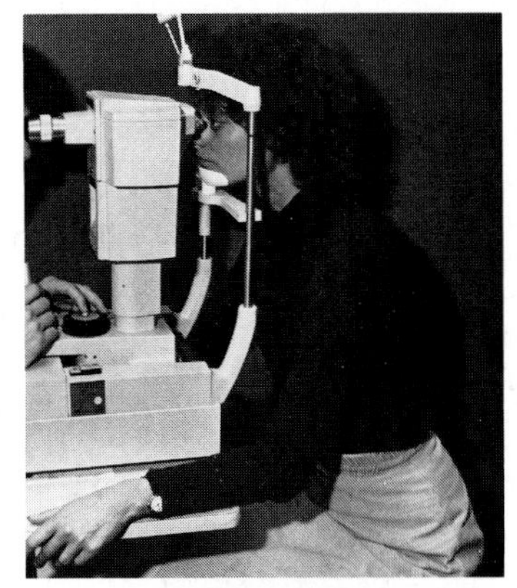

5 Tell your patient to open her eyes and look for a red dot in the eyepiece. (If necessary, adjust the Rx knob until she can see the dot. If her vision's normal, position the knob so its two black marks align vertically.) Ask her to stare at the dot.

Make sure *both* her eyes are open and that her mouth's closed. Also, instruct her to breathe normally. Otherwise her intraocular pressure (IOP) may be falsely high.

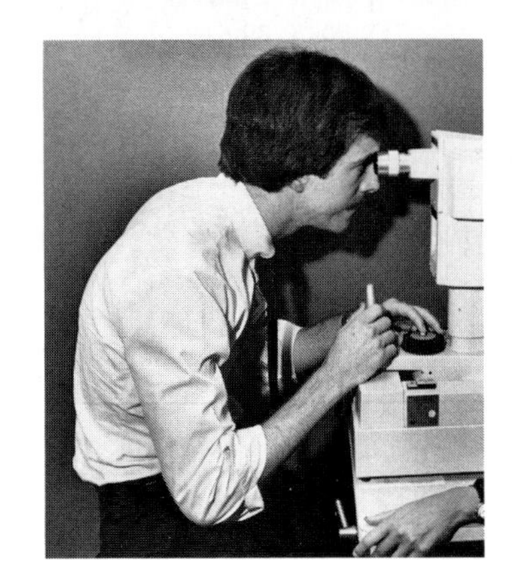

6 Now, look into the examiner's eyepiece. You'll see a circle and a moving red dot. (This dot is a reflection from the patient's cornea.) Use the joystick and elevation control knob to maneuver the dot into the circle. When you've done so, release an air puff by depressing the air pulse button.

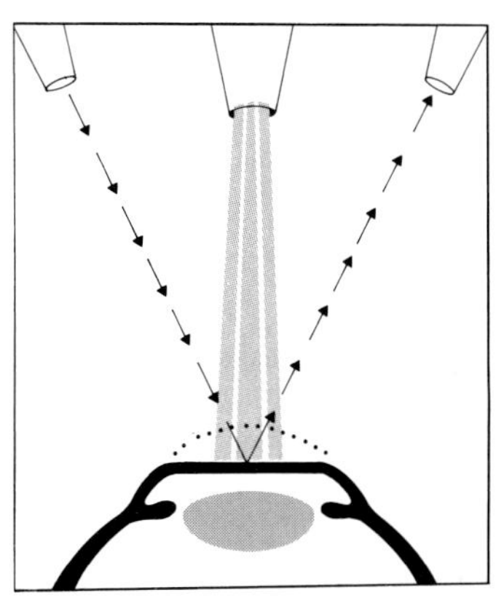

7 The air puff flattens the cornea, as shown here. The tonometer then calculates IOP and shows the measurement on the display screen.

Record the result. Repeat the procedure twice; then continue the test on the right eye. Document all your findings.

Special tests

Understanding glaucoma medications

Depending on the type and cause of your patient's glaucoma, the doctor may order one of four medication types to relieve intraocular pressure. Read the following chart to learn about them.

Cholinergic

carbachol topical (Isopto Carbachol*)
pilocarpine hydrochloride (Isopto Carpine*)

Action

Constricts the pupil and ciliary muscle and dilates conjunctival vessels of outflow tract, increasing aqueous humor outflow

Possible side effects

- Sensitivity reaction to succinylcholine
- Blurred or diminished vision
- Hyperemia
- Eye congestion (redness)

Nursing considerations

- Administer topically to patients with primary open-angle glaucoma, as ordered.
- Minimize systemic absorption by pressing on inner canthus for 1 or 2 minutes after instilling the drops.

Adrenergic

epinephrine bitartrate (Epitrate*)
epinephrine hydrochloride (Epifrin*)

Action

Decreases aqueous humor production and dilates the pupil, increasing aqueous humor outflow

Possible side effects

- Severe stinging sensation
- Dotted conjunctival pigmentation secondary to drug oxidation
- Sensitivity reaction
- Tachycardia
- Palpitations
- Increased blood pressure
- Severe allergic conjunctivitis after long-term use

Nursing considerations

- Administer topically.
- Use cautiously in a patient with both primary open-angle glaucoma and a shallow anterior chamber.
- Use cautiously in a patient with hypertension or cardiovascular disease.
- Protect solution from heat and light. Don't use discolored medication.

Carbonic anhydrase inhibitor

acetazolamide (Diamox*)
dichlorphenamide (Daranide*)

Action

Inhibits transport mechanisms across the ciliary epithelium, reducing aqueous humor production

Possible side effects

- Metabolic acidosis
- Paresthesias of the face and extremities
- Metallic taste
- Anorexia
- Nausea and vomiting
- Diarrhea
- Formation of renal calculi
- Dehydration, electrolyte imbalance

Nursing considerations

- Administer P.O.
- Give to patients with open-angle or acute closed-angle glaucoma, as ordered.
- Give alone or with a cholinergic or adrenergic medication, as ordered.
- Obtain periodic complete blood counts and serum electrolyte measurements from patient on long-term therapy.
- Contraindicated as long-term treatment of certain types of noncongestive closed-angle glaucoma.
- Warn patient of medication's diuretic effects, especially if he's elderly.

Osmotic

anhydrous glycerin (Ophthalgan)
mannitol (Osmitrol*)

Action

Produces intravascular or local hyperosmolarity, reducing aqueous humor production. Works quickly to relieve acute attacks of primary closed-angle glaucoma.

Possible side effects

- Increase in serum glucose
- Nausea and vomiting
- Dizziness
- Headache
- Fever
- Rhinitis
- Urticaria
- Fluid volume shift
- Dehydration, electrolyte imbalance (except for local medications)

Nursing considerations

- Administer certain medications, such as mannitol, I.V. Administer others topically; for example, anhydrous glycerin.
- Use an in-line filter when administering mannitol.
- As ordered, give a topical anesthetic, such as tetracaine hydrochloride (Pontocaine*) or proparacaine hydrochloride (Ophthetic*), before anhydrous glycerin administration. Because anhydrous glycerin rapidly absorbs eye fluids, this medication causes eye pain.
- Warn patient that eye drops may temporarily blur his vision.
- Closely monitor fluid intake and output. Systemic forms have an osmotic diuretic effect that may cause dehydration and electrolyte imbalance.

*Available in both the United States and Canada

Reviewing glaucoma surgery

Will the doctor decide to treat your patient's glaucoma surgically? The answer depends on the type of glaucoma your patient has and on his condition.

If he has chronic open-angle glaucoma, the most common type, the doctor will probably prescribe only medication. But expect the doctor to treat this type of glaucoma surgically if:

- the medication fails to control intraocular pressure (IOP) or the patient fails to maintain medication therapy.
- the patient develops a sensitivity or toxicosis from the medication.
- a cataract develops.

If your patient has closed-angle glaucoma, the doctor will probably perform surgery immediately after treating the symptoms with medication. Keep in mind that surgery may produce such complications as hemorrhage and infection. Cataract formation is a common long-term surgical complication.

To learn more about surgical procedures for glaucoma, study the following information and illustrations.

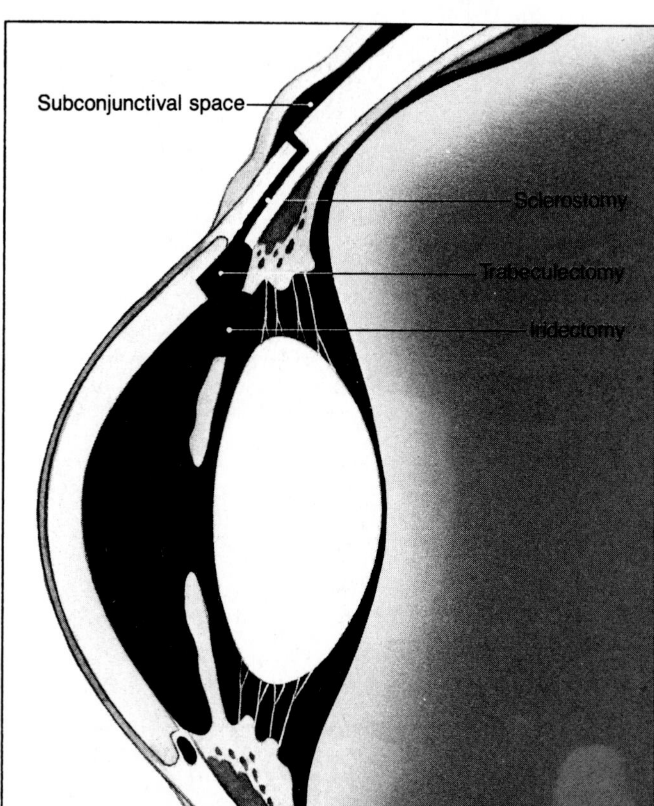

Trabeculectomy and thermal sclerostomy

These two procedures are similar and are used primarily in treating chronic open-angle glaucoma. To establish an artificial drainage route for aqueous humor, the doctor creates a channel through the sclera (sclerostomy). This channel permits the aqueous humor to drain from the anterior chamber into a space between the conjunctiva and the sclera called the subconjunctival space (see illustration above). By draining aqueous humor, the new channel relieves elevated IOP. About 80% of patients treated this way recover normal IOP. Some patients, however, continue to need drug therapy after surgery.

Iridectomy
Used to treat chronic closed-angle glaucoma, this procedure provides direct access for aqueous humor from the posterior chamber to the anterior chamber. The doctor makes an incision in the anterior chamber and excises part of the iris (see illustration below). The incision remains the same size, because a hole in the iris doesn't heal or close. As a preventive measure, the doctor may perform a prophylactic iridectomy in the opposite eye.

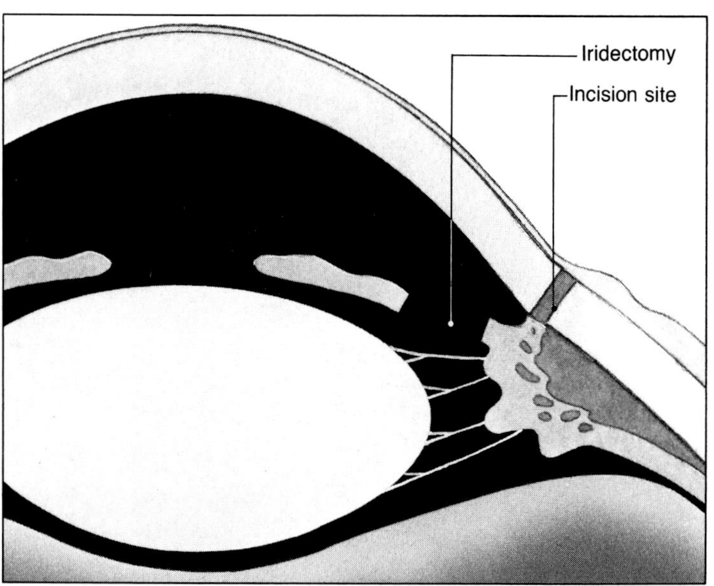

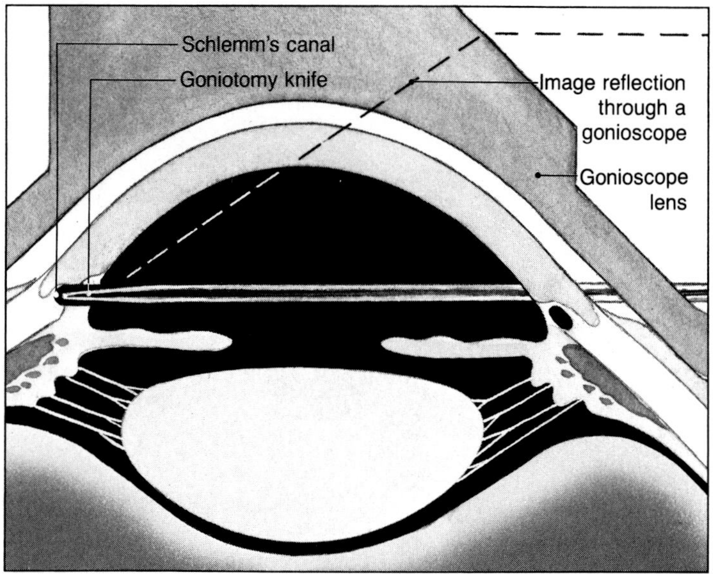

Goniotomy
This procedure is the traditional treatment of developmental glaucoma. During this surgical procedure, the doctor first examines the eye's anterior compartment with a specially designed lens and mirror, called a gonioscope. He uses this lens to locate an appropriate incision site along Schlemm's canal. Then, he cuts across the anterior chamber (see illustration above) and makes a bowlike 120° incision in the trabecular meshwork. The aqueous humor follows this route to Schlemm's canal. To maintain normal IOP, the doctor may make two or three incisions.

Trabeculotomy
This procedure has become popular in treating developmental glaucoma. To perform it, the doctor incises the conjunctiva and sclera and cuts into Schlemm's canal. He then lacerates the inner wall of Schlemm's canal with a surgical instrument called a trabeculotome (see illustration below). The laceration, which never heals, permits aqueous humor to flow into Schlemm's canal. Except in rare instances, this surgery cures developmental glaucoma.

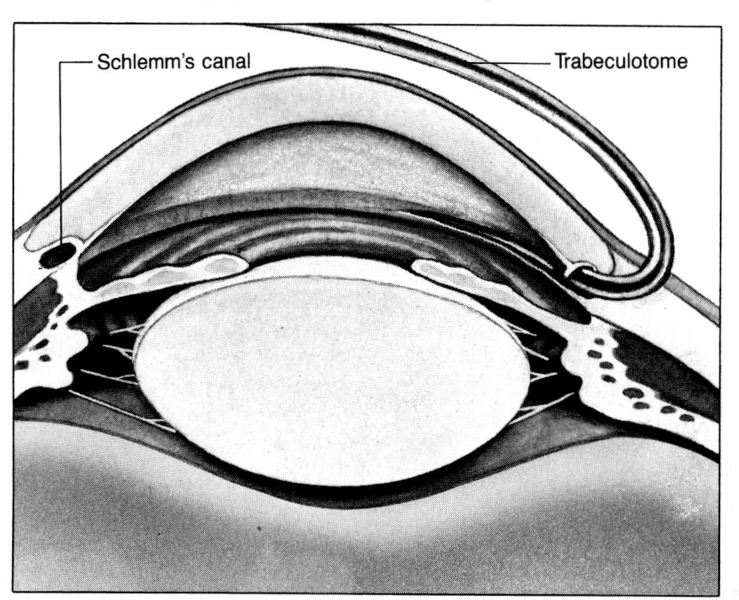

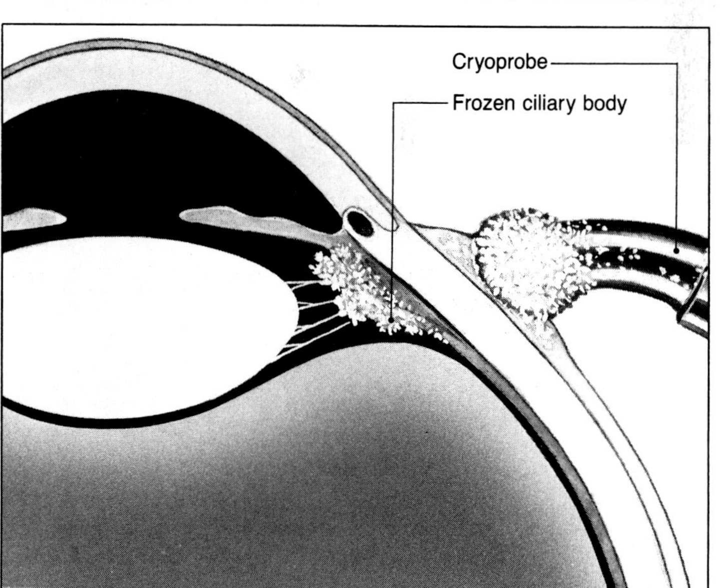

Cyclocryotherapy
This procedure decreases aqueous humor production. It's helpful for a patient with chronic open-angle or chronic closed-angle glaucoma and may be used as a last resort if other surgical procedures fail. For 45 to 60 seconds, the doctor holds a cryoprobe against several sites overlying the ciliary body (see illustration above). This probe temporarily freezes each site. The resulting ciliary body atrophy reduces aqueous humor production. A possible complication is overreduction of aqueous humor production, resulting in softening of the eyes.

Special tests

Understanding edema

A small amount of fluid in the interstitial space is normal. But when a lot of fluid accumulates, edema results. Edema may affect a local area (for example, an arm or leg) or a general area (for example, the entire back or sacrum). Fluid can also accumulate in large body cavities, such as the chest and lungs, causing serious complications. Hypoxia, for example, may result from pulmonary edema.

On these two pages you'll learn more about specific types of edema. As you read, keep in mind that all edema types affect the body in at least one of the ways described below.

Change in capillary wall permeability. Damage to a capillary vessel's wall increases the wall's permeability, allowing fluid to escape into the interstitial space. Causes of increased capillary wall permeability include:
- anoxia
- shock
- allergic reaction
- crushing injury
- some types of snake venom.

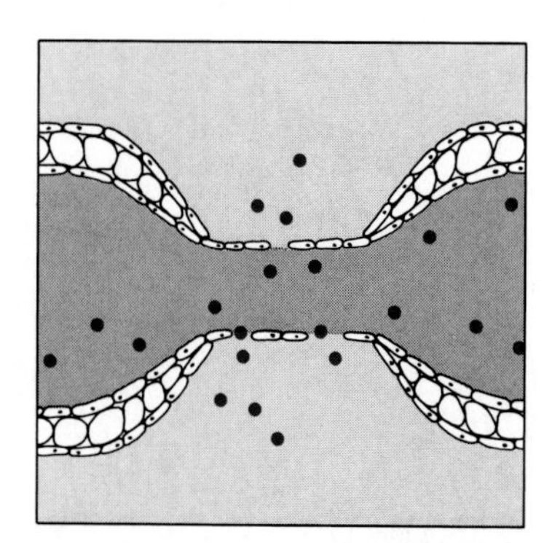

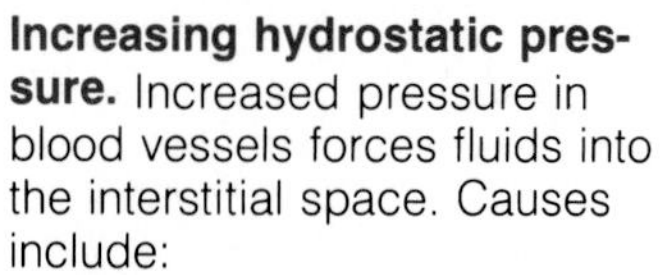

Increasing hydrostatic pressure. Increased pressure in blood vessels forces fluids into the interstitial space. Causes include:
- congestive heart failure (which increases pressure in the venous system)
- prolonged standing (which raises pressure in the legs and feet)
- overhydration.

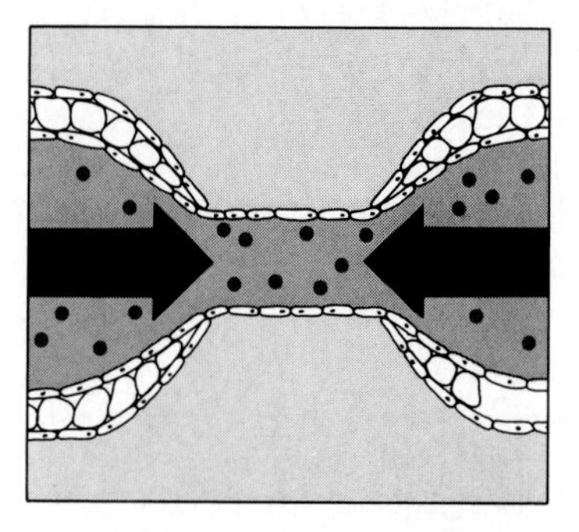

Decreasing osmotic pressure. A decrease of osmotic substances (chiefly protein) in the vessels causes fluid to shift toward the interstitial space, where osmotic pressure is higher. Causes include:
- kidney disease (causing large quantities of protein to be excreted in the urine)
- liver disease (which prevents albumin from being synthesized normally)
- starvation
- malnutrition.

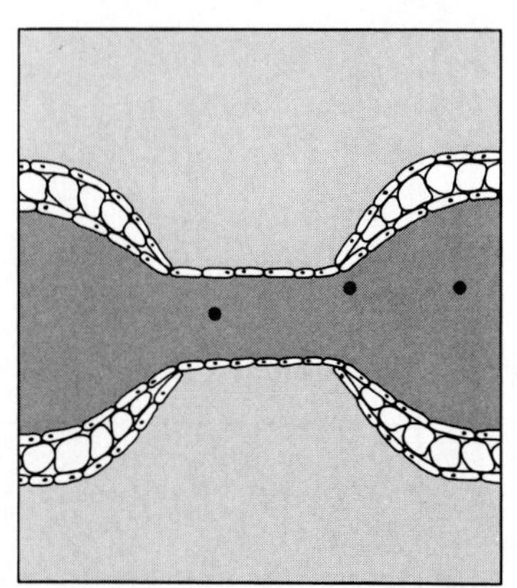

Lymphatic or vascular blockage. Blockage of lymph system or blood vessels prevents normal fluid circulation. Causes include:
- surgical removal of lymph glands (as in mastectomy)
- tumor
- tight girdle
- elastic stockings.

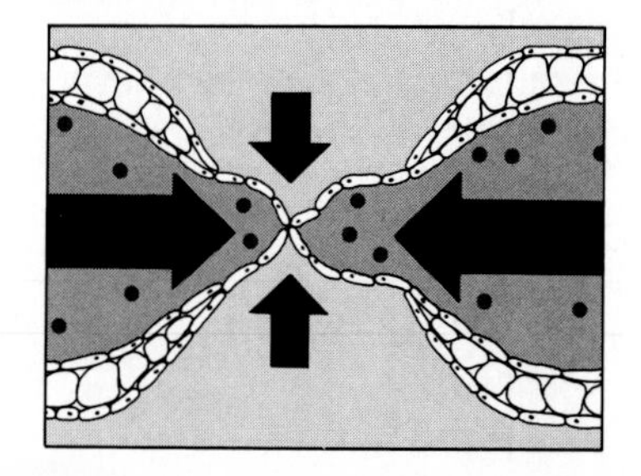

Assessing edema

Does your patient have edema? Consider inspection and palpation your most valuable assessment techniques.

Because gravity helps determine where fluid collects, closely inspect the patient's most dependent areas (feet and ankles of ambulatory patients; sacrum, back, and hips of a patient on bed rest). Do you see swelling? Use your thumb to firmly depress the tissue over a bony prominence for at least 10 seconds. When you release thumb pressure, the depression should return to normal contour immediately. If it doesn't, *pitting edema* is present.

If you identify an area swollen by pitting edema, continue assessing the area until you determine how far the edema extends. Document your findings.

Note: Not all localized swelling is edema, so take care to palpate for the crackling feeling of subcutaneous air or the firmer feel of an arthritic nodule.

Be sure to carefully monitor your patient's weight, using the guidelines on page 38. Fluctuations in a patient's daily weight may provide a clue to developing fluid collection.

Documenting edema

After determining that your patient has edema, you're ready to classify it on a scale of trace (least severe) to +4 (severest). Use the information below as a guide.

Edema value	Finding
Trace	Pressure causes a visible indentation that quickly disappears after pressure release.
+1	Pressure causes an indentation that remains for about 5 seconds after pressure release.
+2	Pressure causes a moderately deep indentation that remains for about 15 seconds after pressure release.
+3	Pressure causes a moderately deep indentation that remains for about 30 seconds after pressure release.
+4	Pressure causes a deep indentation that lasts for longer than 1 minute after pressure release.

Identifying third-space edema

Third-space edema occurs when fluid accumulates in a large body cavity, such as the abdomen. Or, it may develop deep in an arm or leg muscle compartment. A trauma patient is particularly prone to this condition, called *compartment syndrome.* (You'll learn how to monitor compartment syndrome in this book's third section.)

As third-space edema progresses, it may cause life-threatening complications; for example, hypotension, severe dehydration, and pulmonary edema.

How can you detect it?

One reliable sign of third-space edema is an imbalance in your patient's fluid intake and output. For example, if your patient's intake far exceeds his output and your assessment doesn't reveal peripheral edema, suspect third-space edema. Also, look for sudden weight gain, indicating an increase in body fluids.

Has it been a while since you assessed a patient for third-space edema? If so, review the chart below.

Anasarca
(generalized massive edema)

Signs and symptoms
- Increase in pitting edema values
- Progressive increase in extremity circumference

Treatment
- Determine cause and correct it, if possible. (May be associated with end-stage kidney disease or cancer.)
- Administer mannitol (Osmitrol*) or albumin I.V., as ordered, to encourage controlled fluid shift from third space into intravascular space. *Note:* Give diuretics other than mannitol with caution. They may cause hypovolemia, while having little effect on third-space edema.
- Restrict fluid and salt intake, as ordered.
- Give analgesics, as ordered.

Special considerations
- Elevate dependent body parts.
- Turn patient frequently; massage sacrum, hips, and other affected body areas.
- If patient's face is affected, warn him that his eyes may swell shut.
- If his neck is affected, frequently check for a compromised airway. Keep a tracheotomy tray on hand.
- Remove rings, bracelets, or tight clothing. Make sure the patient's identification bracelet is nonconstrictive.
- Don't give injections in edematous areas.

Compartment syndrome
(muscle compartment edema)

Signs and symptoms
- Increase in pitting edema values
- Increase in extremity circumference
- Cool skin distal to compartment
- Possible sensation loss

Treatment
- Determine cause and correct it, if possible.
- Give analgesics, as ordered.

Special considerations
- Promote venous and lymphatic draining by keeping extremity at heart level.
- Remove rings, bracelets, and tight clothing.
- Measure extremity circumference at least every 2 hours.
- Monitor compartment pressure with pressure monitoring equipment, if ordered.
- Periodically, check patient's pulses, color, temperature, and capillary refill distal to edema.
- Don't give injections in edematous areas.

Note: If edema compromises vascular and nerve supply to the affected area, the doctor may perform a fasciotomy. Prepare the patient for this procedure, if indicated.

Hydropericarditis
(pericardial edema)

Signs and symptoms
- Pericardial friction rub
- Progressive increase in central venous pressure (CVP)
- Enlarged heart on chest X-ray
- Jugular vein distention
- Faint heart sounds possible
- Dyspnea
- Orthopnea
- Tachycardia

Treatment
- Determine cause and correct it, if possible.
- Keep patient on bed rest to reduce cardiac demand.
- Give oxygen and analgesics, if ordered.
- If indicated, prepare patient for invasive treatment; for example, partial pericardectomy (which allows fluid to flow into the pleural space) or fluid aspiration with cardiac needle.

Special considerations
- Keep cardiac needle and large syringe handy. Edema may cause pericardial compression.
- Monitor vital signs at least every 30 minutes.
- Monitor for CVP increase (caused by compression of heart's right side).
- Auscultate to detect friction rub.

Pleural effusion
(edema in pleural space)

Signs and symptoms
- Decreased breath sounds
- Dullness over affected area on percussion
- Pleuritic chest pain
- Dyspnea
- Poorly defined intercostal space on affected side
- Tachycardia

Treatment
- Correct cause, if possible.
- Give oxygen, as ordered.

Special considerations
- Monitor arterial blood gas measurements.
- Encourage deep breathing to prevent atelectasis.
- If condition's severe, prepare patient for chest tube insertion or thoracentesis.

Pulmonary edema

Signs and symptoms
- Enlarged heart and congested pulmonary vessels on chest X-ray
- Shortness of breath
- Pink, frothy sputum
- Rales on auscultation
- Orthopnea
- Tachycardia
- Coughing
- Tachypnea

Treatment
- Support respiration and give oxygen, as needed.
- Give bronchodilators, such as aminophylline, as ordered.
- Give diuretics, such as furosemide (Lasix*) or ethacrynic acid (Edecrin*), as ordered.
- If ordered, give morphine sulfate to reduce anxiety and relieve left ventricular workload.
- If ordered, give digitalis to improve myocardial contractility.

Note: As an emergency measure, the doctor may order rotating tourniquets to reduce blood volume returning to the heart.

Special considerations
- Monitor vital signs hourly.
- Place patient in high Fowler's position.
- Monitor arterial blood gases.
- Prepare patient for rotating tourniquets, if ordered. (For more on pulmonary edema, see the NURSING PHOTOBOOK PROVIDING RESPIRATORY CARE.)

Ascites
(abdominal edema)

Signs and symptoms
- Increased abdominal girth
- Umbilicus extroversion
- Prominent abdominal veins

Treatment
- Determine cause and correct, if possible. (May be caused by liver disease or damage; for example, alcoholic cirrhosis.)
- Increased intravascular osmotic pressure by administering albumin I.V., as ordered. Increased osmotic pressure helps draw fluid from the third space into the blood vessels, for elimination by the kidneys.
- Administer diuretics cautiously. Diuretics rapidly decrease intravascular volume (possibly causing hypovolemia) but have little or no effect on ascites.
- Restrict fluid intake, as ordered.
- Provide oxygen, if ordered.

Special considerations
- Assess for numbness and tingling of lower extremities from pressure on inferior vena cava.
- Place patient in semi-Fowler's position or help him sit upright in a chair to relieve pressure on his diaphragm.
- If indicated, prepare patient for invasive treatment; for example, LeVeen shunt insertion to allow one-way flow of ascites fluid from abdomen to the superior vena cava.

---

*Available in both the United States and Canada

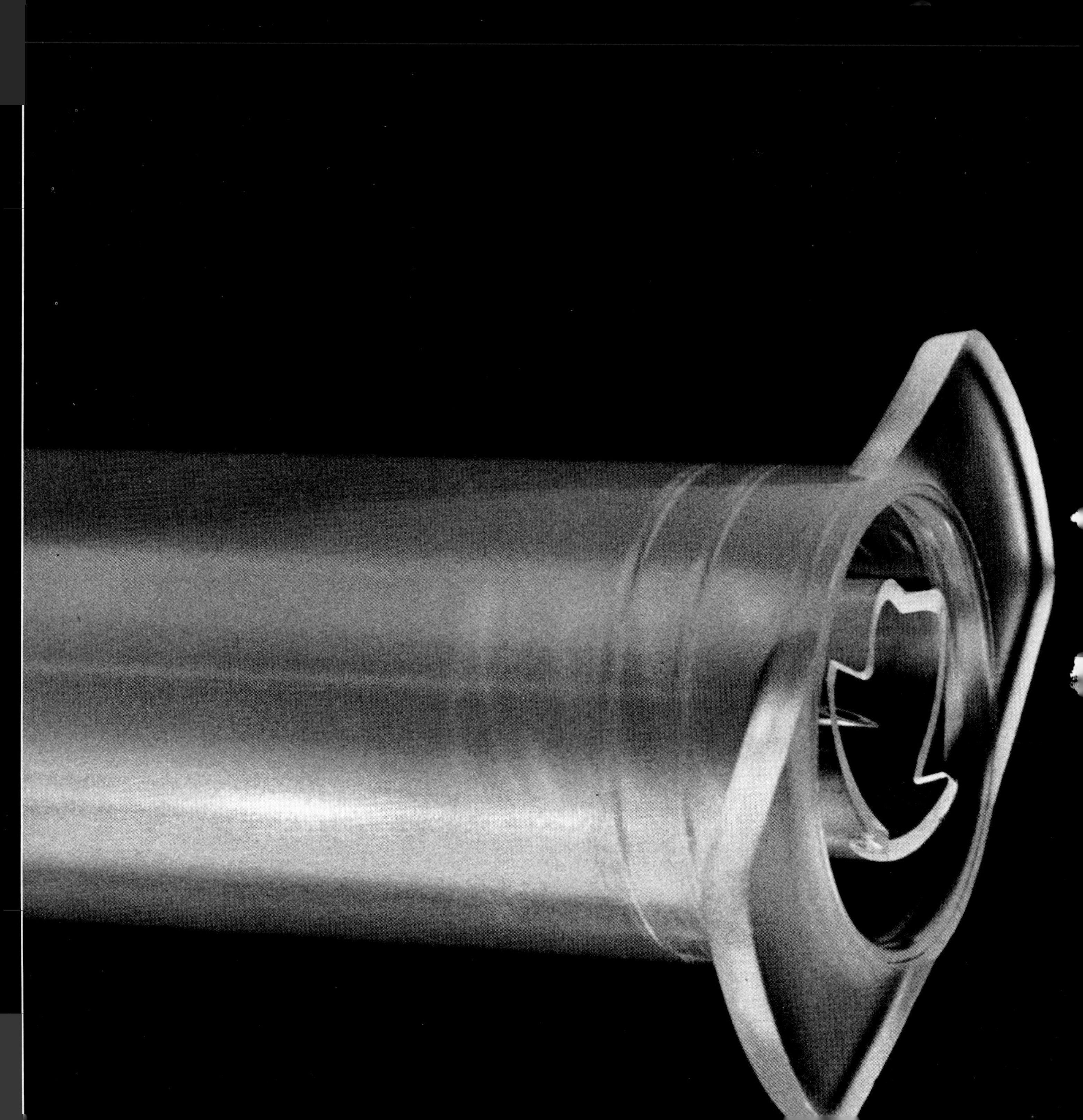

Using Special Equipment

Respiratory

Cardiovascular

GI and endocrine

Intravenous

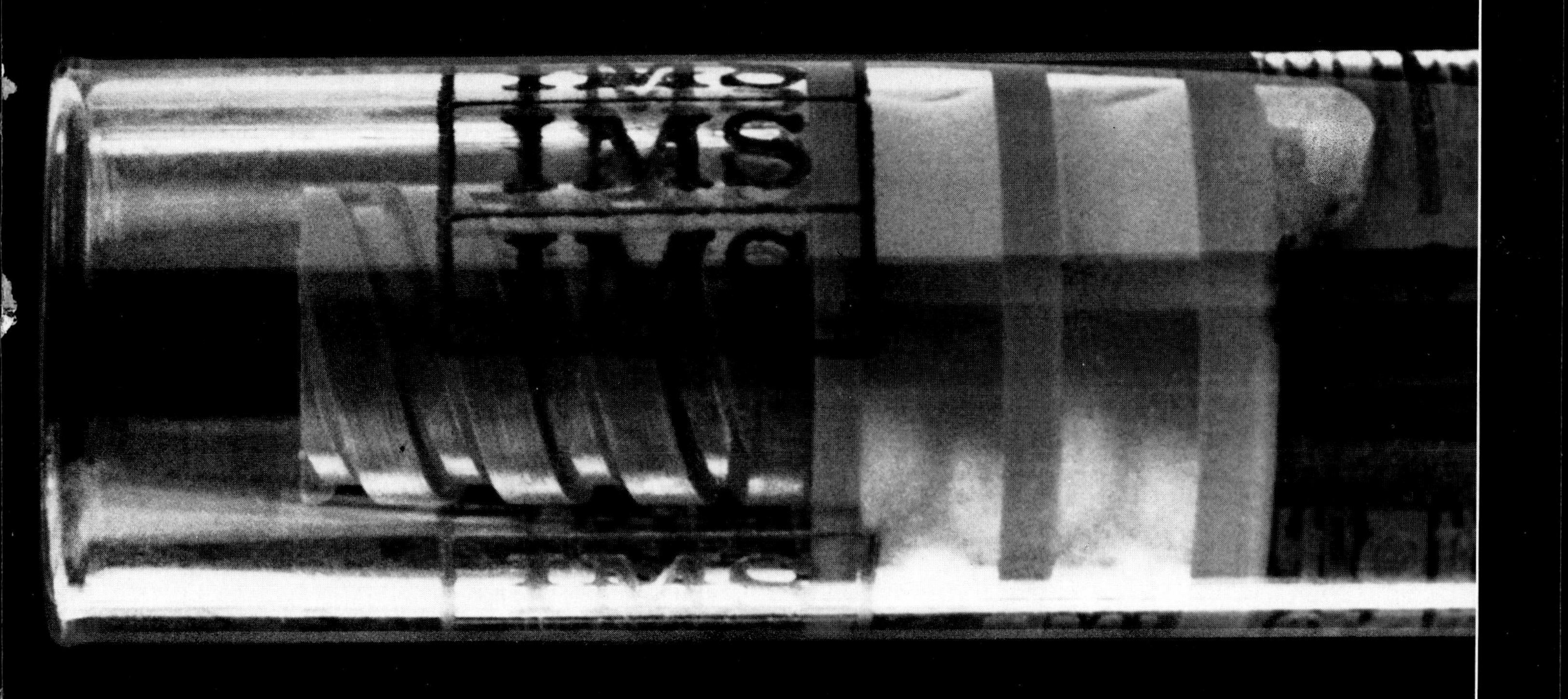

Respiratory

Does your patient have a respiratory condition? Depending on his specific problem, the doctor may order one of the two procedures featured in this section: bronchoscopy or continuous positive airway pressure (CPAP).

On the next three pages, you'll find out how to prepare a patient for either procedure and how to care for him during therapy. In addition, you'll learn:

- what a bronchoscope looks like and how it works.
- how to prevent complications after bronchoscopy.
- how therapy with CPAP can help your patient.

Reviewing bronchoscopy

In the past, bronchoscopy was routinely performed in the operating room. But now, thanks to today's more sophisticated equipment, bedside bronchoscopy's a safe alternative for some patients.

If your patient's scheduled for this procedure, do you know your responsibilities? Can you clearly explain the procedure to him and answer his questions? If you're not sure, review the information on these two pages.

Learning about the bronchoscope

A bronchoscope like the one illustrated at right is made of flexible plastic and equipped with a fiber-optic lens that enables the doctor to visually examine your patient's tracheobronchial tree. When fitted with accessory instruments, the bronchoscope can also be used to remove polyps and other lesions, as well as excessive secretions or mucous plugs; to collect tissue specimens; and to photograph or film the tracheobronchial tree.

The fiber-optic bronchoscope has four cylindrical channels. One channel connects the eyepiece to the distal end, enabling the doctor to inspect the tracheobronchial tree. (By using a sidearm lens attachment, an assistant or student can observe tracheobronchial anatomy along with the doctor.) Light fibers are contained in two other channels, to illuminate the area. These light fibers are attached to a high-intensity light source that's enclosed in a specially designed box. The fourth channel is open, to provide a passageway for removal of tissue or secretions or for anesthetic administration.

Not all bronchoscopes are made of flexible plastic. Some are made of rigid metal; these cause more discomfort during insertion and increase the risk of trauma to the tracheobronchial tree.

Performing bronchoscopy

After anesthetizing the patient's nostrils and pharynx, the doctor inserts the bronchoscope through either a nostril or the mouth. (If he's using a metal bronchoscope, mouth insertion is the only option.) He then advances the bronchoscope's distal end to a point just above the vocal cords.

Next, to prevent coughing and gagging from laryngeal and carina tracheae stimulation during insertion, he introduces a few drops of anesthetic through the bronchoscope's open channel. Then, he continues to advance the distal end down the patient's tracheobronchial tree.

After performing an inspection, the doctor may decide to collect a specimen. To do so, he passes biopsy forceps or a cytology brush through the bronchoscope's open channel. To remove secretions (or a foreign object), he connects suction equipment to this channel.

Now, learn how to prepare your patient for this procedure and care for him afterward by reading the following information.

Note: Bedside bronchoscopy's contraindicated for a patient who needs mechanical ventilation. If necessary, the doctor gives the patient a general anesthetic and performs the procedure in the ICU or operating room.

SPECIAL CONSIDERATIONS

Caring for a patient undergoing bronchoscopy

Although the doctor performs bronchoscopy, your role's important, too. Of course, you're responsible for your patient's care, both before and after the procedure. But that's not all. Before the procedure, you gather the necessary equipment. And during the procedure, you closely monitor your patient's condition and provide continuous reassurance. Become familiar with all your responsibilities by studying the following points.

Preprocedure

- Don't permit your patient to eat or drink anything for 6 to 12 hours before the bronchoscopy, as ordered.
- Tell him what to expect during the procedure. For example, inform him that he'll be positioned either sitting or lying flat. Assure him that he'll receive medication to minimize discomfort, and advise him to relax as much as possible. Answer his questions.
- Tell him the doctor will spray an anesthetic into his throat before inserting the bronchoscope and that this medication may have an unpleasant taste.
- Tell him that he can still inhale and exhale after bronchoscope insertion. If the doctor chooses nose insertion, advise the patient to take slow, deep breaths through his mouth. If the doctor chooses mouth insertion, advise the patient to breathe through his nose. Tell him the procedure takes from 30 minutes to 1 hour.
- Administer the prescribed sedative or anxiolytic (for example, morphine sulfate) 30 minutes to 1 hour before the procedure, as ordered. Tell the patient that the medication will help him relax and suppress his cough reflex.
- Administer atropine sulfate I.M. 30 minutes before the test, as ordered. This medication controls oral and tracheal secretions and prevents bradycardia and other arrhythmias. Warn the patient that his mouth will be dry.
- Document baseline vital signs and chest auscultation findings.
- Make sure the patient's signed a consent form, if required by hospital policy.
- Remove the patient's dentures, if he's wearing any. Inform the doctor about loose teeth, caps, or bridges that may become dislodged if the doctor inserts the bronchoscope in the patient's mouth. Also report any signs of oral disease;

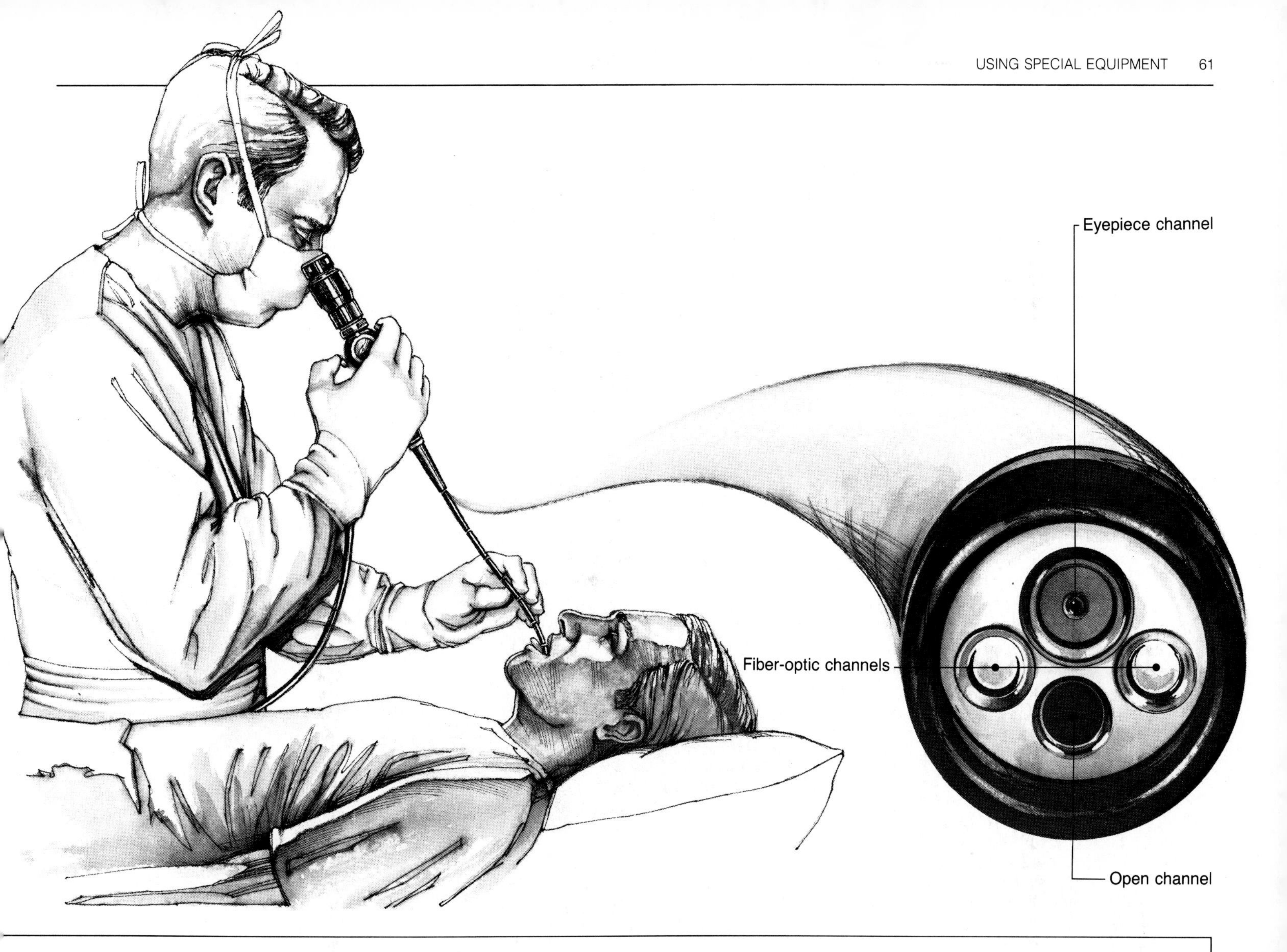

for example, inflammation or sores.

• Gather this equipment: bronchoscope and accessories (including suction machine), 30-ml syringe, sterile saline solution, glass slides and fixative, specimen container with formaldehyde, local anesthetic (as ordered), and topical lidocaine hydrochloride (Xylocaine Jelly 2%) to lubricate the bronchoscope's tip and anesthetize the lower trachea.

• Obtain resuscitative and suctioning equipment and tracheotomy tray. Keep this emergency equipment in the patient's room for 24 hours after the procedure. *Note:* You'll need *two* suction machines—one for the bronchoscope and another for emergency use.

During the procedure

• Frequently assess your patient's vital signs. Inform the doctor of any abnormality.

• Explain each step. Remember, your patient will remain awake throughout the procedure.

• Provide continuous reassurance. By holding your patient's hand, you can restrain him, relieve his anxiety, and prevent him from grabbing the bronchoscope.

• Refill the syringe with sterile saline solution, as needed.

• Carefully label each specimen according to its source, and note whether the doctor obtained it with or without a saline lavage.

• Prepare bronchial brushings on a lab slide, and immediately immerse the slide in fixative.

• Put specimens in a formaldehyde container; label it, and send it to the lab.

Postprocedure

• Place your patient on his side or in semi-Fowler's position, as ordered. To minimize the risk of his choking before his gag reflex returns, tell him not to attempt swallowing. Provide tissues or an emesis basin to catch secretions. *Note:* If the patient's unconscious, position him on his side, with the head of the bed slightly elevated.

• Post a sign over the patient's bed indicating that he's to take nothing by mouth.

• Monitor your patient's vital signs and be alert for cardiac arrhythmias (possibly caused by vagal stimulation during the procedure) or other signs of myocardial infarction.

• Auscultate his chest and compare results with your preprocedure findings.

• After about 1 hour, test his gag reflex. If no response occurs, wait 30 minutes and try again.

• When the gag reflex returns, remove the sign from over the patient's bed and offer liquids. After 8 hours, he may eat soft foods; unless complications occur, he may resume his normal diet within 24 hours.

• Watch for adverse medication reactions.

• Observe for signs and symptoms of tracheobronchial trauma or perforation; for example, blood-tinged sputum, hypoxia, cyanosis, laryngeal stridor, dyspnea, and neck edema.

• If a biopsy was performed, instruct the patient to avoid coughing and clearing his throat.

• Observe and palpate for any subcutaneous crepitus around the patient's face and neck. Report such findings immediately.

• If necessary, provide comfort measures for his throat, such as an ice collar.

• Encourage deep breathing.

• According to hospital policy, wipe the bronchoscope's exterior and flush the open lumen with alcohol and sterile water before returning it to its proper storage place.

• Document everything.

Respiratory

Understanding continuous positive airway pressure

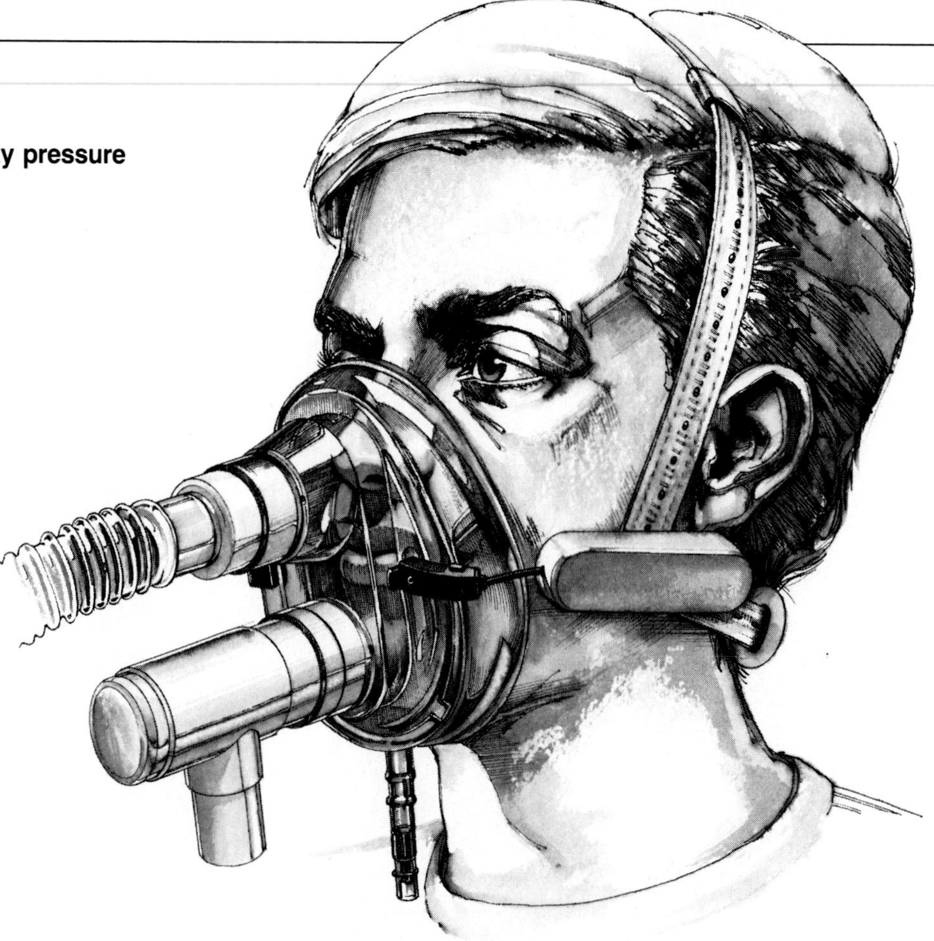

Carl Rhoden, a 52-year-old engineer, has had pneumonia for 3 weeks. Although you've been administering antibiotics and oxygen (through a humidified mask), his condition hasn't improved. In addition, arterial blood gas measurements show that Mr. Rhoden now has hypoxia.

To reverse the condition, the doctor has ordered continuous positive airway pressure (CPAP) therapy. As you know, CPAP therapy provides more oxygen for a patient who can breathe without mechanical assistance. To administer CPAP, you'll use a tight-fitting mask with a humidifier and a valve system, as illustrated at right.

How CPAP works

Before we discuss why CPAP therapy is so valuable for a patient like Mr. Rhoden, take a moment to consider some basic physiology. As you know, a healthy person's alveoli close almost completely each time he exhales; alveoli in a dependent position actually *do* close completely. But during inhalation, the alveoli reopen.

Pneumonia produces secretions that accumulate in the alveoli. These secretions are thick and tenacious and prevent the alveoli from reopening. With fewer alveoli functioning, the lungs have less surface area available for sufficient oxygen exchange.

By administering CPAP therapy, you maintain positive pressure in the patient's airway and alveoli—even after exhalation. As a result, the alveoli never close completely. This, in turn, increases functional residual capacity (FRC), the amount of air remaining in the lungs after normal expiration. By increasing FRC, arterial oxygenation and lung compliance improve. (For more information on how CPAP works, see the NURSING PHOTOBOOK ENSURING INTENSIVE CARE.)

CPAP therapy is contraindicated in patients with chronic obstructive pulmonary disease, such as emphysema. This is because these patients already have high FRC. Treating them with CPAP therapy may cause alveolar distention and rupture.

Caring for your patient during CPAP therapy

Let's assume you're preparing to administer continuous positive airway pressure (CPAP) therapy to Mr. Rhoden. Before you start, explain to him what you'll be doing. Stress the importance of wearing the mask at all times for as long as therapy's in progress. Also, tell him to concentrate on maintaining a normal breathing pattern during therapy, to prevent hyperventilation.

What are your responsibilities during CPAP therapy? Consider the following points. *Caution:* Never leave your patient unattended during therapy. Closely monitor his condition and the equipment.

- Prepare your patient to experience some discomfort from his inability to exhale completely. The tight-fitting mask may also be uncomfortable. But assure him that CPAP therapy isn't painful.
- If ordered, administer a mild sedative to reduce anxiety and decrease oxygen needs.
- Keep suction equipment on hand throughout therapy for use if the patient vomits.
- Maintain water at the indicated level in the humidification reservoir. Otherwise, your patient will breathe dry oxygen, which can damage his delicate respiratory tract.
- Drain condensed water from the tubing, as necessary.
- Maintain compressed air and oxygen flow at the ordered level.
- Closely monitor compressed air and oxygen pressure; make sure it remains within the ordered parameters. Pressure that's too high overdistends the alveoli, causing respiratory distress. Pressure that's too low (for example, from a leak in the system or an incorrect pressure setting) causes shortness of breath.
- Interrupt therapy every 2 to 4 hours and remove your patient's face mask. Wipe moisture from his face and the mask, and examine his skin for signs of irritation. Provide padding with gauze pads, if necessary.
- Every 1 to 2 hours check the skin under the mask's straps for signs of irritation. Readjust the straps or pad the skin with gauze pads, if necessary.
- If the patient has a nasogastric tube in place, regularly inspect the area where the mask presses the tube against his face. Remember, this area's a pressure point; it also may be the source of a leak in the system.
- Regularly assess vital signs and breath sounds and monitor arterial blood gas measurements, as ordered. Stay alert for these possible complications: oxygen toxicosis, pneumothorax, and gastric distention. If complications develop, stop therapy and notify the doctor at once.
- Carefully monitor fluid balance by keeping meticulous fluid intake and output records and by weighing the patient daily.

Cardiovascular

Ever feel overwhelmed by all the new equipment, techniques, and drugs available for your cardiovascular patients? Read this chapter to learn more about a few recent advances in this rapidly growing—and vitally important—nursing field. You'll learn how to:

- perform special assessment procedures using a stethoscope or a Doppler ultrasound device.
- give new cardiovascular drugs safely and effectively.
- use a special computer to take noninvasive cardiac output measurements.
- teach your patient to check pacemaker function by telephone.

Sound helpful? Read on for details.

Your stethoscope: A special piece of equipment

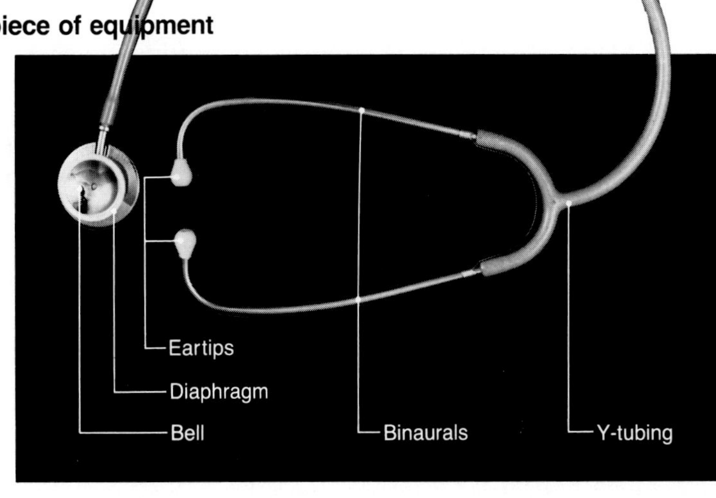

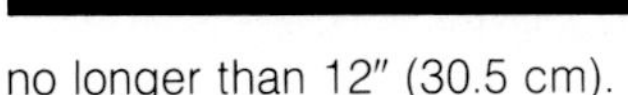

Do you think there's anything special about your stethoscope? Probably not—it's too familiar. You use it many times a day without giving it a second thought. At the end of a shift, you may wad it up and stuff it in a pocket. And if it's disposable, you don't think twice about discarding it.

But consider for a moment how special your stethoscope really is. You use it to auscultate at least three major body systems: cardiovascular, respiratory, and gastrointestinal. As you know, you can learn a lot by listening. That's why your stethoscope's quality is so important.

In the next few pages, you'll learn techniques that help you assess your patient's cardiovascular system by auscultating limb vessels. Your stethoscope's an indispensable tool. Let's take a moment to consider what makes it special.

Examining a stethoscope

Your stethoscope probably resembles the one shown above. Although all stethoscopes are similar, the quality of the sound they transmit varies. As we examine a stethoscope's parts, you'll see why.

Eartips. For best sound transmission, the eartips should fit snugly enough to prevent air leaks but comfortably enough to wear for 5 minutes. Choose a size that occludes the external ear's opening without entering the external ear canal.

Binaurals. This curved metal tubing leading to the eartips has either an internal spring or an external bar to hold the eartips in your ears and prevent the tubing from kinking. An external bar affords best sound transmission.

Y-tubing. Your stethoscope's tubing should be made of flexible, but thick, plastic or vinyl. Thick tubing filters out external noise. In addition, its lumen should be smaller at the bell than at the binaurals.

Keep in mind that the longer the tubing, the greater the sound distortion. So for best results, make sure the tubing is no longer than 12″ (30.5 cm).

Note: Straight tubing offers the shortest, most direct route for sound, although it's sometimes clumsy to use.

Diaphragm. Use the diaphragm to assess high-frequency sounds; for example, vascular and respiratory sounds and the first and second heart sounds.

Bell. Use the bell to assess low-frequency sounds; for example, certain heart murmurs and the third and fourth heart sounds.

Using correct technique

Suppose your stethoscope meets all the criteria for high-quality sound transmission. Now, make sure you use it correctly by reviewing these reminders:

- Always place the chest piece (bell or diaphragm) directly against the patient's skin.
- For good contact, apply the chest piece with enough pressure to leave a slight depression in the skin when you remove the chest piece. But avoid excessive pressure, especially when listening to vascular sounds. You may obstruct blood flow, causing sound loss or false bruits.
- During auscultation, keep the finger holding the chest piece straight and still. Bending your knuckles may produce the phenomenon called *knuckle squeak.* Finger movement across the chest piece also causes interfering noise. *Note:* Moving the chest piece over hair may also cause sound interference.
- During auscultation, move close enough to your patient to avoid stretching the tubing.

Care guidelines

Keep your stethoscope in top working order by following these care guidelines:

- Clean the diaphragm between patients, using a damp washcloth. If the stethoscope becomes very dirty, unscrew the diaphragm holder and carefully wash the diaphragm with soap and water; then, thoroughly dry it. Check the tubing opening for dirt or debris that may obstruct sound; clean the opening, if necessary.
- At least once a week, wipe the tubing with a damp cloth and dry it. Don't use soapy water, unless the tubing's very dirty. (If you wash the tubing with soapy water, take care to thoroughly rinse and dry it afterward.) *Note:* Never clean tubing with alcohol, because alcohol may dry and crack it.
- Periodically, clean your stethoscope's eartips by soaking them in soapy water. Clean the ear holes with a cotton-tipped applicator. Rinse and dry them before replacing them. *Caution:* Don't use someone else's stethoscope without first cleaning the eartips; you may contract an ear infection.
- Don't identify your stethoscope with a name band or tape; it'll interfere with sound transmission. If you wish, have your name engraved on the diaphragm's back instead.
- Inspect the tubing regularly for cracks. Avoid stuffing your stethoscope in a pocket; this promotes cracking.

Cardiovascular

Learning about peripheral auscultation

Chest auscultation is a familiar part of your assessment routine. But does it ever occur to you to listen to the arteries in your patient's neck or limbs? You may be surprised to learn that this assessment technique (called peripheral auscultation) can provide valuable information about your patient's arteries—and help you evaluate his risk of developing heart disease or suffering a cerebrovascular accident.

How? By auscultating major peripheral arteries, you may be able to detect arterial bruits (abnormal sounds caused by turbulent blood flow). In general, arterial bruits signify moderate to severe arterial stenosis from arteriosclerosis.

Accurately identifying and evaluating arterial bruits takes practice. You must learn, for example, to distinguish false (or functional) bruits from clinically significant bruits. False bruits may result from functional heart murmurs or from sounds outside the heart that are unrelated to stenosis. False bruits may become louder if the patient's nervous or excited.

You may inadvertently create a false bruit by pressing too hard on the artery during auscultation. Knowing how much pressure to apply takes practice.

As always, your assessment must include a thorough history and physical examination. Peripheral auscultation is only *part* of your assessment; these findings alone are rarely diagnostic. But if you detect a bruit from one of your patient's arteries, consider it strongly suggestive of arterial disease if he also has one or more of the following:

- weak pulse distal to the bruit
- clinical signs and symptoms suggesting arterial disease
- a history of arterial disease.

Problem solving

In the next photostory, you'll learn how to perform peripheral auscultation. As you work, you may encounter the following problems. Here are some tips to help you deal with them.

- *You think you hear a bruit, but you're not sure.* Try asking the patient to exercise moderately for about 2 minutes. For example, if you're listening to a leg artery, ask him to flex his foot up and down about once per second. By increasing blood flow, such moderate exercise may amplify the bruit. But don't ask the patient to exercise strenuously, because this may cause a false bruit. *Note:* If exercise fails to amplify the bruit, don't assume the artery's disease-free. Keep in mind that pronounced stenosis may limit blood flow so severely that turbulence never occurs. Consider the patient's history and clinical signs before drawing a conclusion.
- *The patient's obese, making auscultation of deep vessels difficult.* To assess a patient who's obese, press the stethoscope's chest piece firmly against his skin, until you hear a sound. As you know, this sound may be a false bruit caused by stethoscope pressure. To determine if you're hearing a false bruit, gradually lessen the pressure on your patient's skin, until the pressure equals approximately what you'd use for a thinner patient. If you no longer hear the bruit, assume it was false.

Performing peripheral auscultation

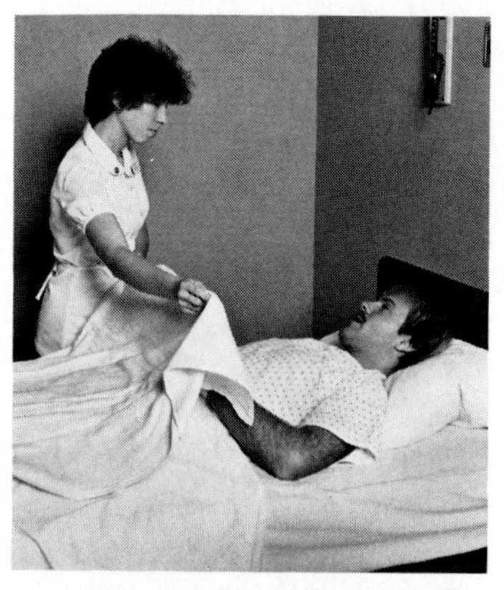

1 Planning to perform peripheral auscultation? If possible, ask your patient to lie down and relax for 30 minutes before you begin. Cover him with a blanket for warmth, if necessary. By encouraging him to relax, you minimize interference from false (functional) bruits, which may be aggravated by nervousness.

Explain the procedure to him, and tell him he'll remain supine throughout the procedure.

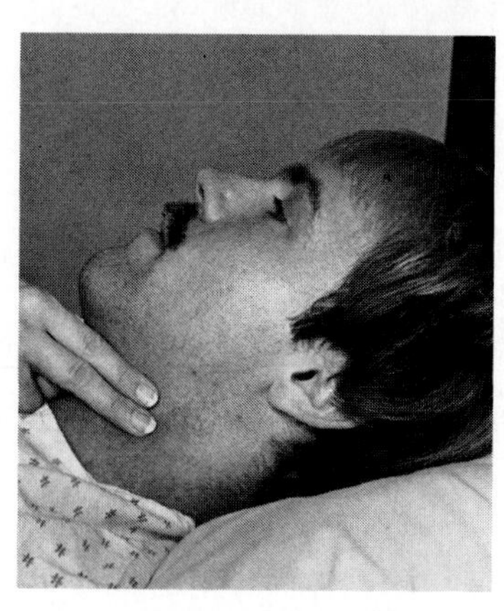

2 As part of your physical exam, document the rate, rhythm, and amplitude of these peripheral pulses: carotid, brachial, radial, femoral, popliteal, posterior tibial, and dorsalis pedis. (Remember to assess all pulses bilaterally.) Also, palpate each artery to determine the wall's condition; a tortuous artery that feels ropelike may be arteriosclerotic. Finally, note whether bilateral arms and legs are equally warm.

Getting acquainted with a Doppler device

Ever had difficulty obtaining an accurate blood pressure measurement from a patient with hypotension? If so, you know one of the limitations of auscultation by stethoscope. When vascular sounds are hard to hear, a Doppler ultrasound device can be an asset.

How it works

The Medasonics Ultrasound Stethoscope Blood Flow Detector, shown at right, is a continuous-wave, audio-output Doppler device. This type of equipment consists of a transmitter crystal, which transmits sound waves, and a receiver crystal, which receives the echos. A moving target, such as circulating blood cells, alters the frequency (or pitch) of returning sound waves. Their frequency is directly related to blood flow velocity.

The difference in frequency between the transmitted sound and the received sound is called *Doppler shift.* Because Doppler shift is usually within human auditory range, the received sound is simply directed through an audio amplifier to a loudspeaker or headset.

Assessing blood pressure

A stethoscope, as you know, amplifies internal body sounds, including the sounds of blood flow turbulence you listen for when taking a blood pressure measurement. The Doppler works differently; instead of amplifying sounds, it detects blood flow by bouncing ultrasound waves off circulating blood cells. When you're assessing blood pressure, this difference gives the Doppler several advantages over the stethoscope. For one thing, the Doppler enables you to detect blood flow even when turbulence is inaudible by stethoscope. For another, it helps you determine systolic pressure with greater accuracy, even when turbulence *is* audible. Why? Because after you release pressure on the artery, the Doppler alerts you

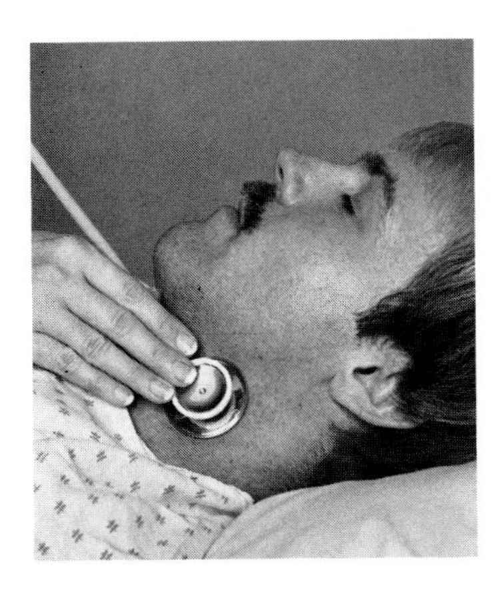

3 Always auscultate bilaterally, from head to toe. First, place your stethoscope's diaphragm over a carotid artery, as shown.

Avoid applying pressure to *both* carotid arteries simultaneously, because you'll impede cerebral blood flow. Also, if your patient has heart disease, examine each carotid artery cautiously. Pressure on it may cause cardiac arrhythmias.

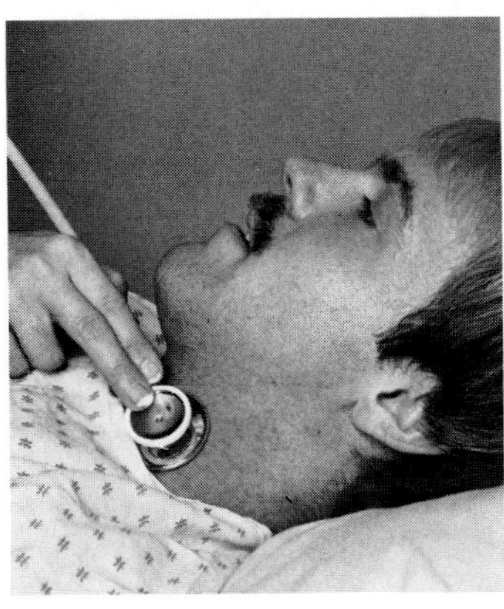

4 If you detect a bruit, determine where it's loudest. Keep in mind that the carotid artery divides near the lower jaw; a bruit at this site suggests arterial disease that may affect the brain.

Also auscultate the carotid artery near the collarbone, as the nurse is doing here. A bruit audible at this point may signify turbulence in the heart or the aortic root (the portion of the aorta located just above the aortic valve).

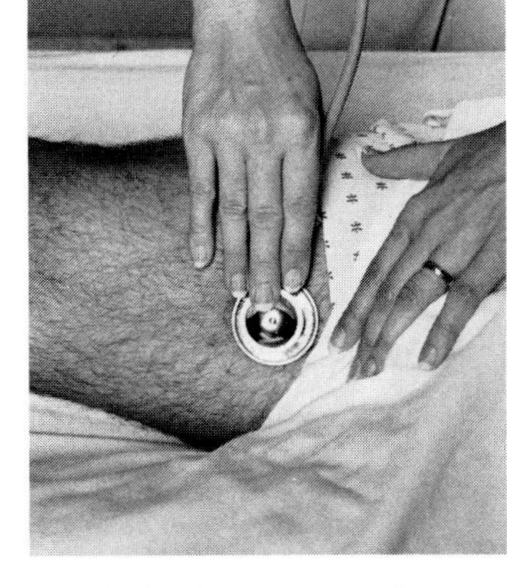

5 Now, check the femoral artery. Place the stethoscope's diaphragm against the adductor canal, where the femoral artery is situated. As shown here, the femoral artery is located at the lower thigh's inner aspect. Bruits from this location may indicate lower-extremity arteriosclerosis.

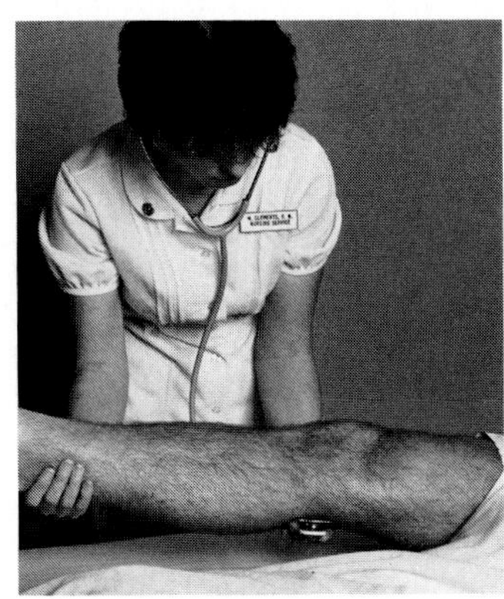

6 Don't neglect to check behind the knee. But take special care as you work. Because the arteries here are so close to the surface, stethoscope pressure may create a false bruit. Minimize this possibility by cupping a hand under the patient's ankle and slightly lifting his leg off the bed, as the nurse is doing here. Now, you can apply your stethoscope with minimal pressure.

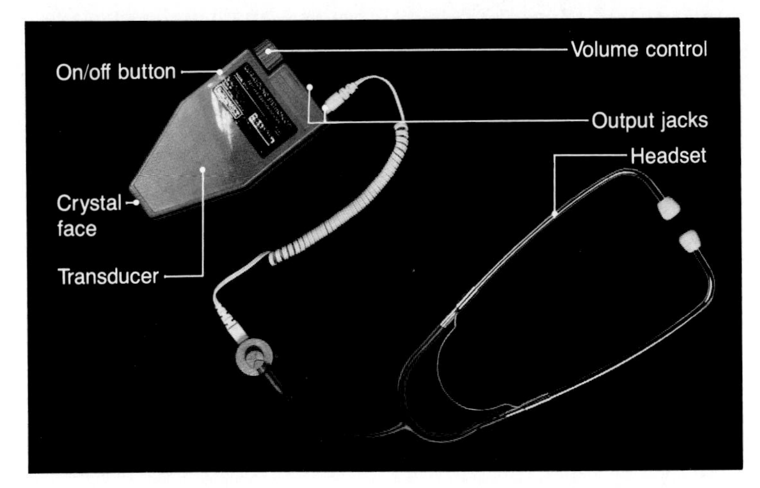

almost immediately when blood flow resumes. The stethoscope, in contrast, alerts you to resumed blood flow only when the flow becomes turbulent enough to produce a sound.

Assessing vascular disease

Suppose your patient complains of periodic pain, coldness, and numbness in his legs and feet—classic symptoms of arterial occlusive disease. By using the Doppler to assess blood flow in his legs, you may be able to determine:

- where the obstructions, if any, are located.
- how long each obstruction is.
- whether arteries distal to the obstructions are patent.

When assessing your patient's vascular status, keep in mind that the Doppler responds to blood flow *velocity,* not volume. (The Doppler signal reflects velocities of 6 cm per second or more.) The Doppler can't help you assess blood flow *volume.* A strong signal, therefore, doesn't mean necessarily that the vessel's transporting enough blood to maintain adequate tissue perfusion. For example, the Doppler returns a strong signal if a patent but severely narrowed artery is transporting a small volume of blood at high velocity. As always, your total patient assessment is essential, and further diagnostic tests (such as arteriography) may be indicated.

As with any assessment tool, the Doppler's value depends on your skill in using it. To obtain a high-quality signal, you must place the transducer precisely over the vessel you're examining. Otherwise, you may mistakenly assess a signal reflected by blood in a collateral vessel.

The way you hold the transducer makes a difference, too, because the strength and pitch of signals vary according to its angle. As a rule, tilt the instrument toward the axis of blood flow.

Other Doppler uses

As you become skilled in using the Doppler, you may also use it to:

- monitor blood pressure in newborn infants (especially low–birth-weight infants), whose vessels are too narrow for successful auscultation.
- verify vessel patency before catheterization or after surgery.
- screen for venous thrombosis.
- measure penile blood pressure as a diagnostic technique to determine the cause of impotence.

Cardiovascular

Assessing pulses with a Doppler device

Your patient, 48-year-old Raymond Kench, has recently undergone a femoral-popliteal bypass graft. Because such a graft predisposes the patient to thrombosis, the doctor expects you to periodically assess graft patency and distal circulation. Use the Medasonics Ultrasound Stethoscope Doppler Blood Flow Detector to assess blood flow in his femoral, popliteal, posterior tibial, and dorsalis pedis arteries. This photostory shows you how to proceed.

In addition to the Doppler transducer and headset shown on the preceding page, obtain ultrasound conductive jelly and an indelible marker. To assure adequate signal transmission, always apply a conductive agent to the assessment site.

Nursing tip: *In a pinch, use a soap solution, water, or water-soluble jelly as a conductive agent. But never use alcohol.*

Explain the procedure to your patient. Assure him that it's painless.

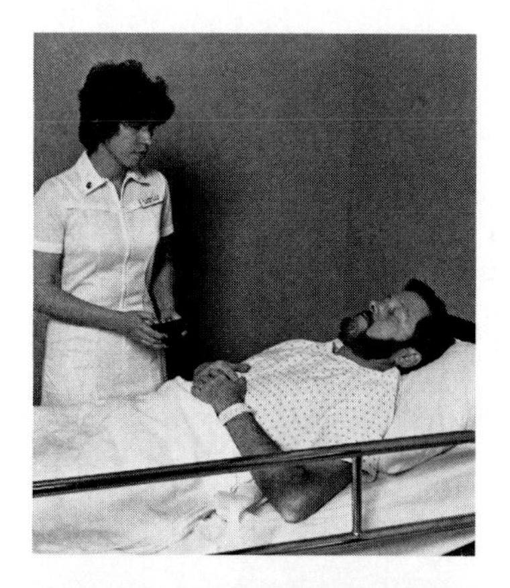

1 Next, place him in the supine position, as shown. *Note:* Position your patient the same way for each subsequent assessment.

Check the patient's affected leg for temperature, color, and sensation. Compare it with the unaffected leg, and note any differences.

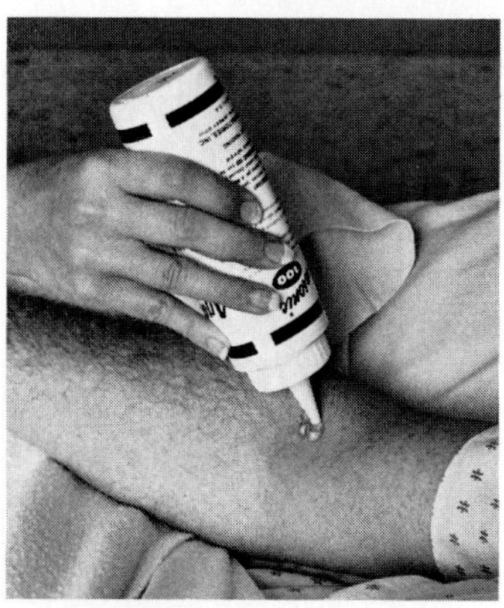

2 If your patient's blood pressure and pulses are normal in his arms, obtain a control signal by assessing one of his brachial arteries. After locating a brachial pulse, apply the conductive jelly to the site, as shown.

Next, plug the headset into either output jack, and set the volume control knob about midway. *Note:* A co-worker can plug another headset into the free jack and listen with you.

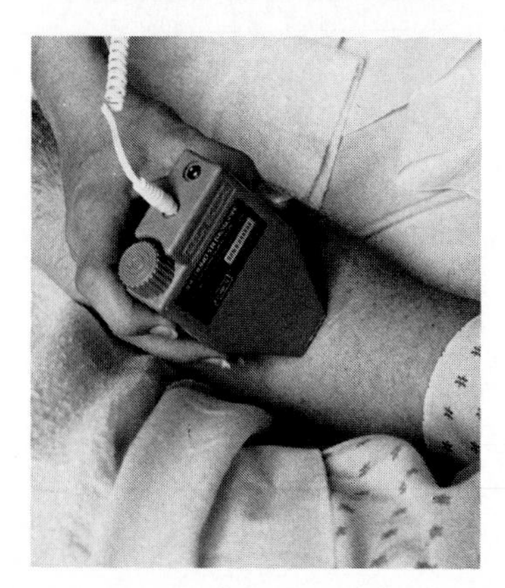

3 Then, gently apply the transducer's crystal face to the site. Take care not to press hard enough to obstruct blood flow. For best results, angle the transducer in the direction of blood flow.

To activate the transducer, depress and hold the on/off button on the transducer's side. The transducer remains active as long as you depress the button and for several seconds after release. Adjust the volume control knob as necessary.

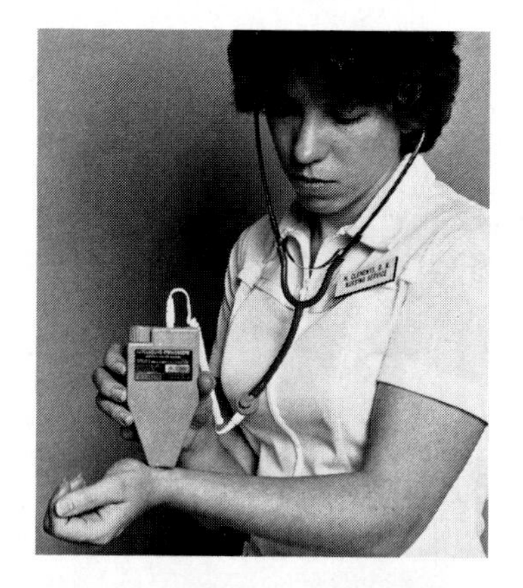

4 Having trouble hearing a signal? Try applying more jelly to the site, and make sure the crystal face is clean. If you still have difficulty, test the transducer by applying jelly over one of your own arteries and listening for a signal. If you still can't hear one, replace the transducer's batteries. If these measures fail, suspect that the headset cord or the transducer is damaged.

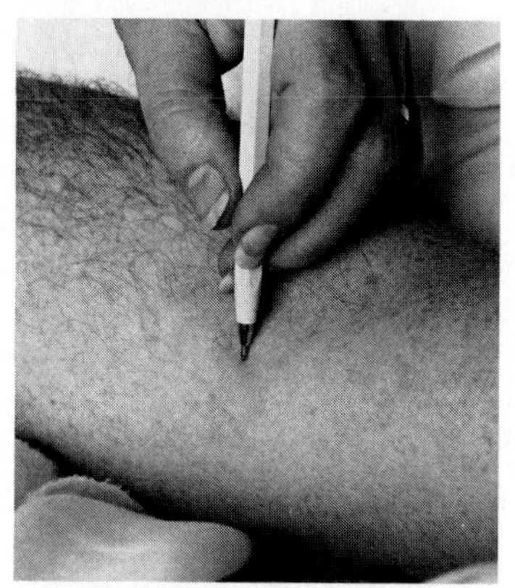

5 When you've located the brachial artery, you'll hear an intermittent, swishing sound with each heartbeat. Note the sound's pitch and amplitude. This sound is normal for your patient. Use it for comparison with lower-extremity sounds.

Wipe off the jelly and mark the pulse point with an indelible marker. Do the same for each artery you assess subsequently, to assure consistency during future pulse checks.

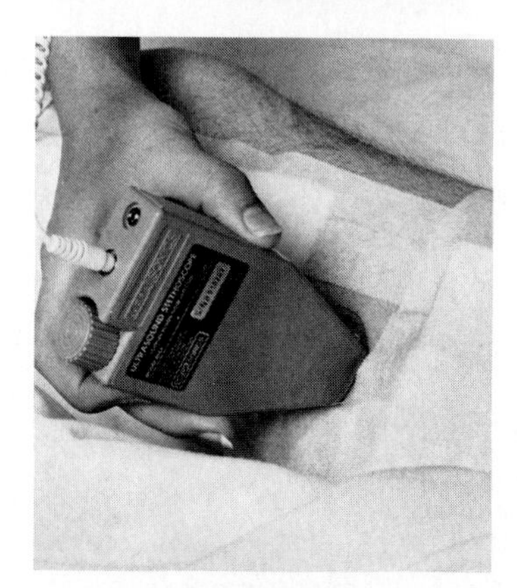

6 If the doctor's left an opening in your patient's dressing, prepare to assess the femoral artery next. Locate it by using the superficial femoral vein as a landmark; the femoral artery's adjacent to it. Or, use the incision as a landmark. Apply conductive jelly over the femoral vein, position the transducer as described above, and press the on/off button to activate it.

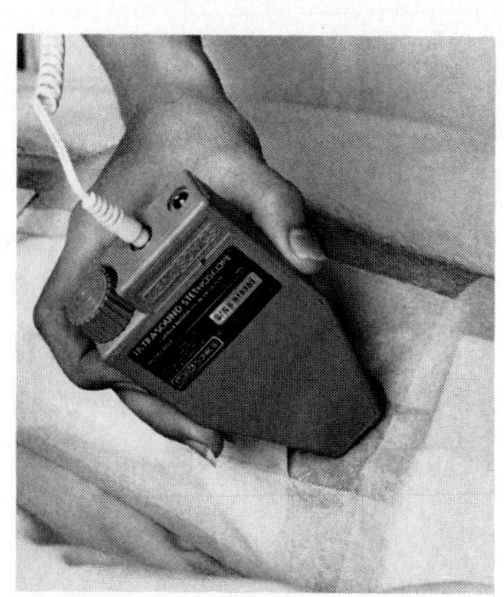

7 When the transducer detects a large vein, such as the femoral, it returns a constant, low rumble that sounds like a windstorm. When you hear this signal, slowly move the transducer from side to side, until you hear the femoral artery signal. If it's similar to the brachial signal, assume that blood is flowing at normal velocity. (If you hear an abrupt change in amplitude and pitch, you may be detecting blood flow in collateral arteries.)

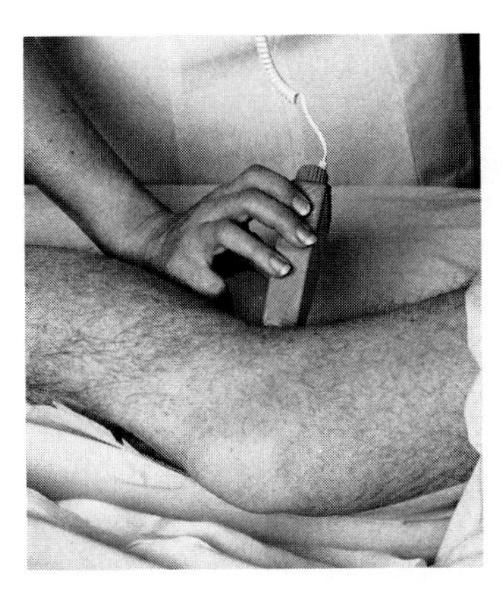

8 Under most circumstances, you'll place your patient in the prone position to assess his popliteal artery. But because the prone position may be uncomfortable for him after arterial graft surgery, place him in the sidelying position. Then, locate the artery, apply conductive jelly, and listen for a signal. Remember to mark the pulse point.

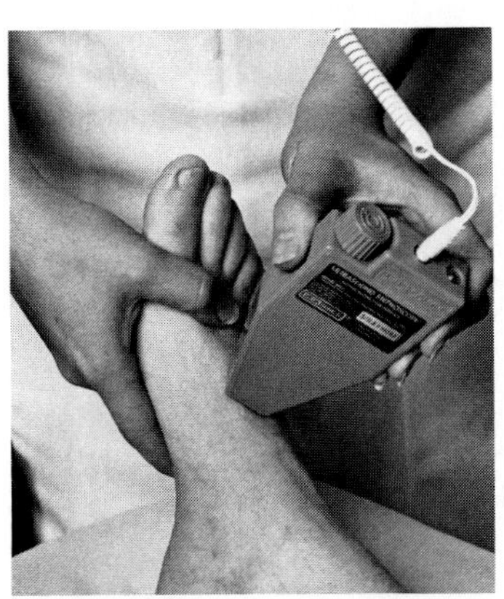

9 Finally, assess the posterior tibial and dorsalis pedis arteries. If you have difficulty locating either artery, slowly move the transducer across the area where you expect it to be, until you hear the arterial signal.

If you can't locate one of the lower-extremity arteries, suspect a vessel spasm or a thrombus or other occlusion in the area above the usual pulse point. Notify the doctor at once.

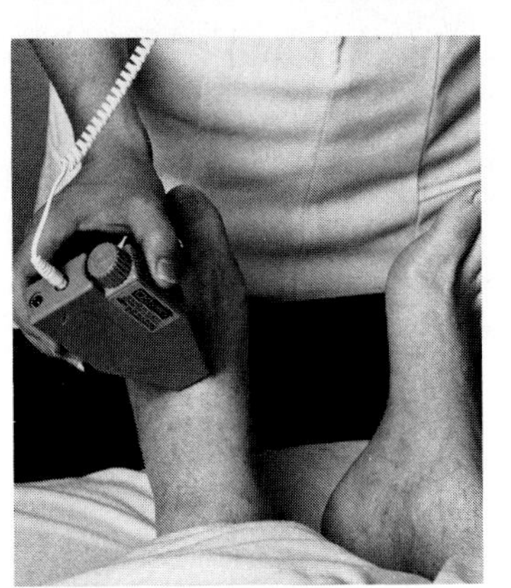

10 Complete your assessment by repeating the procedure on the patient's unaffected leg and foot. Whether or not the signals from this leg sound like those from the postop leg depends on the degree of arterial disease present.

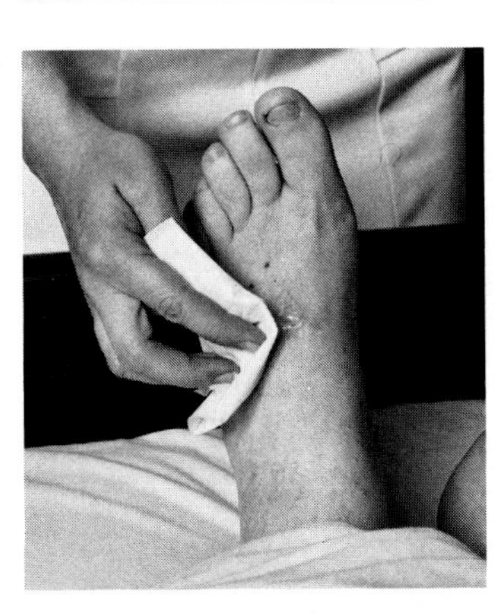

11 Use a tissue to thoroughly cleanse all jelly from your patient's skin, especially around the incision. Then, clean the transducer's crystal face with a tissue. *Caution:* Never clean the transducer with alcohol or another organic solvent. See the manufacturer's recommendations for cleaning and sterilizing.

Document your findings and your patient's positions during the procedure.

Taking ankle blood pressure

As part of your assessment of Mr. Kench, use the Doppler blood flow detector to take periodic blood pressure readings on his ankles. These readings will help you determine whether perfusion pressure is adequate in his lower legs.

As you probably know, systolic blood pressure is normally higher in the extremities than it is near the heart. Why? Because arteries in the extremities are narrower and less elastic. In addition, backward pressure exerted by blood reflected at anastomoses (arterial junctions) increases systolic pressure.

Nevertheless, systolic ankle pressure should approximate systolic arm pressure. If ankle pressure is 30 mm Hg higher or lower than brachial pressure or is lower than the preoperative baseline ankle pressure, suspect a problem and notify the doctor. Important: *Keep in mind that when a patient goes into shock, blood pressure decreases in his legs before his arms.*

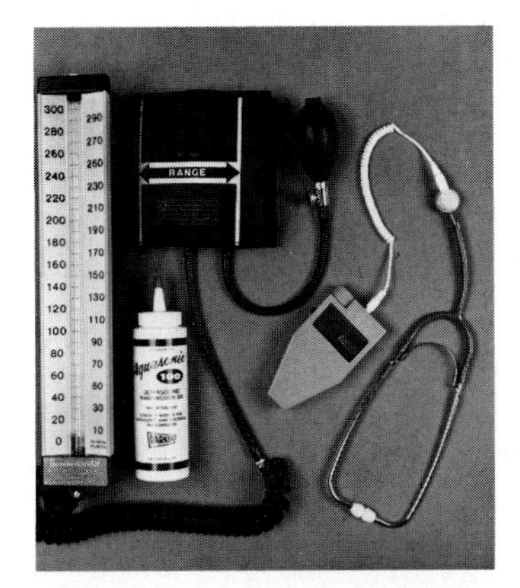

1 First, gather a Doppler transducer and headset, conductive jelly, and mercury sphygmomanometer. Then, establish your patient's brachial pressure. Proceed as usual, using the Doppler device (instead of a stethoscope) to detect returning blood flow. *Remember:* Apply conductive jelly over the site before using the transducer.

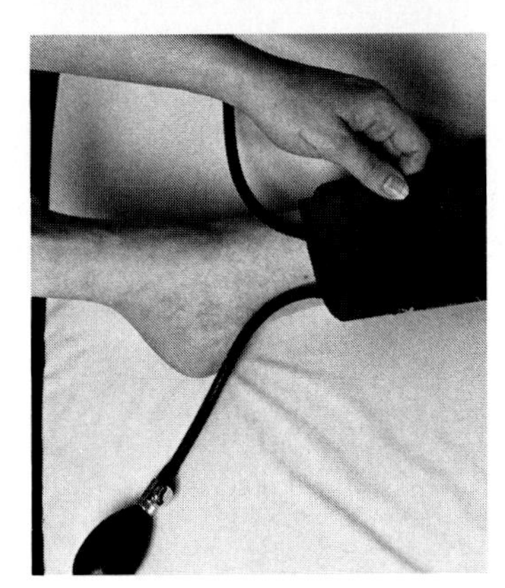

2 Now, apply the sphygmomanometer cuff just above the ankle, as shown here. Apply conductive jelly over the area where you expect to find the dorsalis pedis pulse, and activate the transducer to locate the artery. *Remember:* You marked this spot with indelible ink during your first pulse assessment.

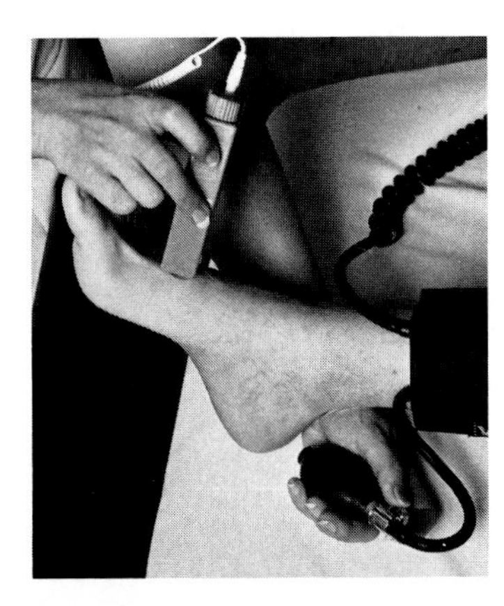

3 To make sure blood flow to the foot isn't hampered by pressure on the leg, *slightly* elevate the patient's foot, as the nurse is doing here. By resting his ankle on your wrist, you avoid applying pressure to an artery that supplies the dorsalis pedis, such as the popliteal. Then, take the systolic blood pressure reading.

Repeat the procedure on the other ankle. Document your findings.

Cardiovascular

Nurses' guide to I.V. emergency cardiovascular drugs

Until recently, the I.V. emergency cardiovascular drugs listed below were rarely administered outside the ICU. But today, if you're a med/surg nurse, you may be responsible for beginning an infusion of one of these drugs before the patient enters the ICU. And some patients may even remain on your unit while receiving the drug.

Of course, you must be fully informed about any drug you administer. Study this chart to learn about four important cardiovascular drugs you may be unfamiliar with. *Note:* All dosages given below are for adults.

dobutamine hydrochloride
(Dobutrex)

Indications
Short-term treatment of cardiac decompensation from depressed contractility caused by organic heart disease or cardiac surgery

Dosage
Dilute powdered drug (packaged in a vial) with 10 to 20 ml of sterile water or 5% dextrose in water. Add the contents of a vial (250 mg) to 250, 500, or 1,000 ml of 5% dextrose in water, sterile normal saline solution, or lactated Ringer's solution. Titrate drip rate to 2.5 to 10 mcg/kg/minute. (If necessary, give up to 40 mcg/kg/minute.)

Intended effects
- Stable blood pressure maintained within normal range
- Increased cardiac output, reflected by increased urinary output

Possible side effects
- Increased heart rate or blood pressure (especially systolic blood pressure)
- Premature ventricular beats
- Angina or nonspecific chest pain
- Nausea or vomiting
- Shortness of breath

Contraindication
Idiopathic hypertrophic subaortic stenosis

Special considerations
- Don't mix dobutamine with sodium bicarbonate injection or other alkaline solution.
- If present, treat hypovolemia as ordered before giving dobutamine.
- Precisely regulate flow rate with an infusion pump.
- Closely monitor vital signs. Prepare patient for transfer to ICU for monitoring of pulmonary artery wedge pressure and cardiac output.
- Document urinary output.
- If severe side effects occur (for example, tachycardia or an excessive rise in blood pressure), reduce the administration rate or temporarily discontinue the infusion, as ordered, until the patient's condition stabilizes.
- Don't give if patient's recently received a beta blocker, such as propranolol or metoprolol. Beta blockers may make dobutamine ineffective.
- May be used with nitroprusside for afterload reduction.
- Oxidation of drug may slightly discolor admixtures containing dobutamine but doesn't affect potency.
- I.V. solutions remain stable for 24 hours.

dopamine hydrochloride
(Intropin*)

Indications
Low cardiac output, hypotension from low cardiac output, poor perfusion of vital organs, and shock or other hemodynamic imbalances resulting from myocardial infarction, trauma, endotoxic septicemia, open heart surgery, renal failure, and congestive heart failure

Dosage
Available in 200- and 400-mg ampuls or in premeasured single-dose disposable syringes. Add the contents of the ampul or syringe to 250 or 500 ml of 5% dextrose in water, normal saline solution, a combination of 5% dextrose in water and saline, or lactated Ringer's solution. Titrate to 2 to 5 mcg/kg/minute, up to 50 mcg/kg/minute. Adjust as necessary for desired hemodynamic or renal response.

Intended effects
- Increased cardiac output, reflected by increased urinary output
- Increased blood pressure
- Improved capillary filling
- Improved skin color and temperature

Possible side effects
- Ectopic heartbeats
- Nausea or vomiting
- Tachycardia
- Angina or palpitations
- Hypotension
- Headache
- Vasoconstriction
- Shortness of breath
- Tissue necrosis with extravasation

Note: Uncommon side effects include bradycardia, widening of QRS complex, conduction disturbances, piloerection, azotemia, and hypertension.

Contraindications
Pheochromocytoma, uncorrected tachyarrhythmias, ventricular fibrillation. Use cautiously in a patient with occlusive vascular disease, cold injuries, diabetic endarteritis, or arterial embolism; in a patient who's pregnant; and in a patient receiving monoamine oxidase (MAO) inhibitors.

Special considerations
- If present, treat hypovolemia as ordered before giving dopamine.
- Give through large vein; for example, an antecubital fossa vein. During infusion, closely monitor site for signs of extravasation. If extravasation occurs, stop infusion immediately and call the doctor. He may counteract effect by infiltrating the area with 5 to 10 mg of phentolamine in 10 to 15 ml of normal saline solution.
- Precisely regulate flow rate with an infusion pump.
- During infusion, closely monitor blood pressure, pulse rate, urinary output, and extremity color and temperature. Titrate infusion rate according to patient response, as ordered.
- If patient has received MAO inhibitors, reduce initial dose by at least one tenth, as ordered. MAO inhibitors potentiate dopamine and prolong its effects.
- Notify the doctor if you observe adverse effects (for example, a disproportionate rise in diastolic pressure); he may adjust dosage or discontinue infusion.
- Don't add any other drug to I.V. container containing dopamine.
- Don't give with alkaline solutions or drugs; for example, sodium bicarbonate or phenytoin sodium.
- If patient receives phenytoin sodium after dopamine has stabilized his condition, closely monitor for blood pressure drop.
- Don't use with ergot alkaloids; extreme blood pressure elevation may occur.
- After discontinuing, closely observe patient for sudden blood pressure drop.
- Discard dopamine solutions within 24 hours after reconstitution; or sooner, if solution becomes discolored.

nitroprusside sodium
(Nipride*)

Indications
Blood pressure reduction during hypertensive crisis; production of controlled hypotension during surgery (to reduce bleeding); reduction of preload and afterload in cardiac pump failure or cardiogenic shock

Dosage
50-mg vial diluted with 2 to 3 ml of 5% dextrose in water and then added to 250, 500, or 1,000 ml of 5% dextrose in water. Infuse at 0.5 to 10 mcg/kg/minute. Average dosage is 3 mcg/kg/minute. Maximum recommended dosage is 10 mcg/kg/minute.

Intended effects
- *For hypertensive crisis:* immediate drop in blood pressure
- *For reduction of preload and afterload:* improvement in shock signs and symptoms, slight rise in blood pressure, reduced heart rate, chest pain relief

Possible side effects
- *From infusing drug too rapidly:* nausea, diaphoresis, muscle twitching, chest or abdominal discomfort, palpitations, dizziness, severe hypotension
- *From overdose:* severe hypotension, metabolic acidosis, signs and symptoms of cyanide or thiocyanate toxicosis (see box on page 70)
- Tissue necrosis with extravasation.

Contraindications
Compensatory hypertension resulting (for example) from coarctation of the aorta or from arteriovenous shunt. In a surgical patient, contraindicated if cerebral circulation is inadequate. Use cautiously in a patient with hypothyroidism, liver disease, or kidney disease and in a patient who's receiving another antihypertensive.

Special considerations
- Choose a large vein for administration.
- Dilute with 2 to 3 ml of 5% dextrose in water *only.* Don't dilute with normal saline solution or water.
- Because drug is light-sensitive, wrap I.V. container in aluminum foil (or other opaque covering). Also wrap I.V. tubing, if required by hospital policy.
- Discard darkly tinted solution (fresh solution has a faint brown tint) and solution that's 4 hours old. Continue the infusion with freshly mixed solution.
- Obtain baseline vital signs before administration, and find out what parameters the doctor wants to achieve. (This depends on whether he's treating the patient for hypertension or for cardiac pump failure or cardiogenic shock.)
- Precisely regulate flow rate with an infusion pump.
- During infusion, check blood pressure at least every 5 minutes at the start of infusion and at least every 15 minutes thereafter. If severe

*Available in both the United States and Canada

hypotension occurs (or you see other signs and symptoms of too-rapid infusion), *immediately* slow or temporarily discontinue infusion (as ordered). Adverse effects associated with rapid infusion should disappear quickly. Resume infusion at a slower rate, as ordered.

- Prepare the patient for transfer to the ICU for continuous blood pressure monitoring and for pulmonary artery wedge pressure and cardiac output measurements.
- Don't administer other drugs through the I.V. line containing nitroprusside.
- Avoid piggybacking nitroprusside with other I.V. solutions, if possible. But keep on hand a 250-ml bag of normal saline solution or 5% dextrose in water and a microdrip infusion set to maintain a keep-vein-open rate if sudden disconnection of nitroprusside is necessary. *Caution:* If you must piggyback nitroprusside, don't adjust the rate of the main I.V. line while the nitroprusside is running. Even a small bolus of this drug can cause severe hypotension.
- Closely monitor the I.V. site for signs of extravasation.
- In long-term use, monitor patient for signs and symptoms of cyanide or thiocyanate toxicosis. Check his acid-base balance at least once daily; metabolic acidosis is the earliest and most reliable indication of cyanide toxicosis. Also, check serum thiocyanate levels daily, especially if the patient has kidney disease or failure. For more details on cyanide and thiocyanate toxicosis, see page 70.

nitroglycerin for injection

(Nitro-Bid I.V., Nitrostat I.V.)

Indications

To treat congestive heart failure associated with acute myocardial infarction, angina pectoris (if patient hasn't responded to organic nitrates and/or a beta blocker), and perioperative hypertension; to maintain controlled hypotension during surgery

Dosage

Add 10 ml of nitroglycerin to a 250-ml glass I.V. bottle of 5% dextrose in water or normal saline solution. Begin infusion at 5 mcg/minute. Increase dosage by 5 mcg/minute every 3 to 5 minutes, until some response is apparent. Then, increase dosage cautiously, if necessary. If patient hasn't responded when dosage has risen to 20 mcg/minute, dosage may be increased in increments of 10, and later 20, mcg/minute. (A patient with normal or low left ventricular filling pressure or pulmonary artery wedge pressure [PAWP]—for example, a patient with angina—may respond fully to the initial dose.) *Caution:* These dosages are calculated for use with minimally absorptive equipment: glass I.V. bottles and specially made I.V. tubing. Dosage adjustments are necessary if drug is given through standard polyvinyl chloride I.V. tubing, because this type of tubing absorbs up to 80% of the drug.

Intended effects

- Reduction in rales
- Improved urinary output
- Chest pain relief
- Decreased blood pressure (when given to treat hypertension)

Possible side effects

- Headache or dizziness
- Tachycardia
- Nausea and vomiting
- Restlessness and apprehension
- Muscle twitching
- Chest or abdominal discomfort
- Palpitations

Contraindications

Sensitivity to nitroglycerin or organic nitrates, hypotension, hypovolemia, increased intracranial pressure, inadequate cerebral circulation, constrictive pericarditis, pericardial tamponade. Use cautiously in a patient with severe liver or kidney disease.

Special considerations

- For accurate dosage delivery, use only glass I.V. containers and specially made, minimally absorptive I.V. tubing; for example, Nitrostat I.V. infusion kit, which absorbs less than 5% of the drug. Nitroglycerin migrates into standard I.V. tubing at an erratic rate, making dosage calculations difficult.
- Precisely regulate flow rate with an infusion pump.
- Closely monitor vital signs.
- Prepare patient for transfer to ICU for PAWP and continuous blood pressure monitoring.
- If you see signs of overdose, such as severe hypotension and reflex tachycardia, notify the doctor and elevate the patient's legs. Slow or temporarily stop the infusion, as ordered, until the patient's condition stabilizes. Because the hemodynamic effects of nitroglycerin normally disappear quickly after the infusion is stopped, the patient probably won't need further treatment. If symptoms persist, be prepared to give an alpha-adrenergic agonist (such as methoxamine hydrochloride) by I.V. infusion.
- Store drug at room temperature.

Protecting Nipride from light

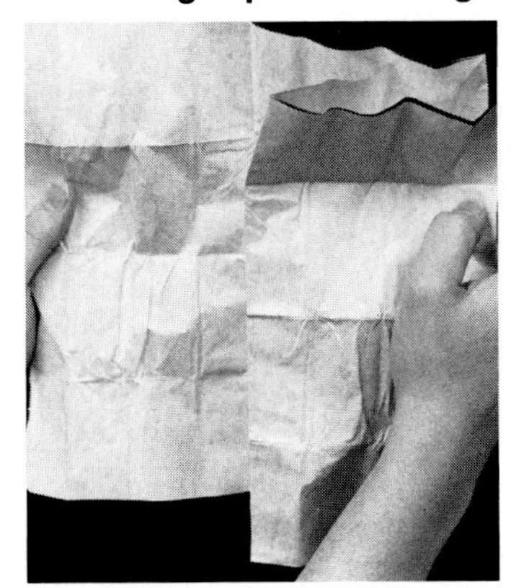

1 As you know, nitroprusside sodium (Nipride*) deteriorates quickly when exposed to light. To protect it, always wrap its I.V. container in aluminum foil (or any opaque material) before beginning the infusion. Follow these steps.

First, obtain enough aluminum foil to cover the container. (The manufacturer of Nipride supplies enough foil to cover a 1,000-ml bag.)

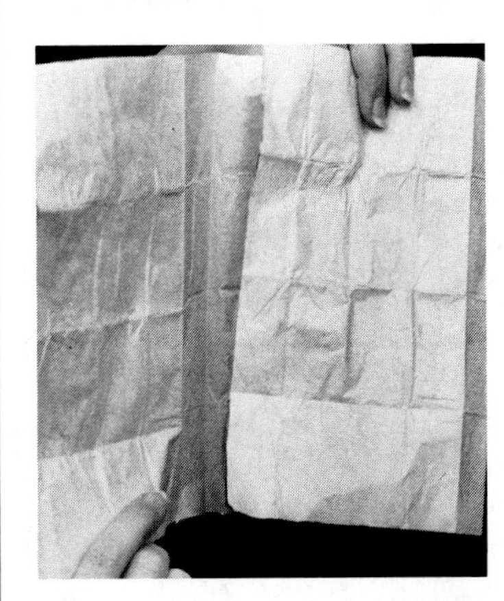

2 If you're using a 250- or 500-ml container, use this easy wrapping system: Fold the foil in half and then in thirds, as shown here. With scissors, cut a slit in the top of the middle portion.

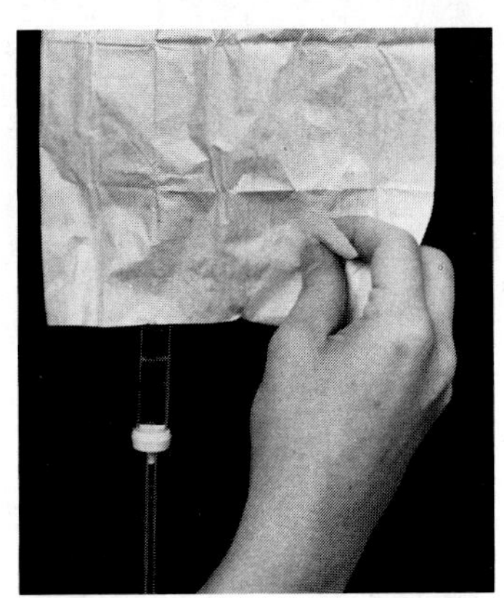

3 Slip the container into the foil so its slot protrudes from the slit. Then, apply a strip of tape on the foil's bottom, as shown, to secure the foil over the bag. Hang the container on the I.V. pole.

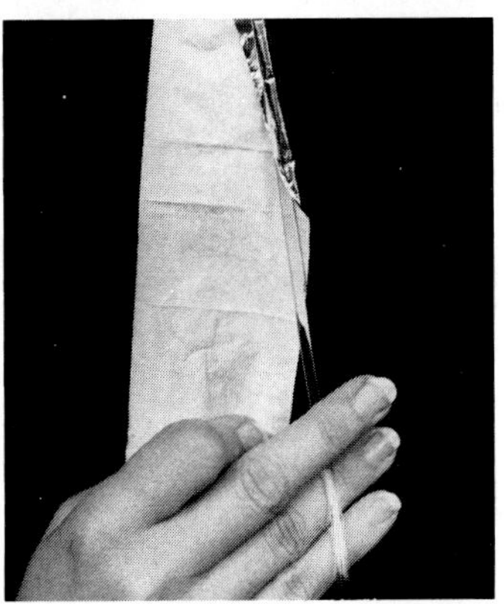

4 If hospital policy dictates, also cover the infusion line with foil or other opaque wrapping. If you're using foil, cut it into 2" (5-cm) strips and pinch it tightly around the tubing. If you're using a piston-action pump (like the IMED 960 featured on pages 70 to 72), also cover the drip chamber. But if you're using a peristaltic pump or an I.V. controller, leave the drip chamber uncovered, so you can easily monitor the drip rate.

*Available in both the United States and Canada

Cardiovascular

PRECAUTIONS

Recognizing Nipride overdose

If your patient's receiving nitroprusside sodium (Nipride*), stay alert for signs and symptoms of overdose. Nipride overdose can cause such life-threatening complications as cyanide toxicosis. Here's why.

Normally, the body rapidly metabolizes Nipride into cyanide. Then, through the action of a liver enzyme and sulfur (usually thiosulfate), it converts the cyanide into thiocyanate.

Because a liver enzyme transforms cyanide into thiocyanate, liver insufficiency may allow toxic levels of cyanide to accumulate. Toxicosis may also occur if the patient's sulfur supplies (especially thiosulfate) are depleted.

Danger signs of cyanide toxicosis

The first sign of Nipride overdose is severe hypotension; other early signs include metabolic acidosis and increasing drug tolerance. Signs and symptoms of cyanide toxicosis include dyspnea, headache, dizziness, vomiting, ataxia, loss of consciousness, imperceptible pulse, absent reflexes, widely dilated pupils, pink skin, distant heart sounds, and shallow breathing.

If you suspect your patient suffers from cyanide toxicosis, take these steps:

- Immediately discontinue the Nipride infusion and notify the doctor.
- Administer amyl nitrate inhalations for 15 to 30 seconds each minute, as ordered, while someone prepares 3% sodium nitrate solution for I.V. administration.
- As ordered, give 3% sodium nitrate solution at a rate of 2.5 to 5 ml/minute, to a maximum dose of 15 ml. Continuously monitor blood pressure during the infusion.
- Next, give an I.V. injection of sodium thiosulfate 12.5 g in 50 ml of 5% dextrose in water over 10 minutes, as ordered. Thiosulfate promotes the conversion of cyanide into thiocyanate.
- After treatment, monitor the patient for return of overdose signs and symptoms. If they reappear, give nitrate and sodium thiosulfate again in one half the previous doses, as ordered.
- If blood pressure drops significantly, give a vasopressor, such as dopamine hydrochloride (Intropin*), as ordered.

Recognizing thiocyanate accumulation

If your patient's liver function and sulfate levels are adequate, long-term Nipride therapy may cause thiocyanate accumulation and toxicosis. Signs and symptoms include tinnitus, blurred vision, and delirium. Prevent these complications by monitoring serum thiocyanate levels once daily; notify the doctor if excessive levels accumulate. *Note:* Elevated thiocyanate levels aren't an indication of cyanide toxicosis.

If your patient has hypothyroidism or severe kidney impairment, use Nipride cautiously, because thiocyanate limits iodine uptake and binding.

*Available in both the United States and Canada

Learning about the IMED Volumetric Infusion Pump

In the chart on pages 68 and 69, you learned about four cardiovascular drugs that may cause serious—even fatal—side effects if infused at an incorrect rate. To minimize this risk, always infuse these drugs with an infusion pump, such as the IMED Model 960 Volumetric Infusion Pump shown below.

The IMED pump is a piston-action infusion pump that provides precision infusion at rates from 1 ml/hour to 999 ml/hour in 1 ml/hour increments. The specially made Accuset pump chamber and infusion set (see lower photo below) aspirates I.V. solution from the I.V. container and then infuses it at the rate you set. If necessary, you can remove the Accuset infusion tubing and replace it with standard I.V. tubing. (For example, to give a viscous total parenteral nutrition solution, replace the Accuset tubing with larger-bore or filtered tubing.)

During the infusion, the display window shows the amount of solution infused. If a problem occurs (or the infusion's complete), a chirping alarm sounds, the red ALARM light lights up, and the problem (for example, occlusion, door open, low battery) is identified in the display window.

Even though this pump is slightly larger and heavier than some other pumps, you can attach it to a standard I.V. pole. When doing so, however, take care not to make the pole top-heavy and unstable. (Special IMED poles are available.)

Because the pump is battery-powered, you can continue to use it while transporting your patient. But when the patient's stationary, plug the pump into an electrical outlet to ensure a constant power source.

Now, learn how to operate the IMED 960 pump by reading the following photostory.

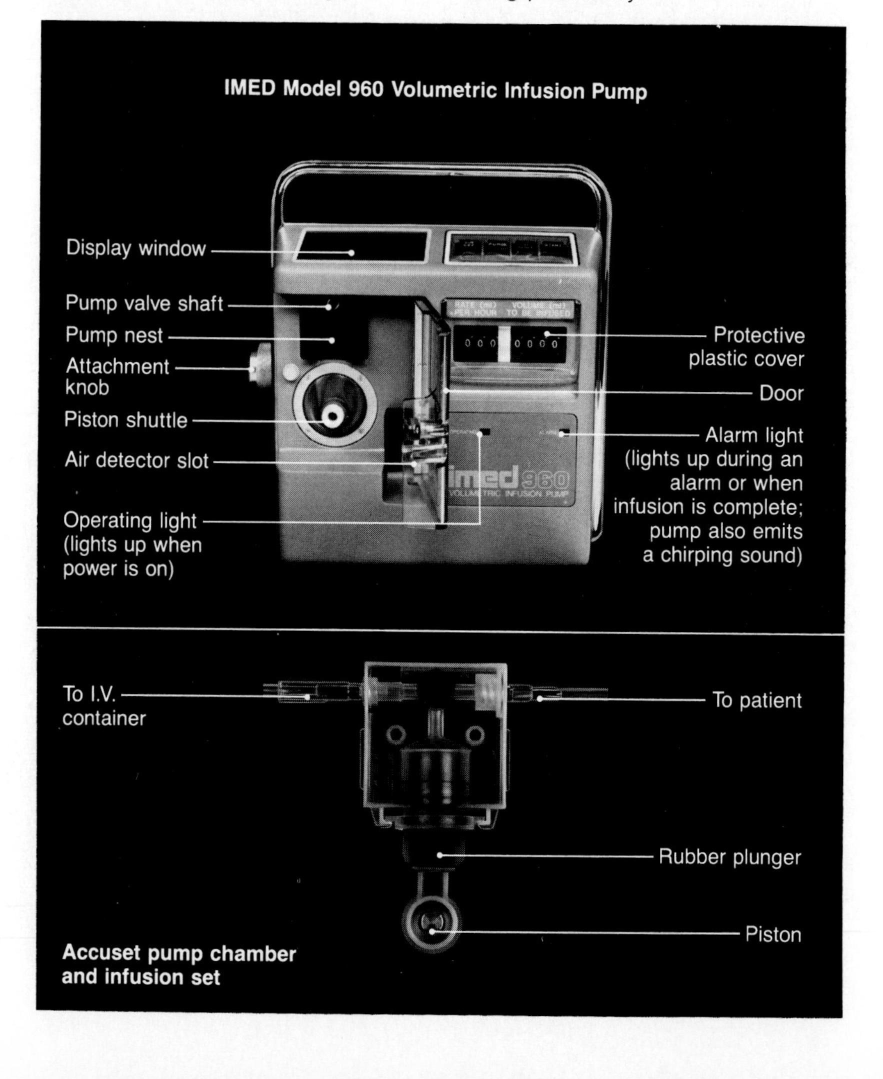

How to operate an IMED Infusion Pump

Using an IMED Model 960 Volumetric Infusion Pump? Read the following photostory to learn how to set it up correctly. Remember: *Thoroughly wash your hands before beginning, and observe aseptic technique throughout the procedure.*

Gather the equipment shown here: I.V. container (as ordered), IMED 960 Infusion Pump, Accuset pump chamber and infusion set, I.V. label, and I.V. pole (not shown). If the I.V. container is a bottle, you'll also need an alcohol swab.

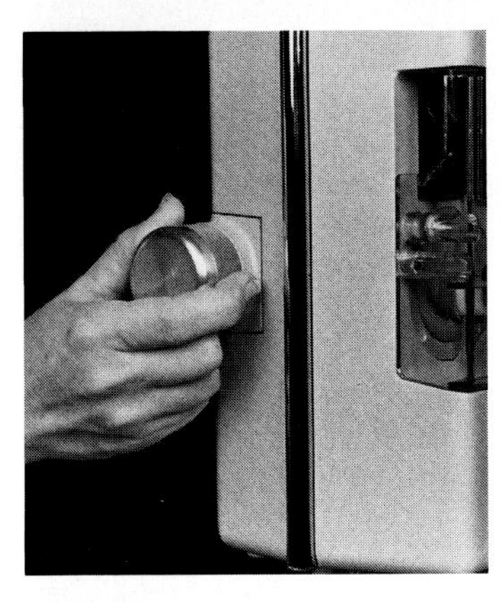

1 Securely attach the pump to the I.V. pole by tightening the attachment knob on the pump's side. Take the equipment to your patient's bedside, and plug the pump into a wall outlet.

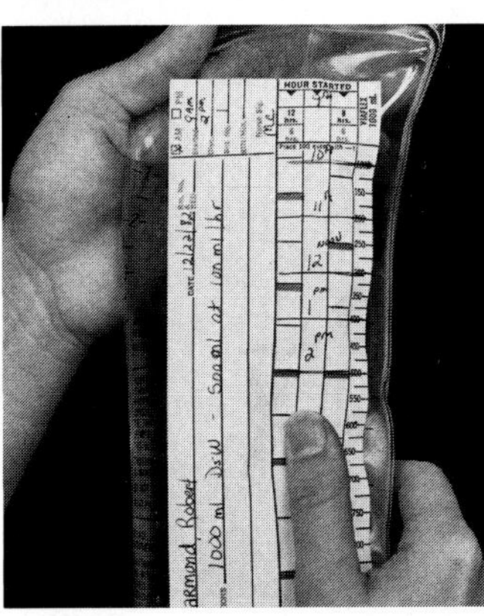

2 Check the I.V. container against the doctor's order, and confirm the patient's identity. Check the container's expiration date to ensure that the solution's fresh. Make sure the container is properly labeled with the patient's name, type of solution and additives (if any), dosage, infusion rate, and date and time you begin the infusion.

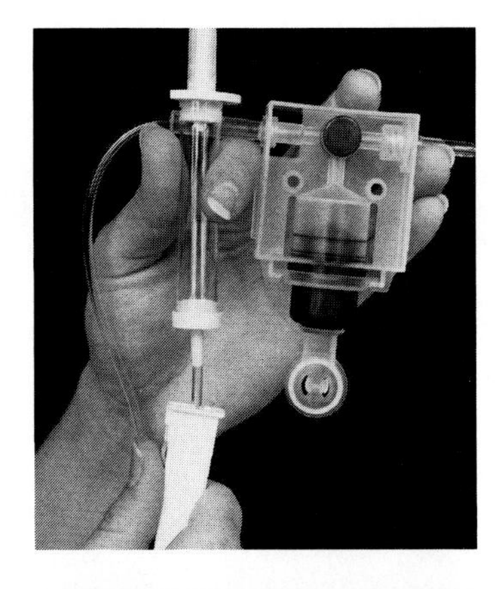

3 Remove the Accuset equipment from its wrapping, and close the flow clamp.

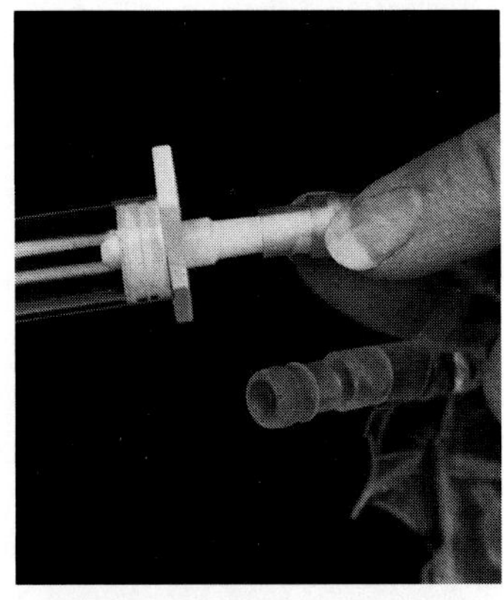

4 If you're using an I.V. bag, remove its port cover. (If you're using a bottle, clean its diaphragm with an alcohol swab.) Then, remove the Accuset's plastic spike protector, spike the container, as shown, and hang it on the I.V. pole.

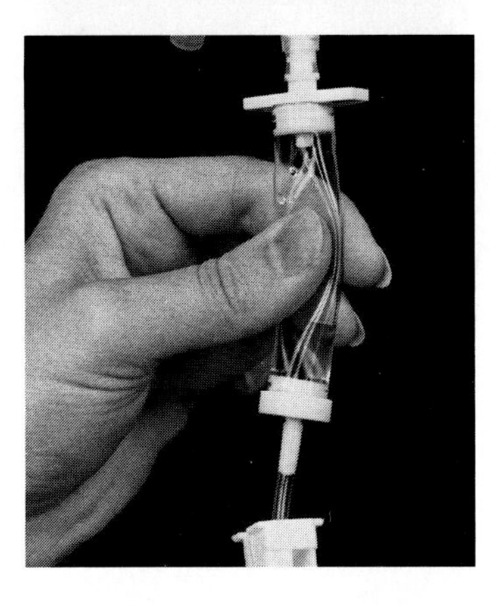

5 Squeeze the drip chamber until it's full. Then, open the flow clamp.

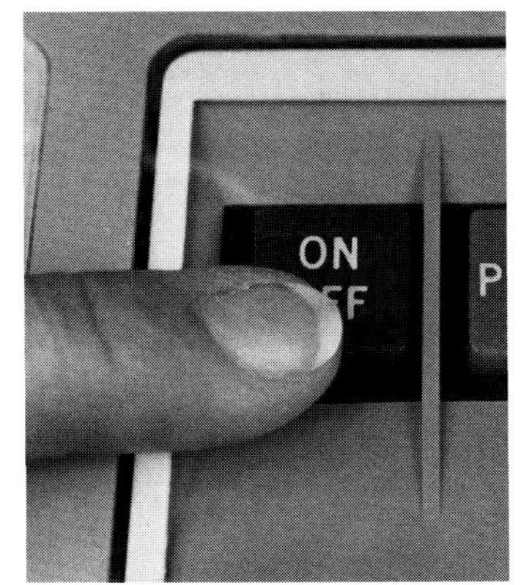

6 Turn on the pump by depressing the ON/OFF button, as the nurse is doing here. *Volume 0* appears in the display window and the OPERATING light shines. Set the RATE (ML) PER HOUR dial at 000 and the VOLUME (ML) TO BE INFUSED dial at 0000.

Cardiovascular

How to operate an IMED infusion pump *continued*

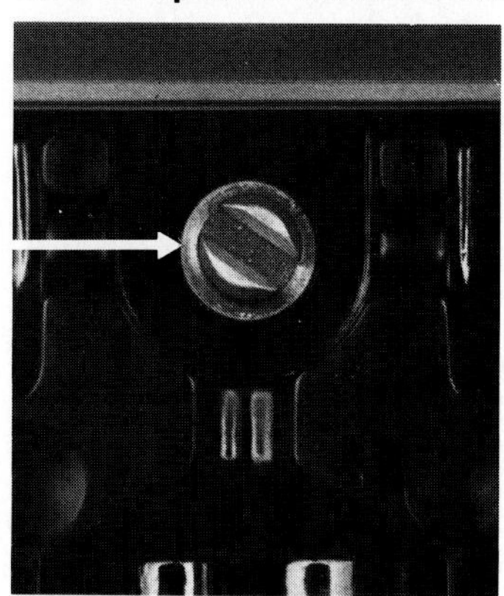

7 Now, open the pump's clear plastic door. Depress the PURGE button and hold it down until the pump valve shaft (see arrow) shifts to a 45° angle, as shown here.

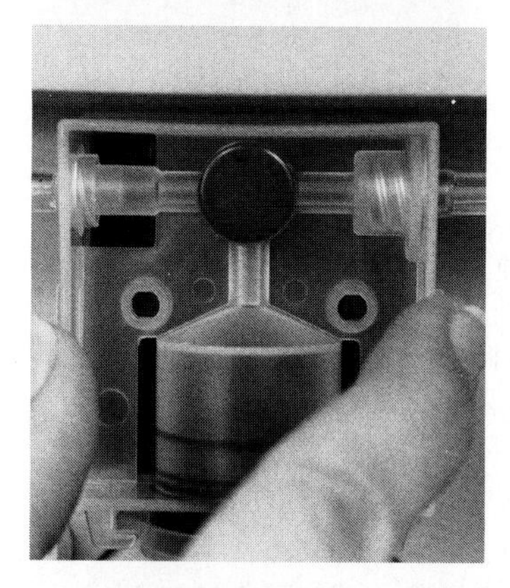

8 Then, snap the Accuset pump chamber into the pump nest, as the nurse is doing here. Firmly press the pump chamber's piston into the piston shuttle, until it's secure.

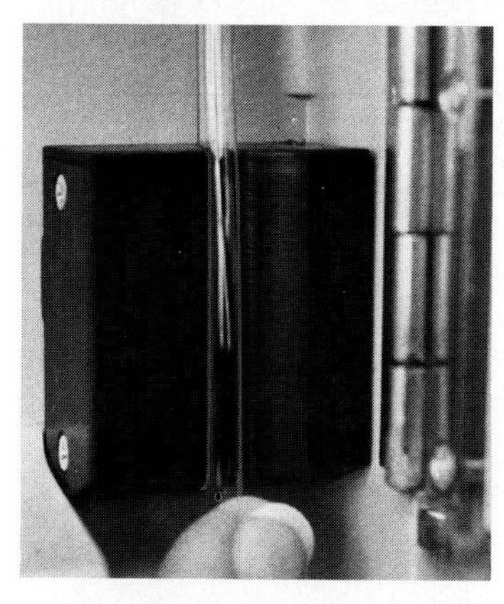

9 Double-check the tubing connections on both sides of the pump chamber. Then, run the tubing extending from the pump chamber's right side through the air detector slot.

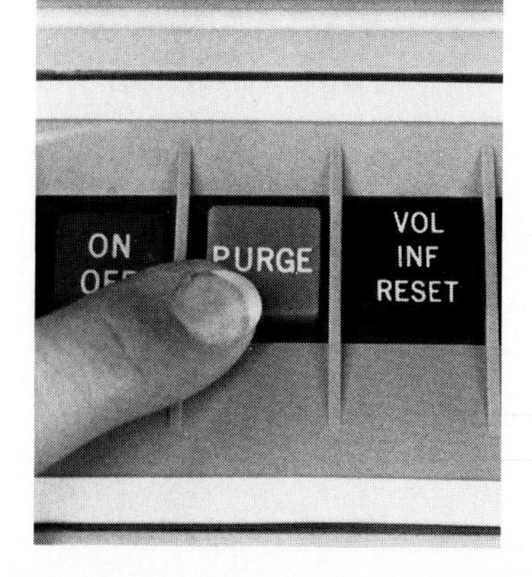

10 Holding the tubing's free end over a wastebasket, purge air from the tubing by again depressing the PURGE button. (The tubing's cap isn't airtight, so you needn't remove it.) Continue to depress the PURGE button until all air is expelled from the tubing and pump chamber. *Caution:* Never use the PURGE button when the infusion set's connected to the patient.

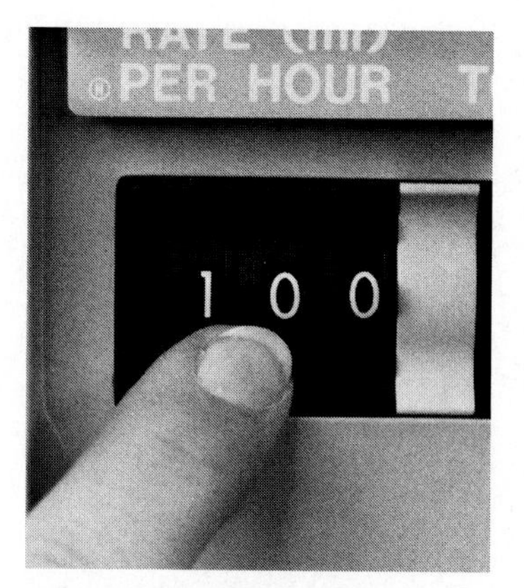

11 Lift the plastic protective cover, and set the RATE (ML) PER HOUR dials, according to the doctor's order. *Note:* If the alarm sounds and the display window signals *Rate not 000,* press the VOL INF RESET button.

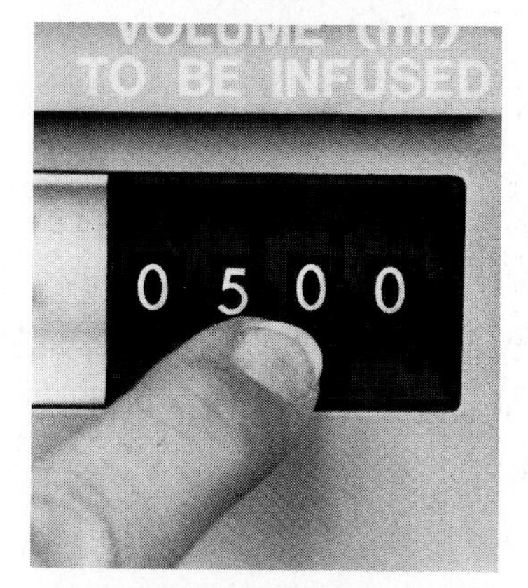

12 Now, set the VOLUME (ML) TO BE INFUSED dials. For example, if the doctor's ordered an infusion of 500 ml, set the dials at 0500, as the nurse is doing here. The pump will stop the infusion after 500 ml have been infused, regardless of whether the I.V. container holds 500 or 1,000 ml.

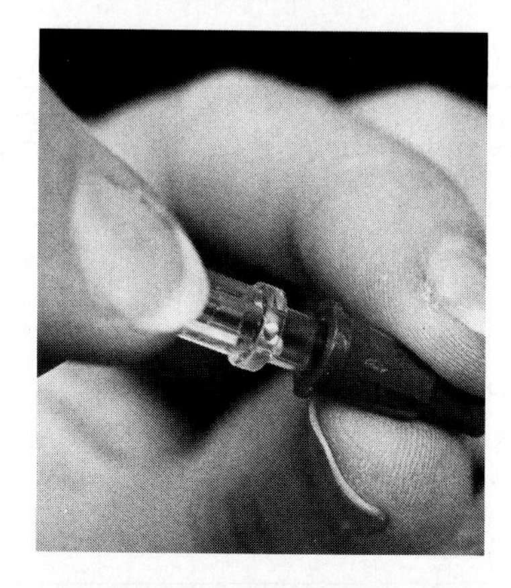

13 Remove the tubing's cap, and attach the tubing to the patient's I.V. catheter or needle.

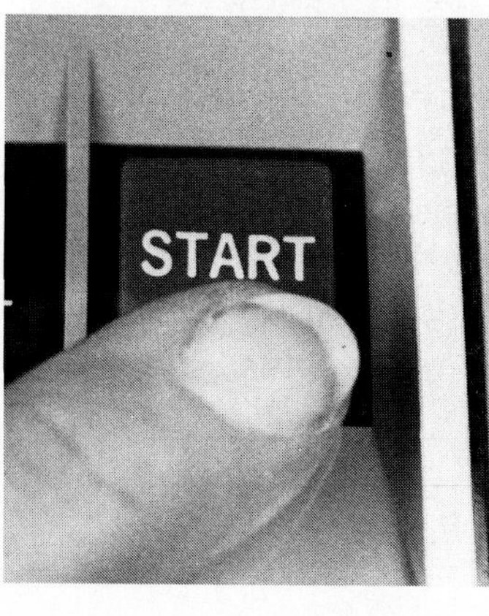

14 Press the START button. A series of dashes will appear across the bottom of the display window, as well as the volume infused. (Keep in mind that the volume number represents the *total* amount infused. When you document fluid intake and output at the end of a shift, subtract the amount infused during previous shifts, if necessary.) If an alarm sounds, locate and correct the problem. Then, press the START button to resume the infusion.

Getting acquainted with UltraCOM

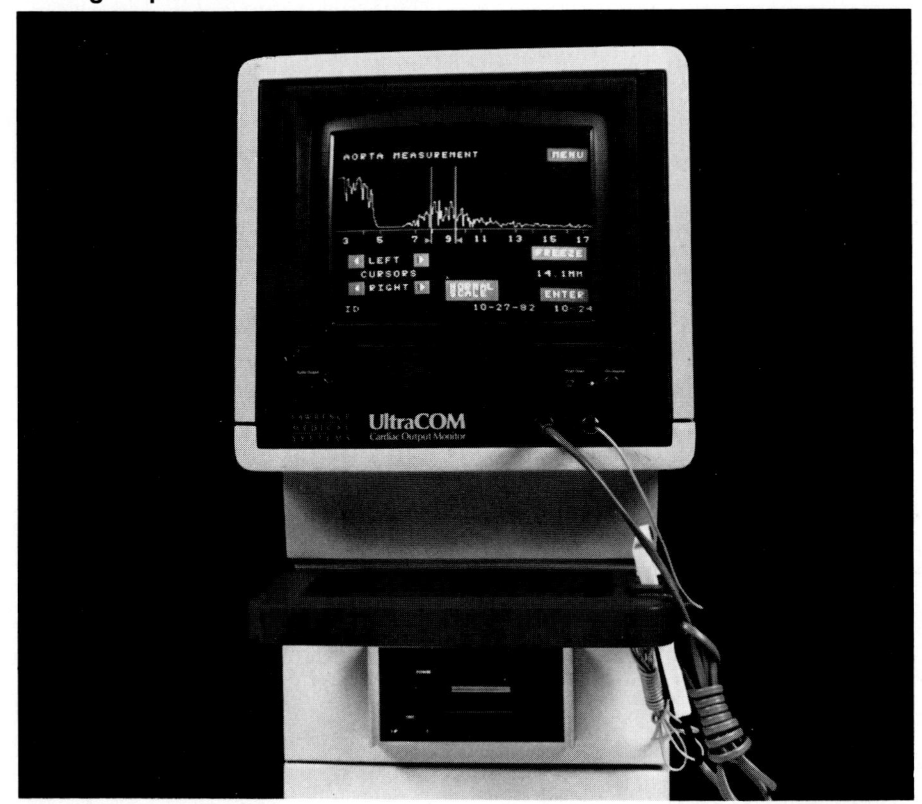

When you think of cardiac output (CO) monitoring, you probably think of a complicated, potentially dangerous procedure necessitating cardiac catheterization. And no wonder. Until recently, only two techniques—thermodilution and dye injection—provided reliable CO measurements. But now, you can obtain accurate measurements with a *noninvasive* technique, using the UltraCOM computer shown above.

The UltraCOM combines ultrasound principles with microprocessor computer technology. Despite its sophistication, the computer's easy to use. Its *touch screen,* which responds to your fingertip's warmth, takes the place of a keyboard or console. Better yet, you don't need to learn complicated computer terminology to use it.

In addition to the UltraCOM computer, the only equipment you need is conductive jelly and two ultrasound transducers supplied by the manufacturer: an echo-ranging transducer and a continuous-wave Doppler transducer.

Using UltraCOM

When you turn on the computer, you'll see a *function menu* on the screen. By pressing the indicated area on the screen, you prepare the computer for one of these functions: receiving patient data (identification number, height, weight, and aortic area), measuring CO, or registering the date and time.

To determine aortic area, hold the echo-ranging transducer on the patient's chest at the third intercostal space, left of the sternum (cardiac window). Angle the transducer until you see waveform spikes like those appearing across the top of the screen in the photo above. These spikes indicate that the sound waves are bouncing off the walls of the heart and aorta. From these returning sound waves, the computer calculates aortic cross-sectional area. Direct the computer to memorize this calculation. *Note:* As a rule, you need do this procedure only once for each patient, because aortic diameter rarely changes.

Next, place the Doppler transducer at the suprasternal notch and angle it toward the aorta. An audible signal guides you. When positioned correctly, the transducer detects Doppler shift caused by red blood cells moving through the ascending aorta. By analyzing this information along with the patient's aortic area, the computer calculates cardiac output.

As this overview suggests, UltraCOM can be an asset on a general unit—and even in a clinic. Learn more about it from the manufacturer, Lawrence Medical Systems.

Checking pacemaker function by telephone

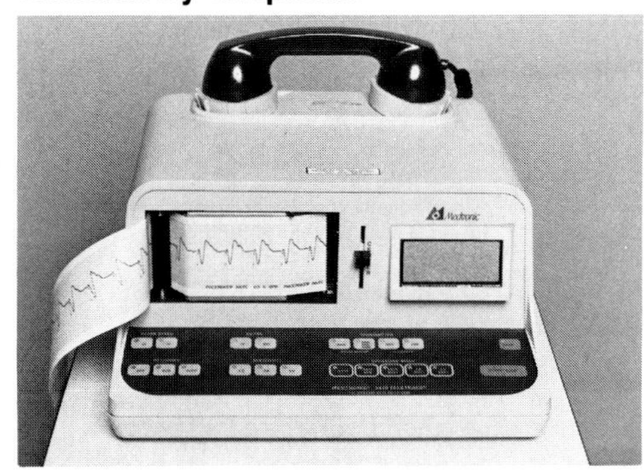

Eleanor Melville, age 77, is in your unit after receiving a permanent cardiac pacemaker. "I'm excited about going home again—but I'm a little worried, too," she tells you. "I don't drive anymore, so I can't get to the doctor's often. How can I be sure my pacemaker's working right?"

Fortunately, you can reassure Ms. Melville that checking her pacemaker function is almost as easy as picking up her phone. Because she has a Medtronic pacemaker, she can use a Medtronic Model 9408 TeleTrace Transmitter to telephone an EKG signal to her doctor's office.

Here's how. At an appointed time, Ms. Melville calls her doctor's office. Then, she rests a small, rectangular transmitter against her bare chest and puts the telephone's mouthpiece against the transmitter's speaker. The transmitter detects electrical signals generated by Ms. Melville's pacemaker and her beating heart and converts them to sound waves. The telephone receiver then sends these sound waves to a receiver in the doctor's office (see photo above), which converts them to an EKG readout strip. By examining the strip, Ms. Melville's doctor can determine whether the pacemaker's maintaining a regular heartbeat.

How often will Ms. Melville have to check her pacemaker? This depends on her condition and the pacemaker's power source. Make sure she understands her doctor's instructions. Also, tell her that her pacemaker will need to be checked more frequently as its power source ages.

Teach her to use the transmitter, and answer her questions. Be sure to show her how to insert a battery in the transmitter, and tell her to replace the battery at least every 3 months. Then, give her a copy of the following home care aid to use as a guide.

Note: The doctor may order finger electrodes instead of a transmitter. These electrodes transmit an EKG signal based on the patient's finger pulses. If necessary, teach your patient how to use them. See the manufacturer's instructions for details.

Cardiovascular

Home care

Checking your pacemaker by telephone

Dear Patient:
Your doctor's prescribed a Medtronic Teletrace Transmitter so he can check your pacemaker by telephone. Your nurse has explained how the transmitter works and has shown you how to operate it. Use this home care aid as a guide after you've been discharged. If you have any questions or problems, call ______________________

1 Here's how the back and the front of your transmitter look. Before using your transmitter for the first time, remove the battery cover and insert the 9-volt alkaline battery supplied by the manufacturer. *Remember:* Replace the battery every 2 or 3 months.

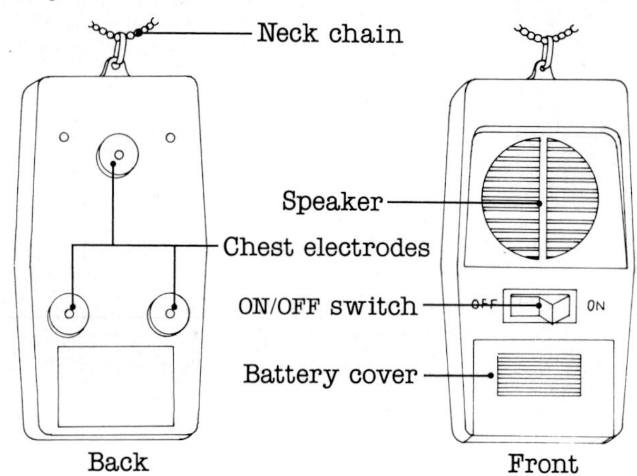

2 When you're ready to use the transmitter, put its chain around your neck, and adjust the chain so the transmitter hangs comfortably at the middle of your chest. Open or remove your shirt and underwear, so the transmitter's chest electrodes rest against your *bare* skin.

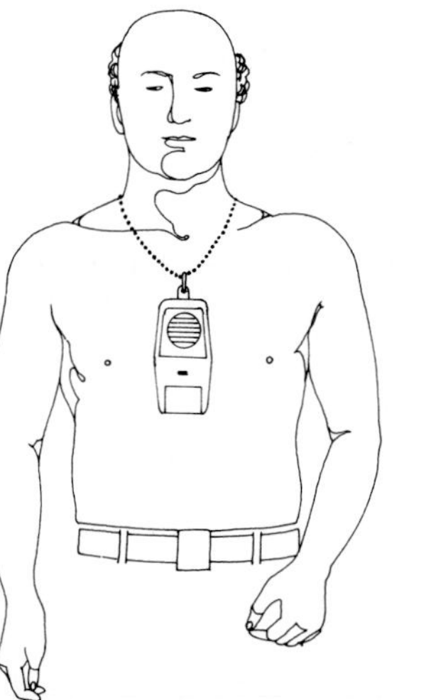

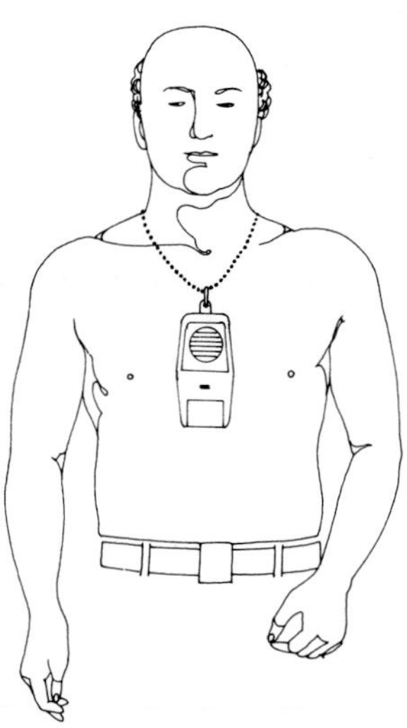

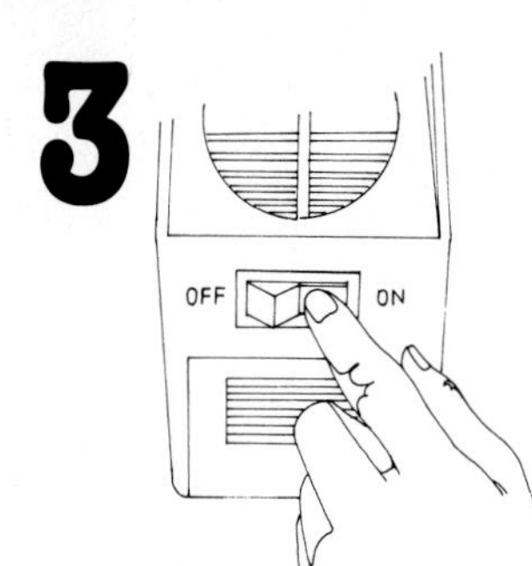

3 When you've contacted your doctor's office by telephone, turn on the transmitter by pressing the ON/OFF switch to the *on* position. Listen for a squealing sound. If you don't hear it, change the transmitter's battery before continuing.

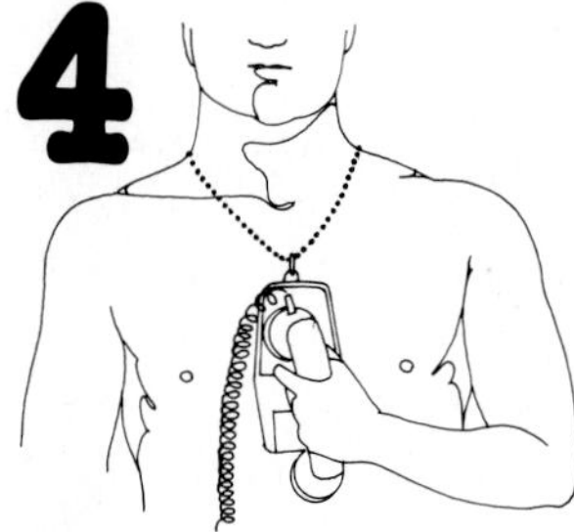

4 When the doctor (or his assistant) is ready to receive your signal, place the telephone's *mouthpiece* against the transmitter's speaker. Hold the telephone as steady as you can, and try to sit still for about 30 seconds.

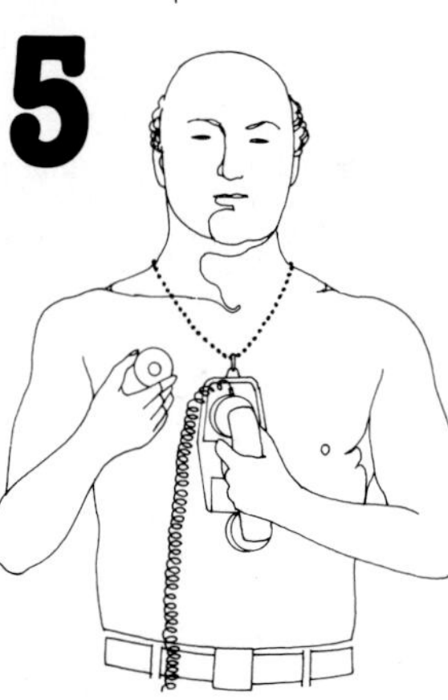

5 After 30 seconds, hold the telephone to your ear, and listen for further instructions. For example, the doctor may want you to repeat the procedure while you hold a special magnet he's given you over the pacemaker. If so, take care to place the magnet *flat* against your pacemaker, and hold it as steady as possible. (If you wish, ask someone to hold it for you.) But don't use the magnet unless the doctor asks you to do so.

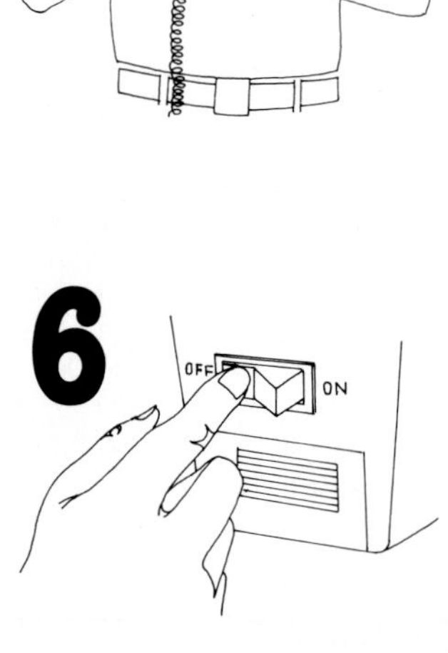

6 If the doctor has no further directions for you, hang up the phone and remove the transmitter from around your neck. Don't forget to switch off your transmitter, and keep it switched off whenever you're not using it.

GI and endocrine

Are you feeding your patient with a nasogastric tube? If so, you probably know how valuable an infusion pump is for maintaining a constant, accurate flow rate. But you may not feel confident using one. To help, this section provides details on the Kangaroo 220 Feeding System.

We also inform you about a new insulin delivery system—the Pen Pump. In the following pages, you'll learn how it works and how to teach your patient to use it.

Finally, we familiarize you with another type of insulin pump—the Auto-Syringe. Read these pages carefully.

Providing tube feedings

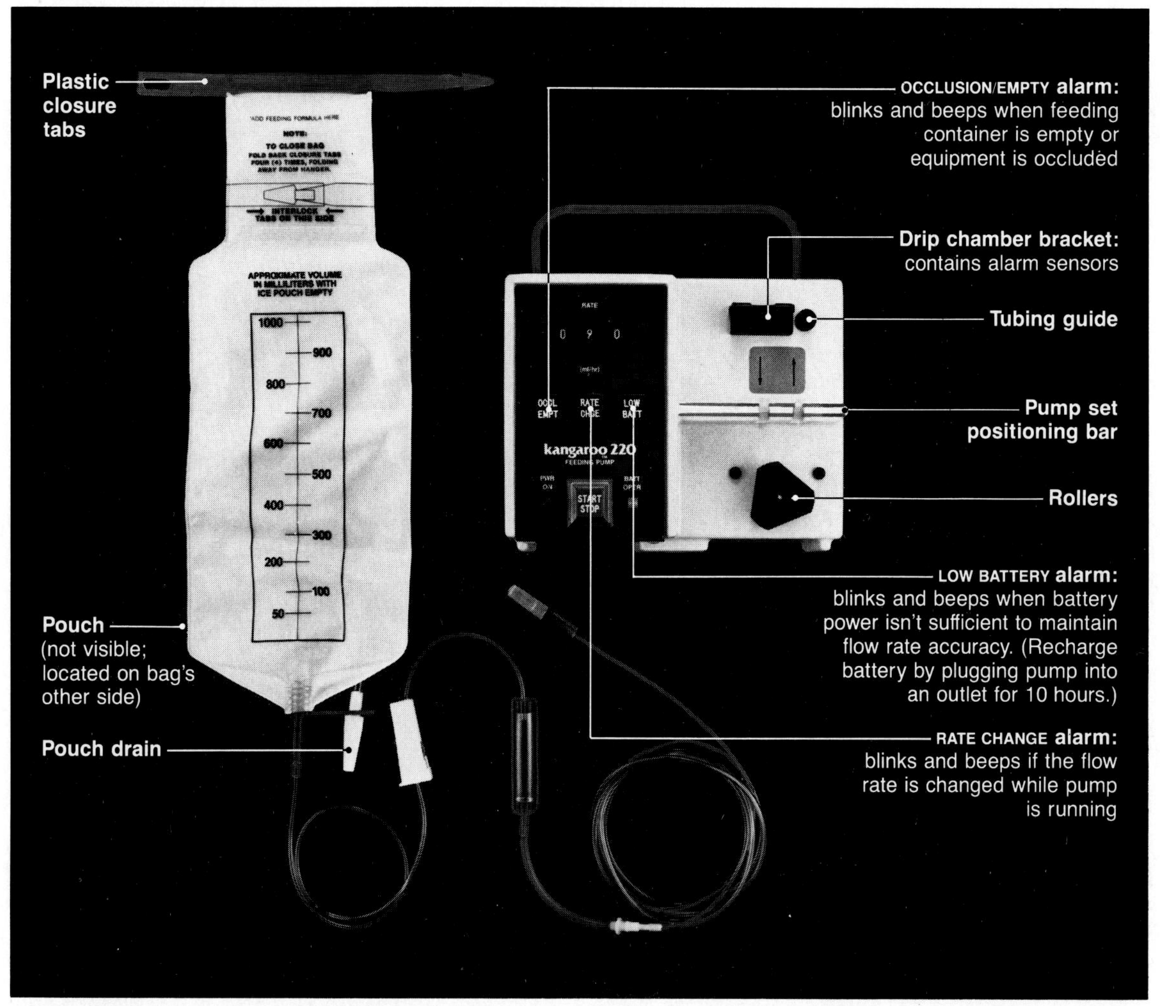

Six months ago, 88-year-old Herman Reingold suffered a cerebrovascular accident that left him severely disabled. Because he didn't receive adequate care at home, he is admitted to your unit malnourished, dehydrated, and with several decubitus ulcers. One of your first priorities is to improve his nutritional status. Because he can't swallow safely, you'll provide nasogastric (NG) tube feedings, as ordered.

Expect a patient like Mr. Reingold, who hasn't eaten normally for months, to be extremely sensitive to the sugar, protein, and fluids he'll receive by NG tube. Try to prevent such complications as diarrhea, cramps, and possibly insulin rebound phenomenon by giving him small, dilute feedings at first.

Depending on the doctor's order and hospital policy, you may dilute his first day's feeding with water until it's one-quarter strength. Each subsequent day, you'll probably decrease the dilution by one quarter, until Mr. Reingold's receiving full-strength feedings. At the same time, you'll gradually increase the volume, as ordered. Of course, you'll modify this schedule as necessary, depending on his condition, how well he tolerates each feeding, and the doctor's instructions.

Using a feeding pump

For a patient like Mr. Reingold, precise volume control is important. To ensure volume control precision, you'll use a feeding pump, like Chesebrough-Pond's Kangaroo 220 Feeding System (see photo above).

The lightweight Kangaroo pump and administration set is specially designed to deliver viscous feeding solutions at consistent, accurate rates. You can use it with any type of enteric feeding tube. And because its flow rate ranges from 5 ml/hour to 295 ml/hour (adjustable in 5-ml/hour increments), you can use it for any patient—even an infant.

The Kangaroo system's administration bag contains a pouch (hence the name *Kangaroo*). If ordered, you can insert ice into the pouch to cool the solution. Doing so delays solution decomposition—an asset if the flow rate's very slow or if additives are ordered.

If the solution needn't be iced, you may warm a feeding solution to room temperature by filling the pouch with warm water. As you know, room temperature solution is less likely to cause abdominal cramping.

As the following photostory demonstrates, the Kangaroo pump is easy to set up and operate. Read on for details.

GI and endocrine

Setting up a Kangaroo 220 Feeding System

Preparing to use a Kangaroo 220 Feeding System? First gather the equipment you need: Kangaroo pump and administration set, I.V. pole, feeding solution (as ordered), measuring cup, and water (if you're diluting the solution). If your patient has a standard-sized nasogastric (NG) tube in place, you may also need an adapter to ensure a good connection between the administration tubing and the NG tube.

Before diluting the feeding solution, determine the amount of solution and water the patient can receive in 8 hours (according to the ordered flow rate). Don't mix more solution than he's scheduled to receive in an 8-hour shift.

Next, calculate the proportion *of water to solution needed to achieve the ordered concentration. (Don't dilute the solution with a liquid other than water. Fruit juices, for example, curdle some solutions.) Then, thoroughly wash and dry your hands.*

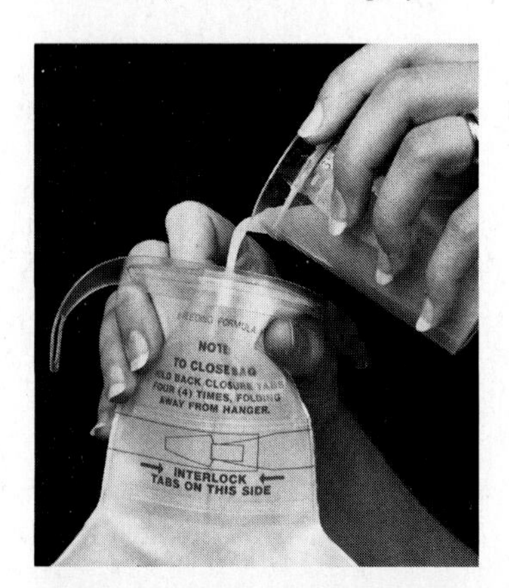

1 Clamp the pump to the I.V. pole and plug the pump into an outlet.

Close the administration set's flow clamp. Next, measure and pour the correct amount of solution into the administration bag, as shown here. (Look for the phrase *add feeding formula here* at the bag's top.) Then, if you're diluting the solution, add the correct amount of water.

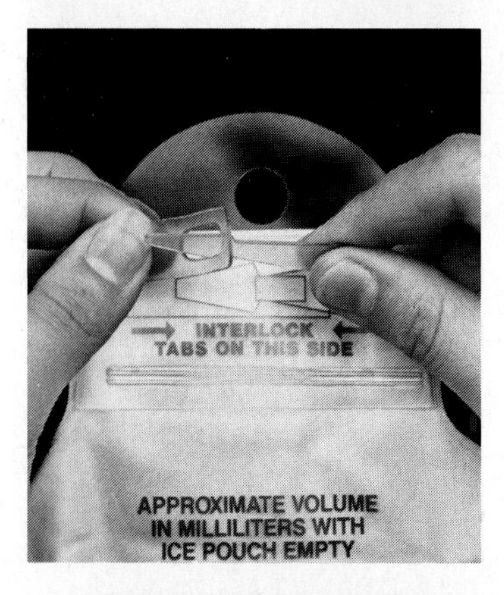

2 To close the bag, fold back the plastic closure tabs four times, so the bag's top rolls away from the hanger tab. Interlock the tabs across the bag's front, as the nurse is doing here.

Then, hang the bag on the I.V. pole. Gently squeeze it several times to mix the solution with the water.

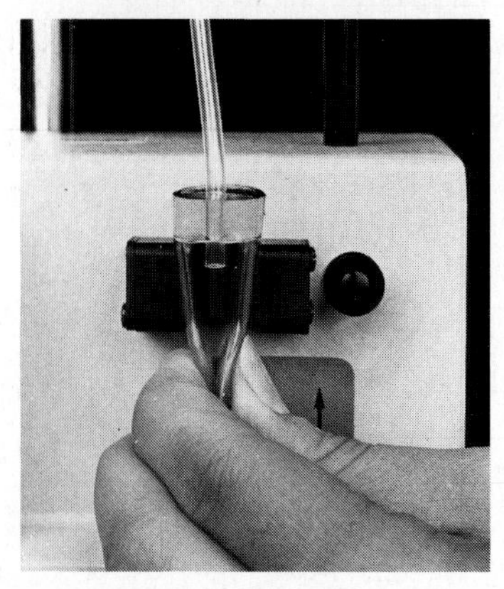

3 Insert the bottom of the administration set's drip chamber into the positioning bar. Then, squeeze and press the drip chamber to insert it into the drip chamber bracket, as shown here.

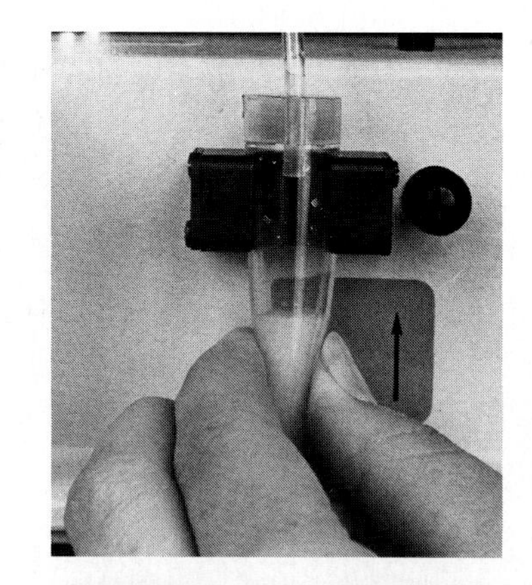

4 Open the flow clamp and squeeze the drip chamber until it's about half full. *Caution:* Don't allow the drip chamber to become more than half full or the occlusion alarm will sound.

Note: Other reasons for the occlusion alarm's sounding are improper placement of drip chamber in pump, coating of drip chamber walls with feeding solution, and spillage on drip chamber bracket.

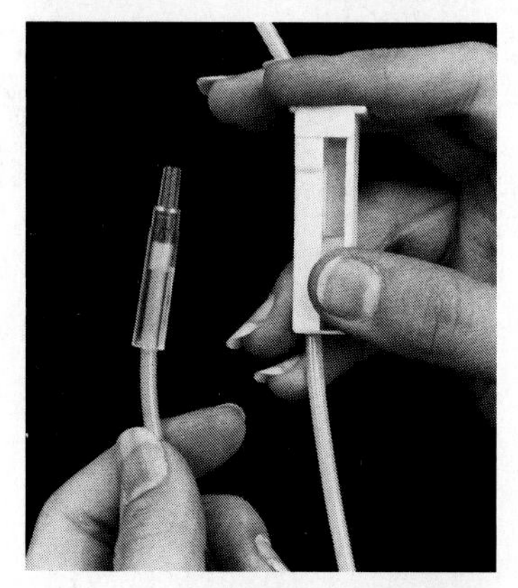

5 Remove the cap at the end of the administration set's tubing and fill the entire line with fluid. When all air's expelled, close the flow clamp.

Connect the tubing to the patient's feeding tube.

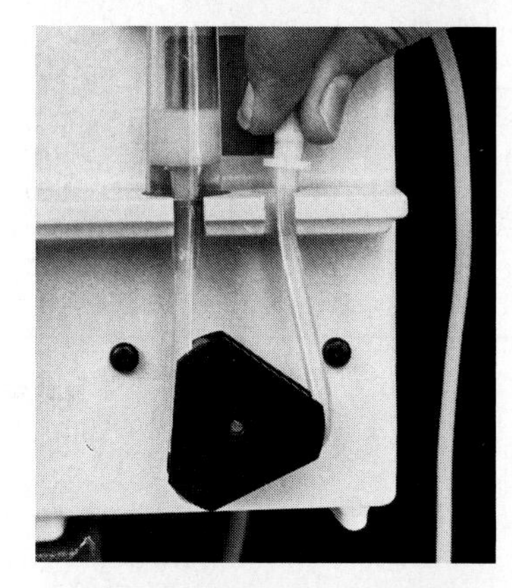

6 Beneath the drip chamber, you'll find a section of stretchable silicone tubing. Extend it around the rollers and through the open notch on the positioning bar. As you see, the flange at the silicone section's end prevents the tubing from slipping back through the notch.

To prevent the tubing from kinking above the shelf, thread it around the tubing guide (the black post beside the drip chamber bracket).

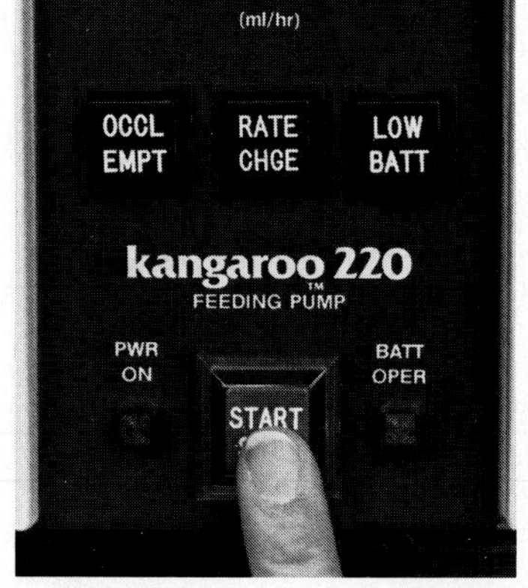

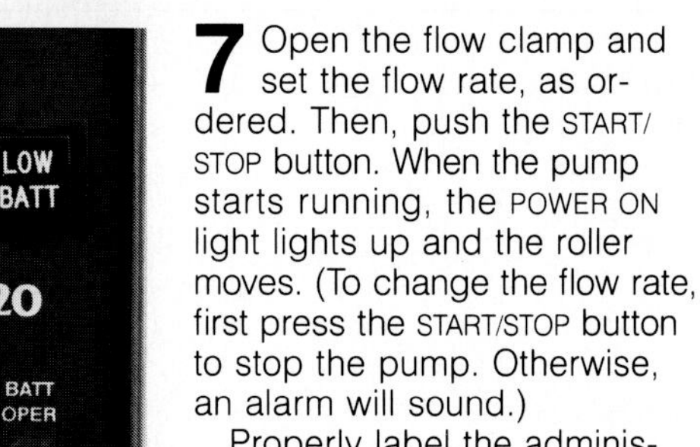

7 Open the flow clamp and set the flow rate, as ordered. Then, push the START/STOP button. When the pump starts running, the POWER ON light lights up and the roller moves. (To change the flow rate, first press the START/STOP button to stop the pump. Otherwise, an alarm will sound.)

Properly label the administration bag, and document the feeding and how your patient tolerated it on his intake/output record.

Learning about the Pen Pump Infuser

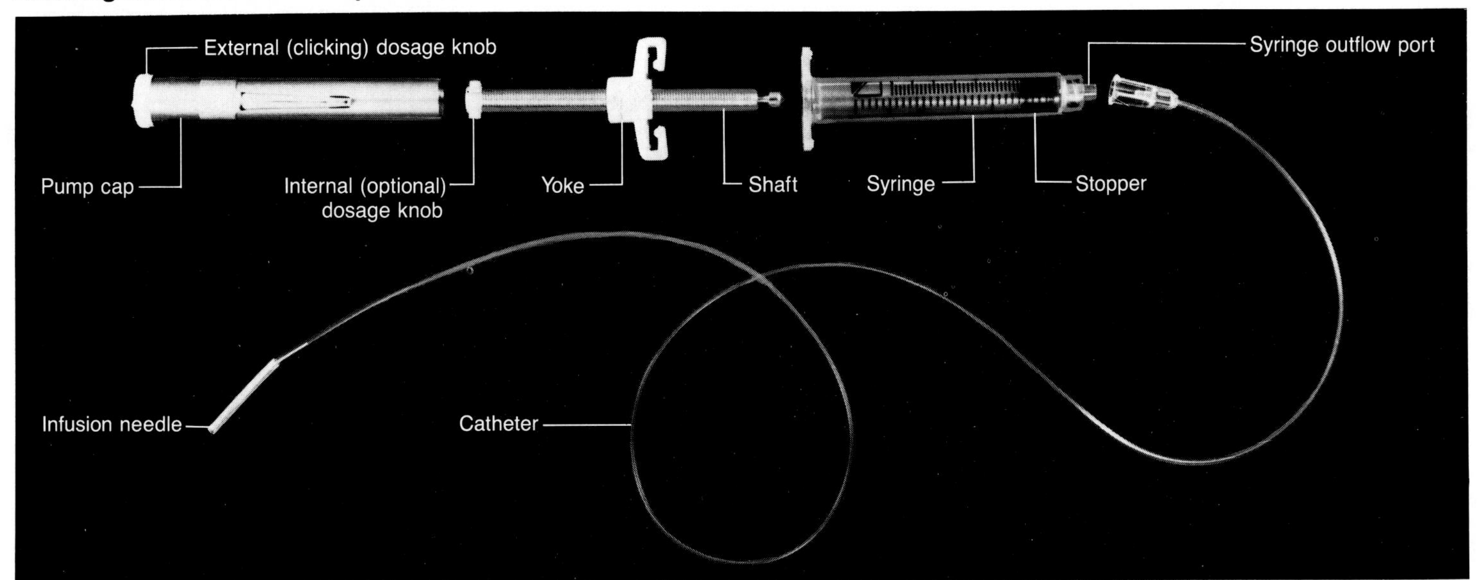

If you've provided care for a patient with diabetes, you know how difficult controlling blood glucose levels can be. For optimum control, most experts recommend multiple daily insulin doses—one dose before each meal or snack—to closely mimic normal pancreatic function. But few patients maintain a multiple-daily-dose schedule because of the added discomfort and problems associated with maintaining acceptable injection sites. Or, they may object to wearing a motorized insulin infusion pump day and night.

The Pen Pump Infuser by Markwell Medical Institute, Inc. may change all that. It enables the patient to receive multiple daily insulin doses at the same site for up to 3 days.

When a doctor prescribes a Pen Pump Infuser, the manufacturer recommends that he hospitalize the patient for several days for comprehensive blood glucose level monitoring and detailed patient teaching. This is where you fit in. Prepare to teach your patient how to use this equipment by reading the following information and photostories.

Getting acquainted with the Pen Pump

The Pen Pump Infuser, shown above, is a fountain pen–sized, lightweight, nonmotorized syringe pump that the patient controls manually. It enables him to receive multiple daily insulin doses at the same site for 1 to 3 days. Then, he replaces the disposable equipment and changes the insertion site. In the next two photostories, you'll find detailed instructions on how to use it.

The Pen Pump is recommended only for the highly motivated diabetic patient. Why highly motivated? Because to use the equipment safely and effectively, he must be willing to closely monitor and record his blood glucose levels six to eight times a day for the first few weeks. Doing so permits the patient and his doctor to determine the patient's insulin needs and precisely calculate daily dosages. After 2 or 3 weeks of intensive monitoring, the patient will continue to regularly monitor his glucose levels but at less frequent intervals.

Your patient can wear his Pen Pump while sleeping and during almost any activity, including showering and swimming. Some patients even wear the equipment while playing contact sports. If your patient chooses to temporarily remove the needle (for example, overnight), he can keep the needle sterile by opening an alcohol swab packet and placing the needle in the packet with the swab.

Initiating therapy

To begin therapy with a Pen Pump, the doctor will probably instruct the patient to test and record his glucose level about 20 minutes before each meal or snack. Then, the patient gives himself a dose of U-100 *regular* insulin. The dosage is based on an estimation of the patient's needs (for example, 10 units before a meal and 4 units before a snack). About 2 hours after beginning the meal, the patient again tests and records his glucose level.

Until the patient's specific insulin needs are determined, he'll also give himself a separate bedtime injection of NPH or lente insulin at another subcutaneous site. Later, the doctor will probably prescribe a mixture of regular and NPH or lente insulin to eliminate the need for a separate bedtime injection.

Patient teaching

While helping your patient learn to use his Pen Pump, emphasize the importance of regular blood glucose level monitoring. Help him set up a calendar for recording his glucose levels before and after meals, and encourage him to maintain intensive glucose self-monitoring for the first few weeks he uses the pump (according to his doctor's directions).

When he begins keeping careful records, your patient may be surprised and alarmed at how poorly his glucose levels are controlled by only one or two daily insulin injections. Assure him that intensive self-monitoring will help him and his doctor stabilize his glucose levels.

Don't assume your patient's well informed about diabetes management—even if he's already managing his insulin therapy. Make sure he understands these important points:

- Never skip a meal or snack after taking insulin.
- Never take insulin if you have symptoms of hypoglycemia; for example, light-headedness, fatigue, nervousness, headache, or trembling. If possible, test your blood glucose level immediately.
- Always carry candy or some other sugar source, in case of hypoglycemia.
- Before taking insulin, ask yourself whether your usual dose needs adjustment. Consider these questions: Is my fasting (premeal) glucose level unusually high or low? Will the meal (or snack) I'm about to eat have more or less than the usual amount of carbohydrates? After eating, will I be exercising more or less than usual?

Following up

After your patient's hospitalization, follow up on his progress with phone contact and outpatient evaluation. Remember, his continued compliance is essential for effective diabetes management.

GI and endocrine

Preparing a Pen Pump Infuser for use

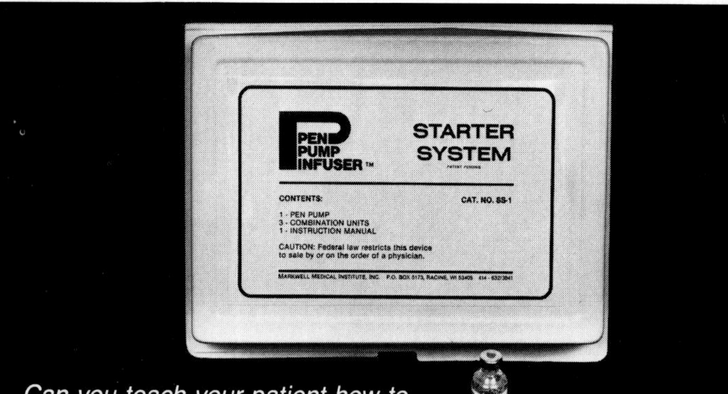

Can you teach your patient how to prepare a Pen Pump Infuser for use? Remember, he'll have to fill it with insulin about twice a week. Make sure you know the procedure by reading this photostory.

First, gather this equipment: a Pen Pump Infuser starter kit (which includes the equipment shown on page 77), U-100 insulin (as ordered), surgical tape (such as Transpore, which is included in the kit) or Op-Site, and two alcohol swabs (not shown). Important: *The Pen Pump Infuser is designed to deliver precise doses of U-100 insulin. Don't use any other insulin concentration.*

If the insulin has been refrigerated, let it warm to room temperature before beginning. This reduces the chance of air bubble formation.

Thoroughly wash and dry your hands. Open the kit and remove the syringe's protective wrapping.

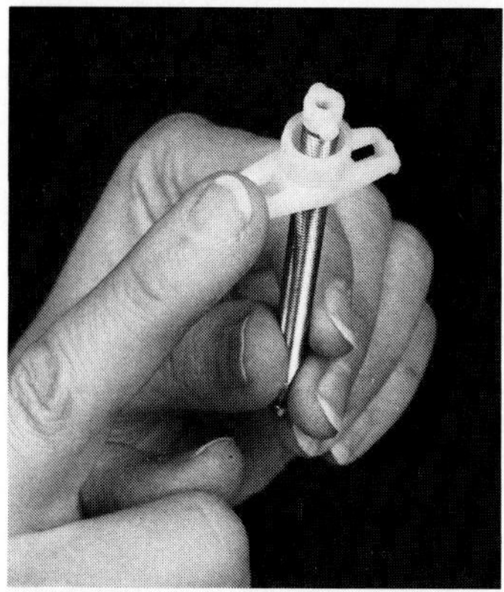

1 To assemble the Pen Pump, spin the white plastic yoke up the screw-threaded shaft, until the yoke reaches the internal dosage knob.

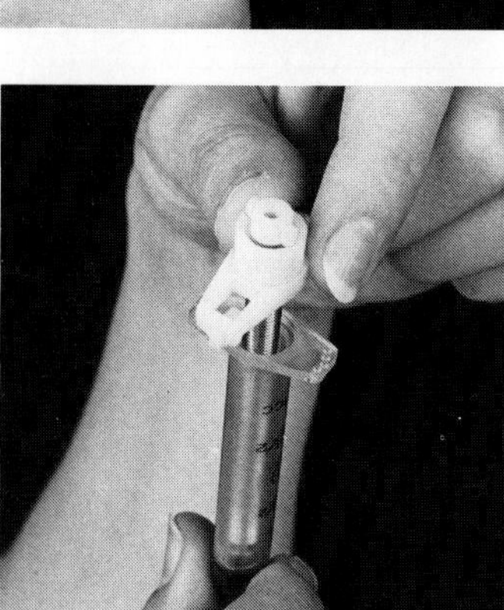

2 Insert the shaft's pointed end into the syringe, and turn the yoke so it's perpendicular to the syringe's flanges.

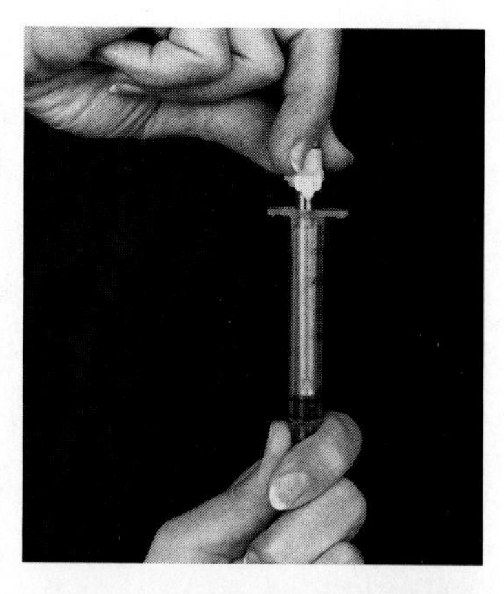

3 Then, firmly depress the shaft until its pointed end snaps into the black rubber stopper.

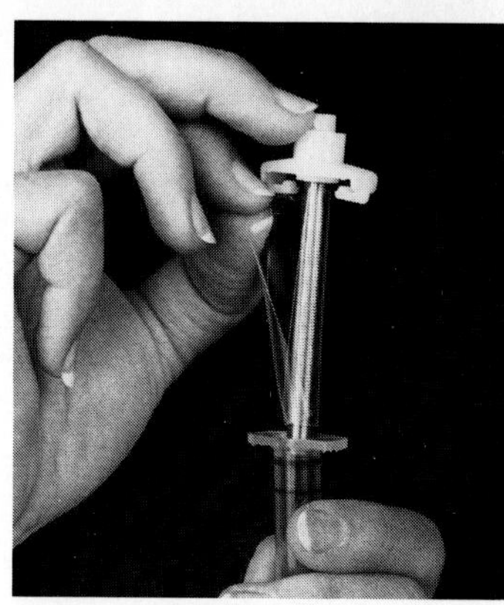

4 Now, pull back the shaft until the stopper rests at the syringe's top. (Take care not to pull the stopper out of the syringe.) As you do so, the syringe's protective plastic sheath will emerge. Remove it, as shown here, and discard it. Then, push the stopper back to the syringe's bottom.

If the patient isn't using an insulin mixture, remove the syringe needle and allow the mixing ball to drop out. Replace the needle.

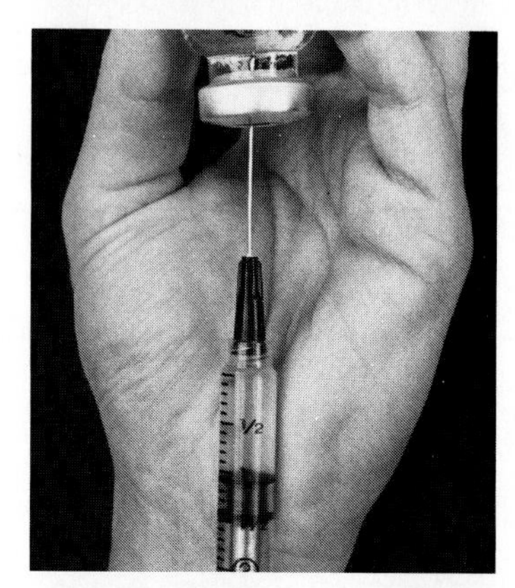

5 Clean the insulin bottle's diaphragm with an alcohol swab, remove the syringe needle's cap, and draw up the ordered amount of insulin. Because the syringe functions as an insulin reservoir between injections, the doctor will probably recommend that you fill the syringe. *Note:* If you're mixing regular insulin with a long-acting insulin, draw up the regular insulin first.

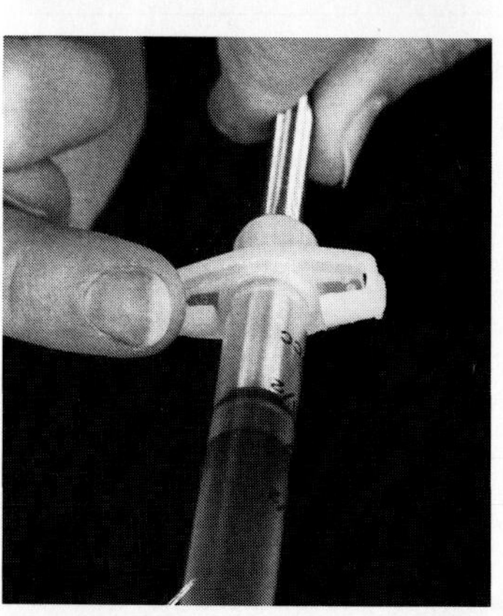

6 Next, spin the yoke clockwise, until it meets the syringe. Lock the shaft in place by snapping the yoke's arms around the syringe's flanges, as shown here. Now, you can move the shaft only by turning one of the dosage knobs.

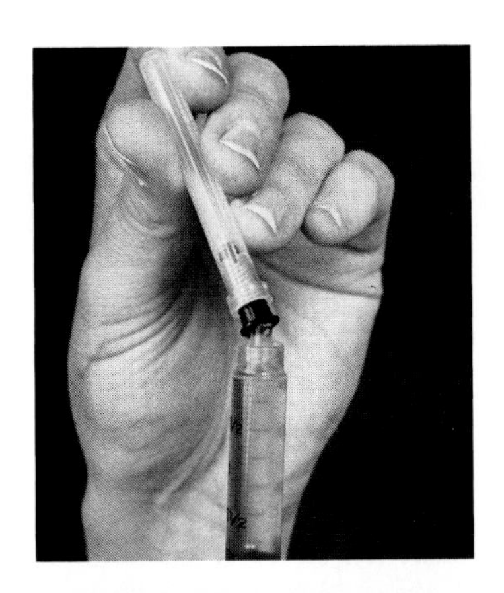

7 Hold the syringe upright and wait for the mixing ball to drop away from the syringe outflow port (unless, of course, you've removed the mixing ball). Recap the needle; then remove and discard it.

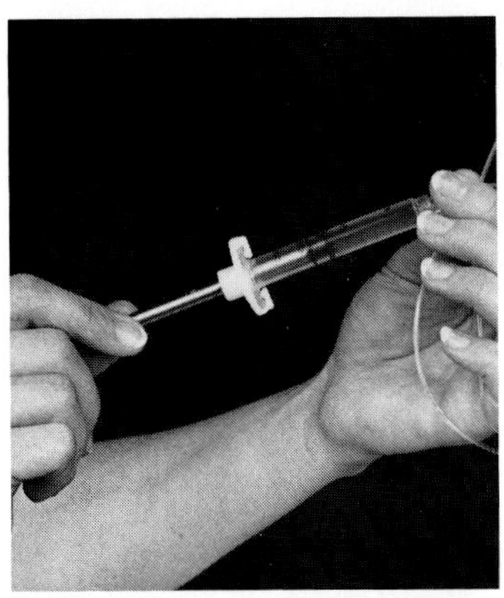

8 Now, attach the infusion catheter to the syringe. Expel air from the catheter and needle by inverting the syringe and turning the shaft's dosage knob (the internal dosage knob) clockwise, as shown here.

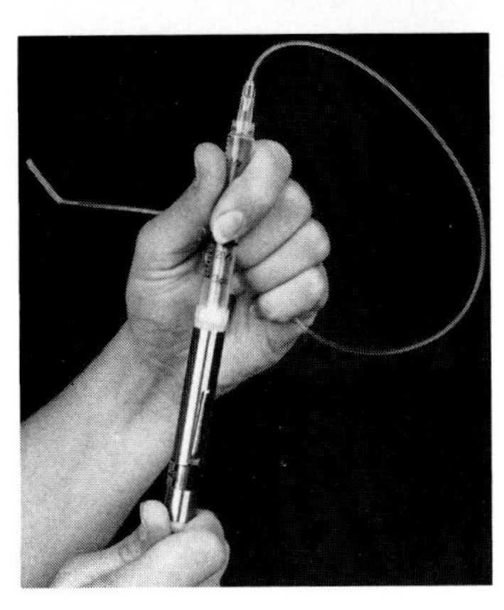

9 Firmly press the pump cap over the shaft, as shown.

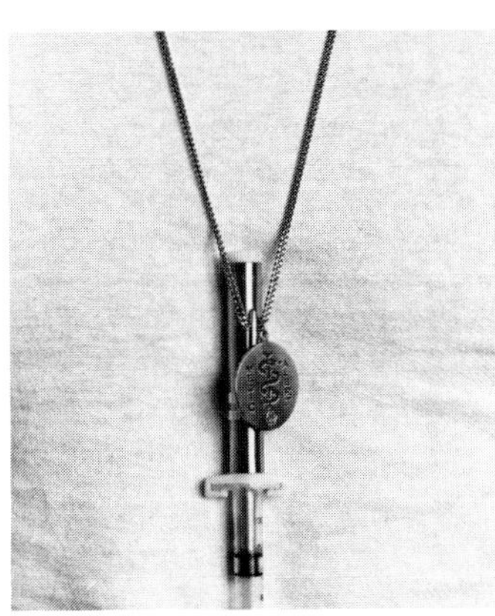

10 Use the clip to attach the pump to the patient's clothing or to a chain around his neck. (This patient's pump is clipped to his Medic Alert necklace.)

Nursing tip: If the syringe contains an insulin mixture, recommend that the patient carry the pump in *cap-down* position. (The manufacturer supplies an optional clip for this purpose.) This position facilitates resuspension of the mixed insulin crystals before injection.

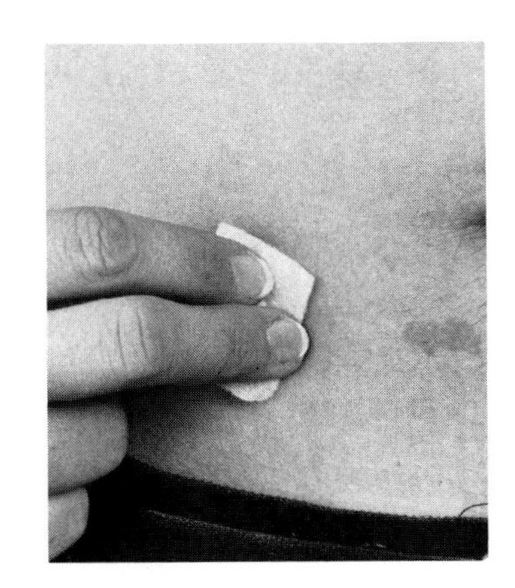

11 Now, you're ready to insert the infusion needle. Choose an appropriate subcutaneous site. (Unless contraindicated, select an abdominal site at the patient's waistline where it won't be disturbed by a belt or waistband.) Cleanse the site with an alcohol swab, and allow the skin to dry.

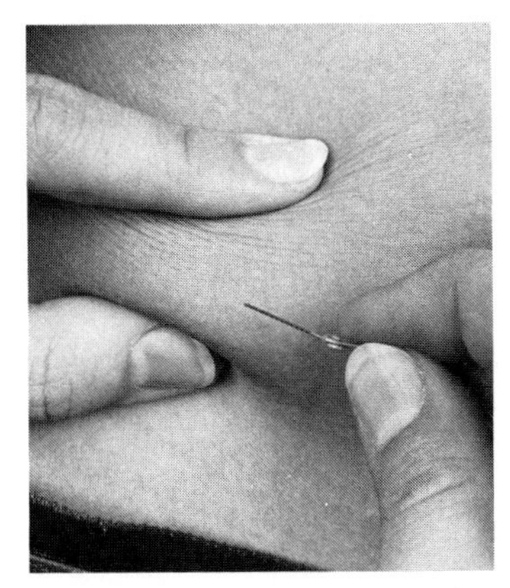

12 Grasp the subcutaneous layer between the thumb and forefinger of your nondominant hand. With your other hand, hold the needle bevel up, so it's angled either upward or perpendicular to the patient's midline. Then, quickly insert it into the subcutaneous layer at a 30° angle.

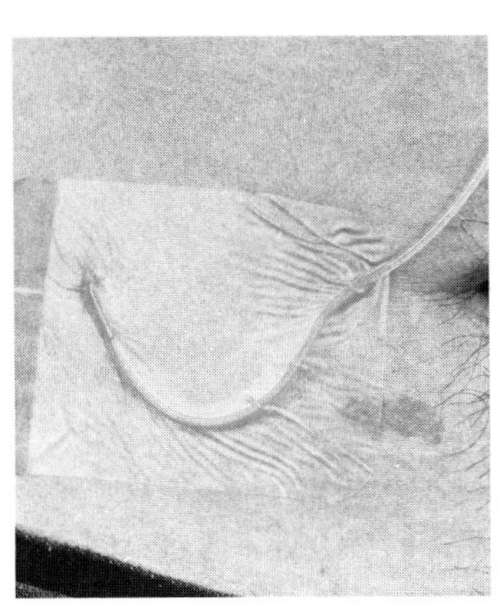

13 Anchor the needle by applying Op-Site over the insertion site (according to the manufacturer's instructions).

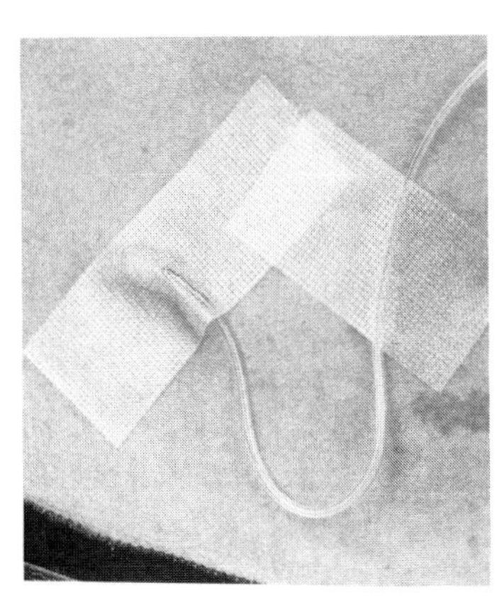

14 Or, secure the needle with surgical tape. Then, form a stress loop below the needle, as shown, and tape it in place. Besides protecting the needle from accidental tugs, a stress loop prevents insulin crystal aggregation in the needle. (If insulin crystals form in the loop, break them up by gently squeezing the loop.)

Now, the Pen Pump's ready for use. To learn how to activate it, read the next photostory.

GI and endocrine

Administering insulin with a Pen Pump

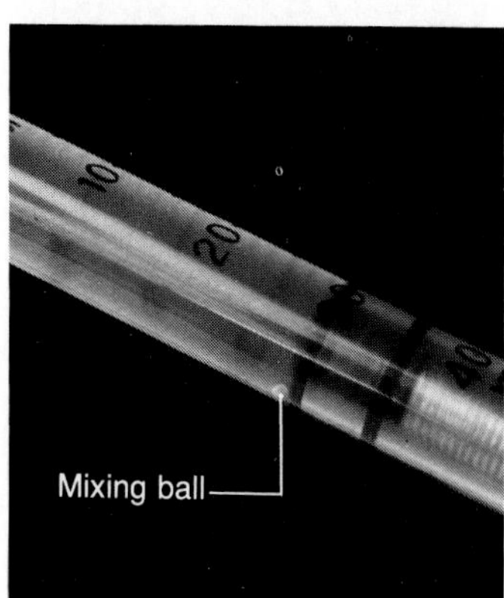

1 Your patient will self-administer insulin from his Pen Pump before each meal or snack. Teach him how to do so by following these steps.

If the syringe contains an insulin mixture, first resuspend the insulin by gently tilting the syringe back and forth. As you do, watch the mixing ball, and make sure it falls in and out of the syringe's outflow port several times.

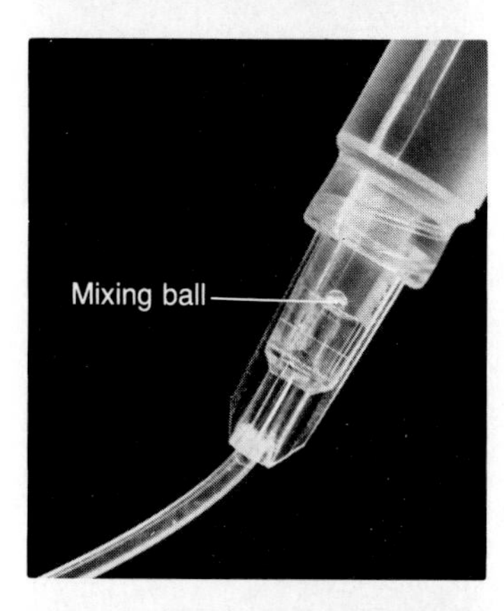

2 When the insulin looks uniformly cloudy, it's ready for injection. Hold the pump at an angle (45° or less). Otherwise, the mixing ball may block the syringe's outflow port, as shown here.

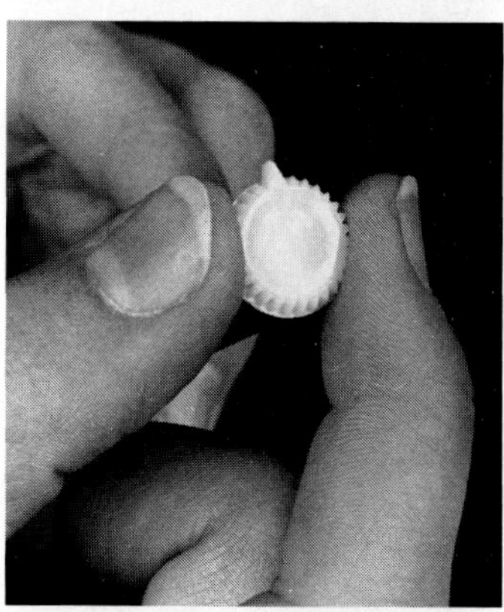

3 To inject the correct amount of insulin, slowly turn the external dosage knob clockwise. You'll hear a click for each quarter turn you move the knob. Each click indicates that you've delivered 1 unit of insulin. To deliver 10 units, turn the knob until you count 10 clicks (two and a half turns). The patient should feel a distinct sensation. If he doesn't, make sure the needle's placed correctly.

Return the pump to the place where it is worn.

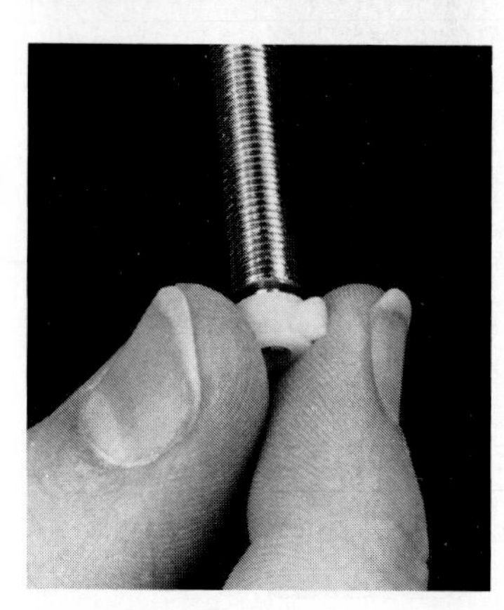

4 If you can't turn the knob, check to see if the mixing ball's wedged in the outflow port. If it is, remove the pump's cap and turn the *internal* dosage knob counterclockwise to relieve pressure inside the syringe. (The external dosage knob won't turn counterclockwise.) Tilt and tap the syringe until the mixing ball rolls free. (If these efforts fail, prepare clean equipment.)

Note: For more details, consult the Pen Pump manual.

Learning about the Auto-Syringe

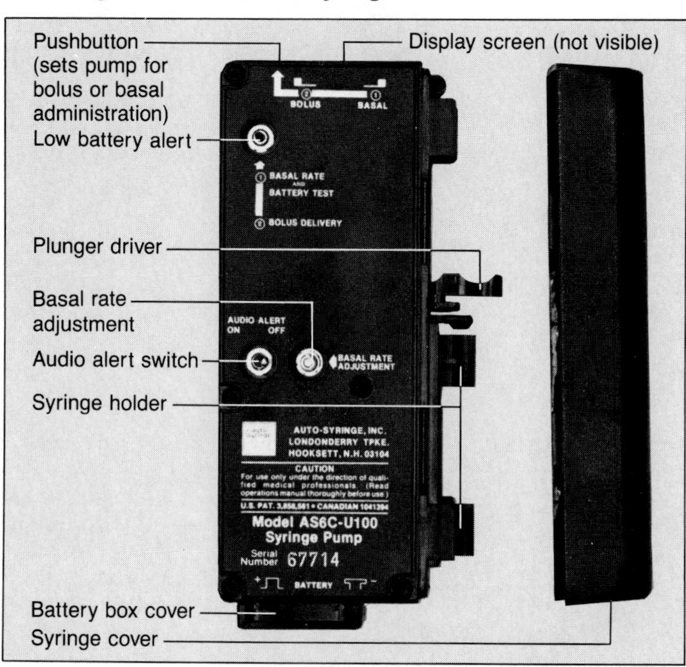

Like the Pen Pump featured on the preceding pages, the Auto-Syringe shown here (insulin infusion model AS6C-U100) is a portable pump that delivers insulin to a subcutaneous site through a needle and catheter. How does the Auto-Syringe compare with the Pen Pump Infuser? Consider these points.

- The Auto-Syringe automatically delivers frequent, intermittent insulin doses at a preset basal rate ordered by the doctor. By doing so, it mimics normal pancreatic function more closely than the Pen Pump. It can also deliver bolus doses, as needed.
- It eliminates the need for mixed insulins; the patient needs only regular insulin.
- A display screen shows either the total number of units to be infused at the basal rate or the number of units being infused as a bolus.
- An alarm system alerts the patient to high pressure in the system (indicating a catheter kink or other obstruction) and runaway infusion. If either of these alarm situations occurs, the pump automatically shuts off.
- An audio alert tone sounds each time the pump infuses one tenth of a unit.

- The Auto-Syringe is heavier and more complicated to use than the Pen Pump.
- It's less durable and must be protected from moisture.
- Because it's designed to infuse daily doses, the syringe must be refilled each day. Also, the manufacturer (Auto-Syringe, Inc.) recommends daily infusion site rotation.
- It operates only on a rechargeable battery supplied by the manufacturer. The battery must be tested daily and recharged as necessary.
- The pump's a potential explosion hazard when near flammable or explosive gases.

Before your patient can safely use the Auto-Syringe, he needs detailed patient teaching. Consult the manufacturer's instruction manual for recommendations.

Intravenous

You're already well versed in the basics of I.V. therapy. After all, you use it regularly to treat a variety of health problems. But you may not be familiar with such specialized I.V. equipment as the Hickman catheter and the heparin lock. On the following pages, we fill you in. We also acquaint you with some simple but effective devices that'll save you time and minimize the risk of complications for your patients. We think you'll find the following section invaluable.

Using a single-dose delivery set

Have you ever used a single-dose drug delivery set? If not, you may be surprised to discover how these disposable, easy-to-use sets facilitate I.V. and I.M. drug administration.

Keep in mind that many types of single-dose delivery sets are available and that each type's slightly different. The information here and on the next few pages will help you sort out the differences.

Look at the Bristoject syringe set shown at right. It includes a vial prefilled with a standard drug dose and a syringe and needle device. The needle, which is beveled at both ends, extends through the syringe barrel. When you screw the drug vial into the syringe barrel, the needle's back end (base) punctures the vial's rubber stopper, making the drug available for injection. (Abboject and Min-I-Jet equipment work the same way.)

Parke-Davis packages phenytoin sodium (Dilantin*) in single-dose Uni/Use glass syringes. On the following pages, you'll learn more details about the Bristoject and Uni/Use systems.

The Tel-E-Ject system consists of a needle and syringe prefilled with diazepam (Valium*). It's ready to use as soon as you remove the rubber needle guard. A word of caution, however: Pull off the needle guard with one quick, firm motion. If you let go of the guard before it's detached, it will snap back against the needle.

Regardless of equipment type, drug dosage and needle length depend on the drug's intended use. For example, a syringe with a 3½" needle accompanies a 10-ml vial of epinephrine hydrochloride (Adrenalin Chloride) intended for intracardiac injection.

Other drugs available in single-dose delivery sets include atropine sulfate; calcium chloride; calcium gluceptate; dextrose; isoproterenol hydrochloride (Isuprel*); lidocaine hydrochloride (Xylocaine*), for either cardiac or local effects; magnesium sulfate; metaraminol bitartrate (Aramine*); and sodium bicarbonate.

Pros and cons

Using a single-dose delivery set has these advantages:

- The equipment is easy to assemble, making drugs available quickly. Because drug, needle, and syringe are packaged together, you needn't collect separate pieces of equipment, which can take valuable time in an emergency.
- Drugs are premixed, so they don't have to be reconstituted.
- Each vial is clearly marked with the drug name and amount. Because the vial's designed for one-time use, you won't encounter worn, hard-to-read labels, as you sometimes do with large drug bottles.
- After an emergency, you can easily document the drugs and doses given by collecting and counting the used vials.
- The equipment stacks well, making it easy to store.

The disadvantage? Only that you may have trouble using a single-dose set correctly in an emergency if you're not familiar with it beforehand. Remedy this problem by reviewing the following pages.

*Available in both the United States and Canada

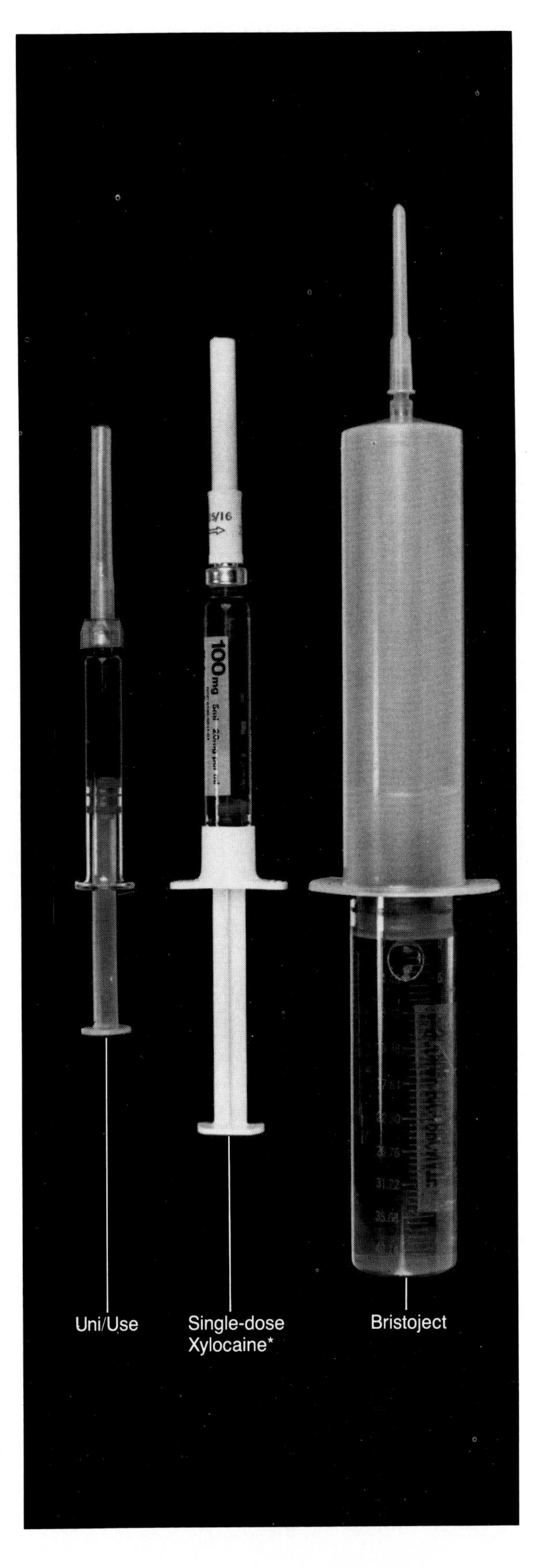

Intravenous

Using a Bristoject syringe set

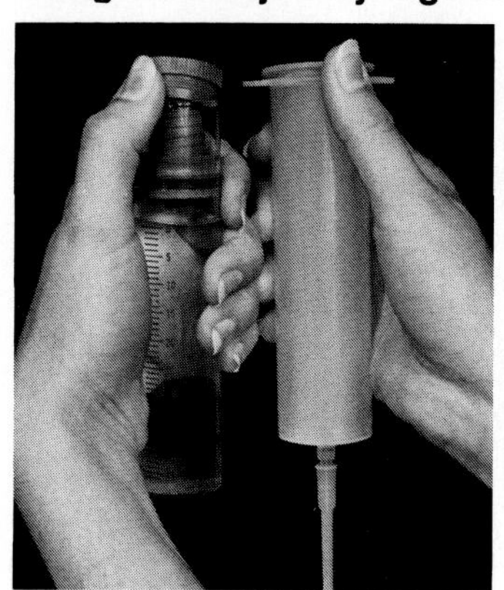

1 To assemble a Bristoject single-dose syringe set, follow these steps: First, remove the drug vial and the syringe with needle from the package. Holding them as shown here, use your thumbs to flip off their protective plastic caps. *Note:* Don't try to pry off the vial's cap with your fingers. The vial's vacuum makes this difficult.

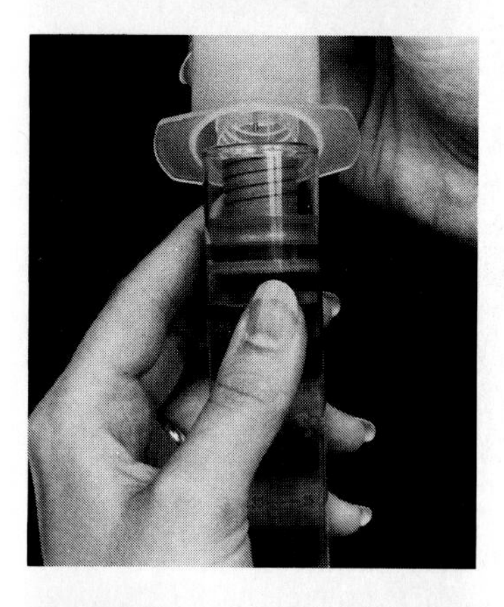

2 Holding the syringe vertically, insert the vial into the syringe barrel. *Important:* Don't touch the needle guard. Doing so may cause the needle to move, preventing it from puncturing the vial stopper properly.

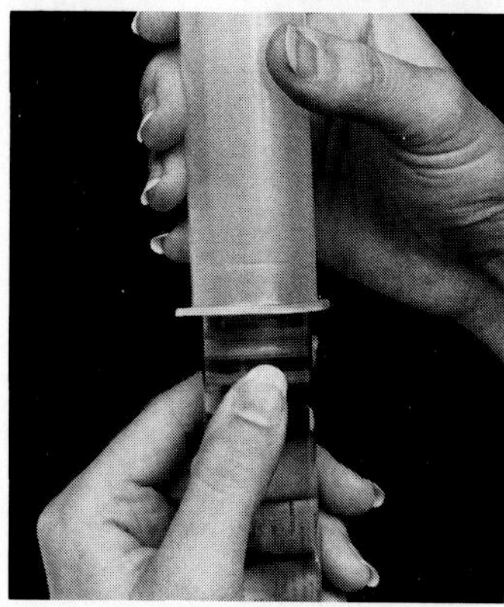

3 Next, rotate the vial clockwise, until you feel resistance. Then, continue one half-turn. The needle's now in contact with the drug.

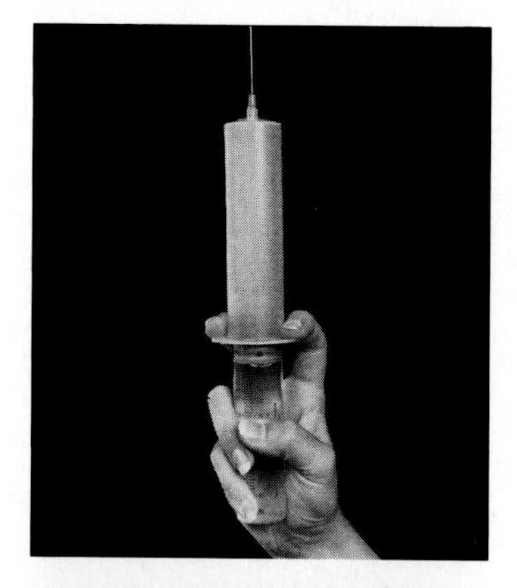

4 Remove the needle guard, expel air (as shown), and inject the drug, as ordered. Avoid rotating the vial during injection or aspiration. Or, rotate the vial in a *clockwise* motion. (Counterclockwise rotation prevents proper needle contact with the drug.)

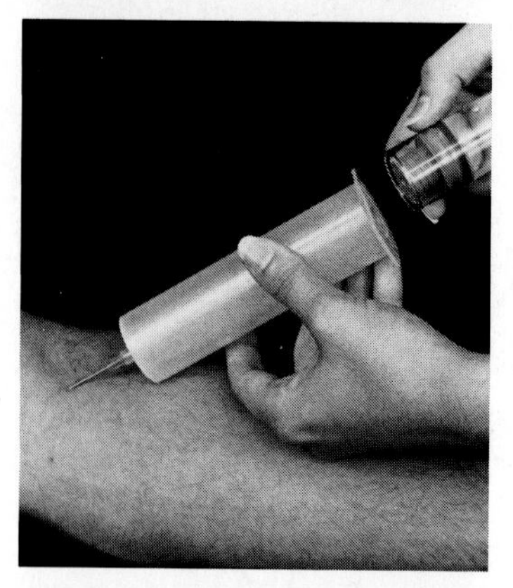

5 Suppose, after drug administration, the patient needs a second dose. Without removing the needle from his vein, remove the empty vial by unscrewing it in a *counter-clockwise* motion. Then, insert a new drug vial in the syringe barrel, following the same procedure described above. *Remember:* You can use only Bristoject vials made to fit this syringe.

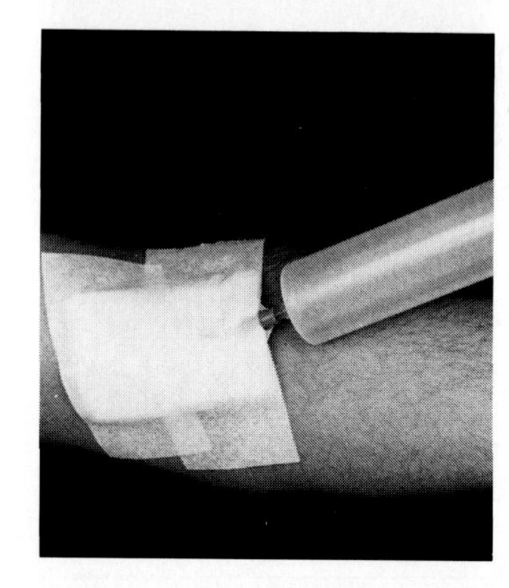

6 As an alternative, you can snap off the needle at the hub, and plug the syringe directly into a stopcock or I.V. catheter, as shown here. Or, you can attach a different-sized needle to the hub.

Using a Uni/Use syringe

To control your patient's generalized tonic-clonic seizure, the doctor orders phenytoin sodium (Dilantin*). If the drug is packaged in a Uni/Use syringe as shown here, proceed as follows:

- Without removing the needle guard, grasp the needle firmly between your fingers and push it toward the syringe. Doing so forces the needle base through the syringe's rubber stopper. *Note:* Don't remove and replace the needle guard before performing this step, or you'll be unable to puncture the stopper.
- When you're ready to give the drug, remove the needle guard and administer the drug, as ordered. *Important:* Don't reapply the needle guard before giving the drug. When you remove it the second time, you may unseat the needle base from the stopper.

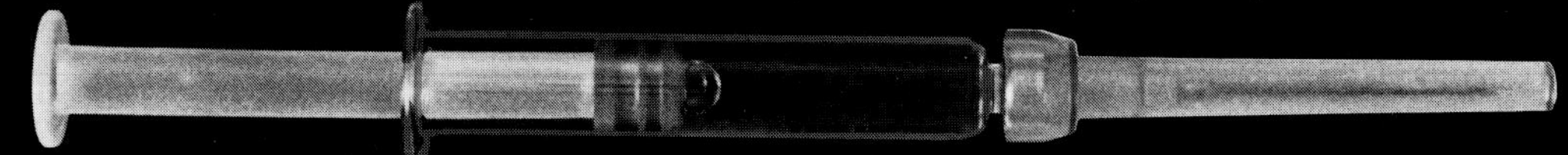

*Available in both the United States and Canada

Giving Xylocaine

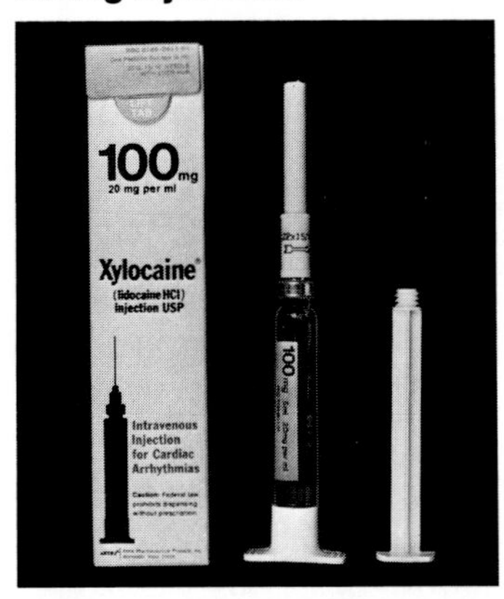

1 You're assisting at a code, when the doctor orders lidocaine hydrochloride (Xylocaine*). On your crash cart, the drug is packaged as shown here. Do you know how to assemble this equipment? Although the procedure's not difficult, you can easily become confused in an emergency. Be prepared by reviewing this photostory.

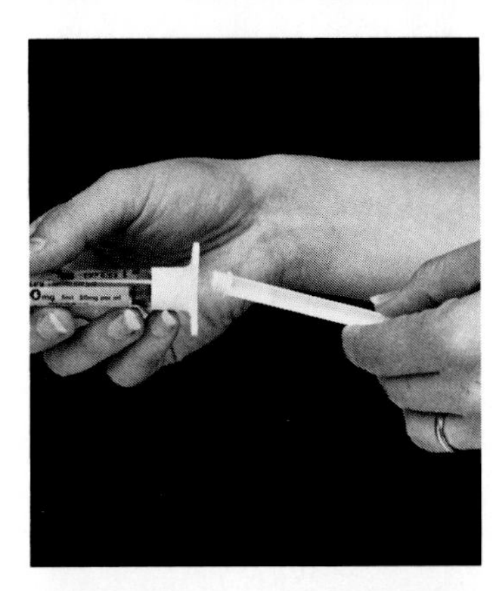

2 First, place the plastic plunger in the back of the syringe, as shown. Gently press and twist the plunger, until it's firmly in place.

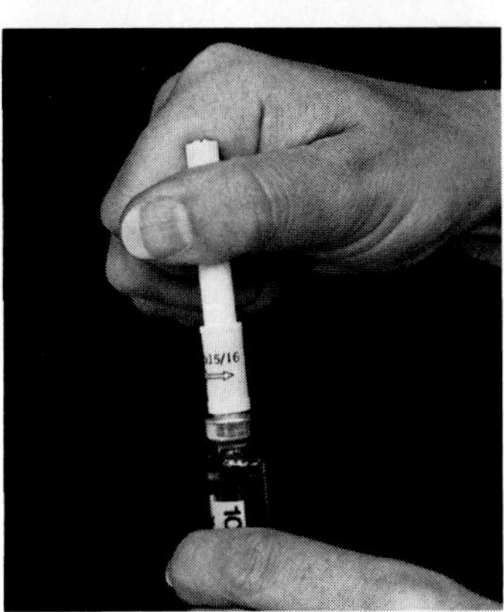

3 Just before giving the injection, turn the needle guard in the direction shown by the arrow on its side (see photo). You'll hear a snapping sound, indicating that the needle has been released from its storage position. When this happens, its base penetrates the syringe's rubber stopper, bringing the needle in contact with the drug.

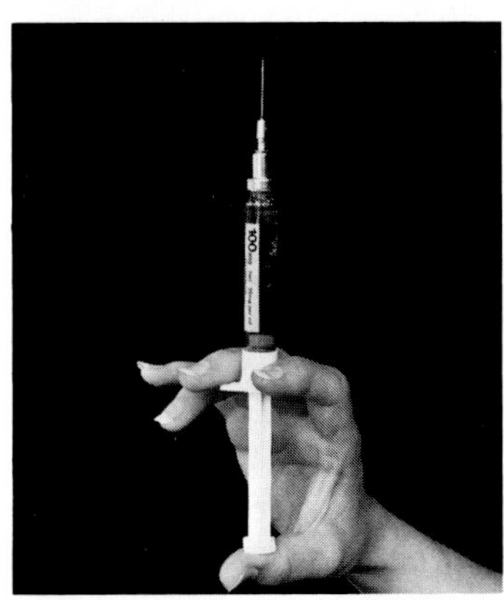

4 The syringe is now ready for use. Remove the needle guard, expel air, and give the drug, as ordered.

*Available in both the United States and Canada

Controlling I.V. flow rate

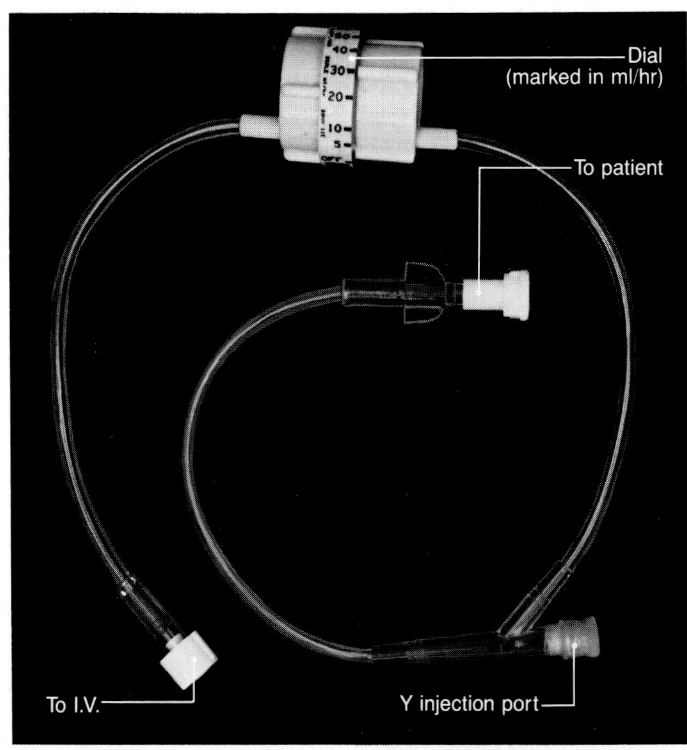

How can you minimize the risk of fluid overload for a patient who's undergoing I.V. therapy? An infusion pump's the most accurate and reliable way to regulate flow rate. But if a pump's not available, consider using an I.V. flow control device like the Sorenson Dial-A-Flo shown here. In the following photostory, you'll see how to use it.

The Dial-A-Flo has these advantages:

- It controls the I.V. infusion at a set rate, reducing the risk of fluid overload when adjusted correctly.
- It's designed for use on both microdrip and macrodrip delivery systems.
- You can use it to give many types of total parenteral nutrition (TPN) solutions or to maintain a keep-vein-open rate on an arterial line.
- You can use its Y injection port to monitor central venous pressure.

A limitation of this device is that it can't infuse blood products or highly viscous TPN solutions. Also, it's designed for use with short, large-gauge needles. A long, small-gauge needle or catheter reduces the I.V. flow rate, making the Dial-A-Flo inaccurate.

This device can help you maintain the ordered flow rate, but don't be lulled into a false sense of security by its use. Remember, it's just a piece of equipment. Continue to regularly monitor your patient's condition and the I.V. flow rate. (For detailed information on I.V. infusion pumps, see the NURSING PHOTOBOOK MANAGING I.V. THERAPY.)

Intravenous

Using a Dial-A-Flo device

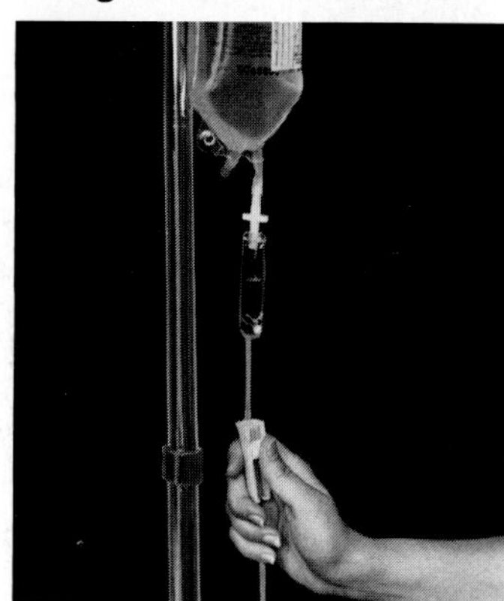

1 Attaching a Dial-A-Flo device to your patient's I.V. line? Make sure you use it correctly by reading this photostory.

After washing your hands, spike the I.V. container, prime the I.V. tubing, and close the flow clamp.

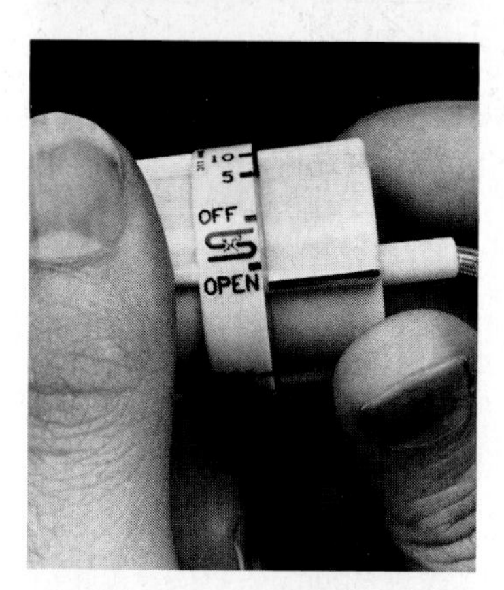

2 Remove the Dial-A-Flo device from its sterile wrapper. Firmly twist the device's dial until it moves freely. Leave the dial in *open* position, as shown.

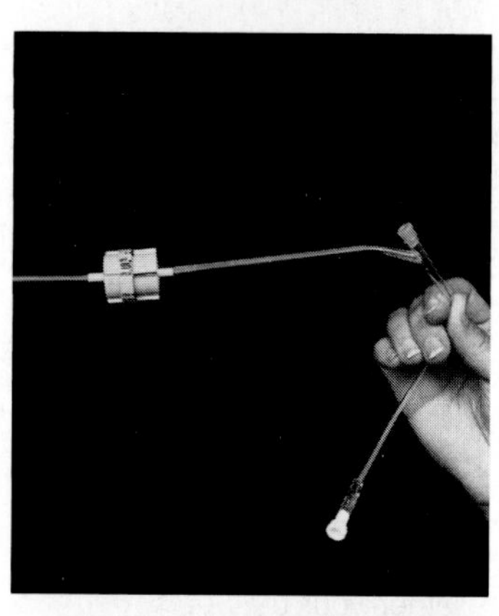

3 Connect the device to the I.V. tubing, so the dial is between the I.V. container and the device's Y injection port. *Note:* To ensure the device's accuracy, don't connect I.V. extension tubing between the device and the container.

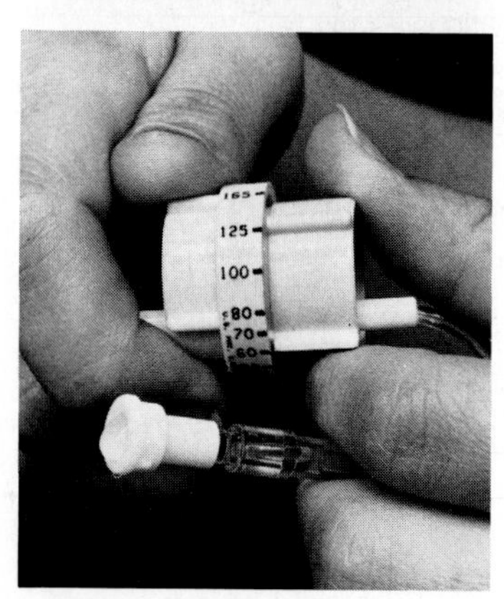

4 Prepare to flush air from the device by positioning its free end over a wastebasket. (Because the cap is perforated, you needn't remove it for flushing.)

Now, fully open the infusion line flow clamp. Turn the device's dial from *open* to *off;* then, turn it back to *open.* When all air's expelled, turn the dial to *off.*

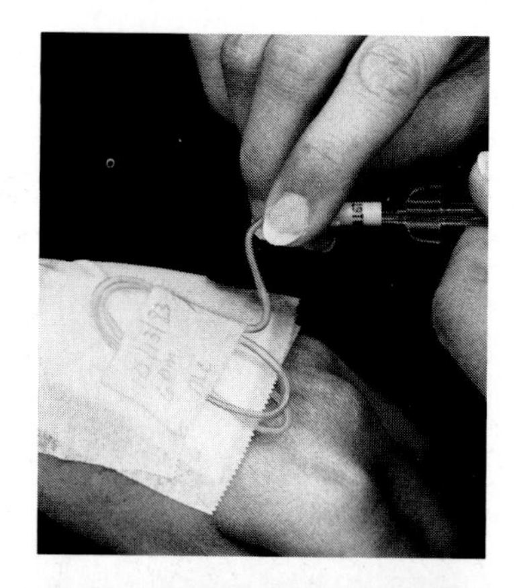

5 Connect the device's free end to the patient's I.V. catheter or needle. Position the I.V. container 30″ (76.2 cm) above the insertion site. *Note:* The manufacturer's package insert measures 30″, to help you position the container at the correct height.

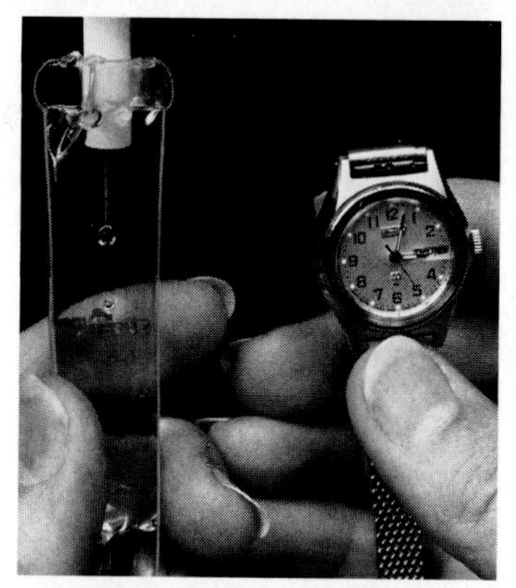

6 Set the device's dial at *60 ml/hour* and count how many drops enter the drip chamber for 1 minute.

If the device is calibrated to the infusion line's drip chamber, the number of drops you count per minute will equal the number of drops per milliliter the drip chamber delivers. For example, if 10 drops equal one milliliter, you should count 10 drops per minute.

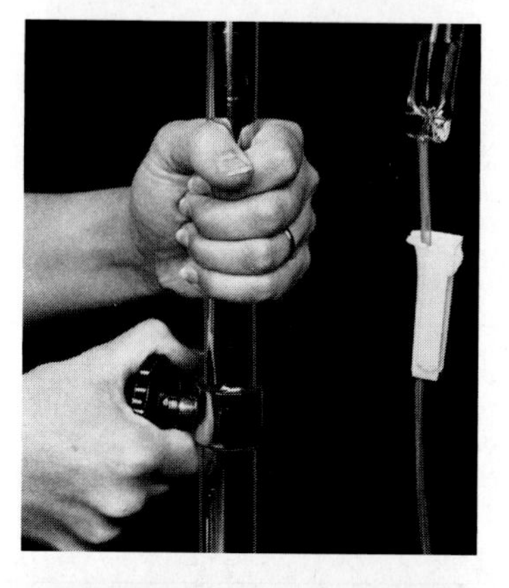

7 Suppose your equipment isn't calibrated. If the flow rate is too fast, lower the I.V. container. If it's too slow, raise the container. When the number of drops per minute equals the number of drops per milliliter for that drip chamber, the device is calibrated to the drip chamber.

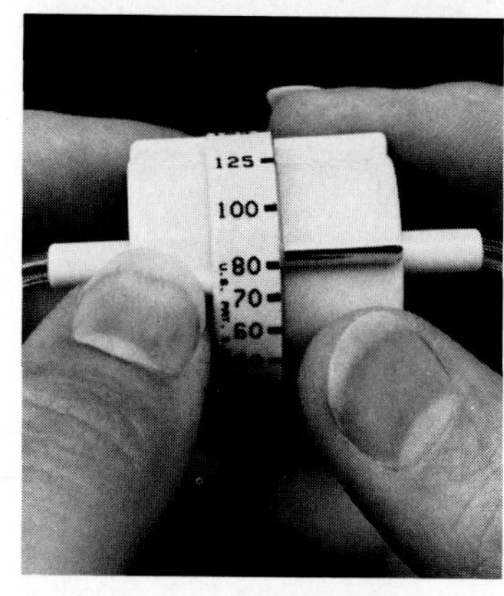

8 Now, turn the device's dial to the number corresponding to the ordered infusion rate. *Remember:* The numbers on the dial indicate milliliters per hour, *not* drops per minute.

Periodically check the infusion rate. It may slow as the container empties. Recalibrate the device if the distance between the insertion site and the container changes. *Caution:* Never leave the dial at or near the *open* position.

Learning about the Hickman catheter

Frank Betz, a 21-year-old college student, recently learned that he has acute myelogenous leukemia. His doctor has recommended insertion of a Hickman catheter to facilitate long-term treatment. Upset by the diagnosis, Frank didn't understand everything the doctor told him about the catheter. Now, he wants to know more. Do you know enough about the Hickman catheter to answer his questions? The information on these pages will help.

As you probably know, the Hickman catheter is a long-term, indwelling I.V. catheter. Although you may be more familiar with the single-lumen type, double-lumen catheters are also available for patients who need large quantities of total parenteral nutrition (TPN) solution or cancer chemotherapy; for example, with doxorubicin hydrochloride (Adriamycin*).

After insertion, the catheter's proximal end rests in the patient's right atrium, as illustrated at right, or in the lower end of his superior vena cava. Its distal end exits from a surgically created subcutaneous tunnel that anchors the catheter and protects the patient from infection.

Its advantages? When maintained properly, the Hickman catheter carries fewer infection risks than other long-term indwelling I.V. catheters. A patient like Frank can receive long-term, intermittent chemotherapy without undergoing repeated venipuncture. Between treatments, he can return home and care for the catheter himself. He'll find that the catheter places almost no restrictions on normal activity.

A Hickman catheter can be inserted in a patient of any size or age and is especially helpful for a patient with poor vascular status, for whom venipuncture is unusually painful. Also, by using a Hickman catheter, a patient who needs TPN (for example, because of Crohn's disease) but who doesn't require hospitalization may care for himself at home.

Besides being used to administer TPN and intermittent chemotherapy, a Hickman catheter can be used to:

- give blood products
- administer medication and I.V. therapy
- perform plasmapheresis or collect blood specimens
- monitor central venous pressure.

Understanding catheter insertion

Most likely, Frank has questions about catheter insertion. Tell him the doctor will probably give him a local anesthetic and that the procedure takes about 1 hour. (If the patient's a child or infant, the doctor performs the procedure with a general anesthetic.) Here's what happens:

If the doctor's chosen to insert the catheter through the cephalic vein (the usual insertion site), he makes an incision in the deltopectoral groove and isolates the vein. Then, he uses long forceps to make a subcutaneous tunnel from the cephalic vein to a predetermined exit point—probably the anterior chest wall, just above the nipple line. After making a small incision at the tunnel's end, he pulls the catheter's distal end through the tunnel.

This part of the catheter has a feltlike polyester cuff around it. In several days, fibrous tissue will attach the cuff to the tunnel walls. Along with the tunnel itself, this tissue growth acts as a barrier to infection. *Note:* Some catheters have two cuffs.

Next, the doctor inserts the catheter's proximal end into the cephalic vein. Using fluoroscopy as a guide, he advances the catheter tip into the lower end of the superior vena cava or all the way into the right atrium (see illustration). Then, he closes the incision at the deltopectoral groove and sutures the catheter's distal end in place at the end of the tunnel. To control bleeding, he applies pressure bandages over each incision.

After catheter insertion, he may immediately begin an I.V. infusion. Or, he may fill the catheter with heparinized solution and apply a heparin injection Luer-Lok cap. For safety, he places a piece of tape around the catheter and a guarded or toothless clamp over it. The clamp prevents air embolism if the cap's dislodged. By using a smooth clamp and protecting the catheter with tape, the doctor reduces the risk of severing the catheter.

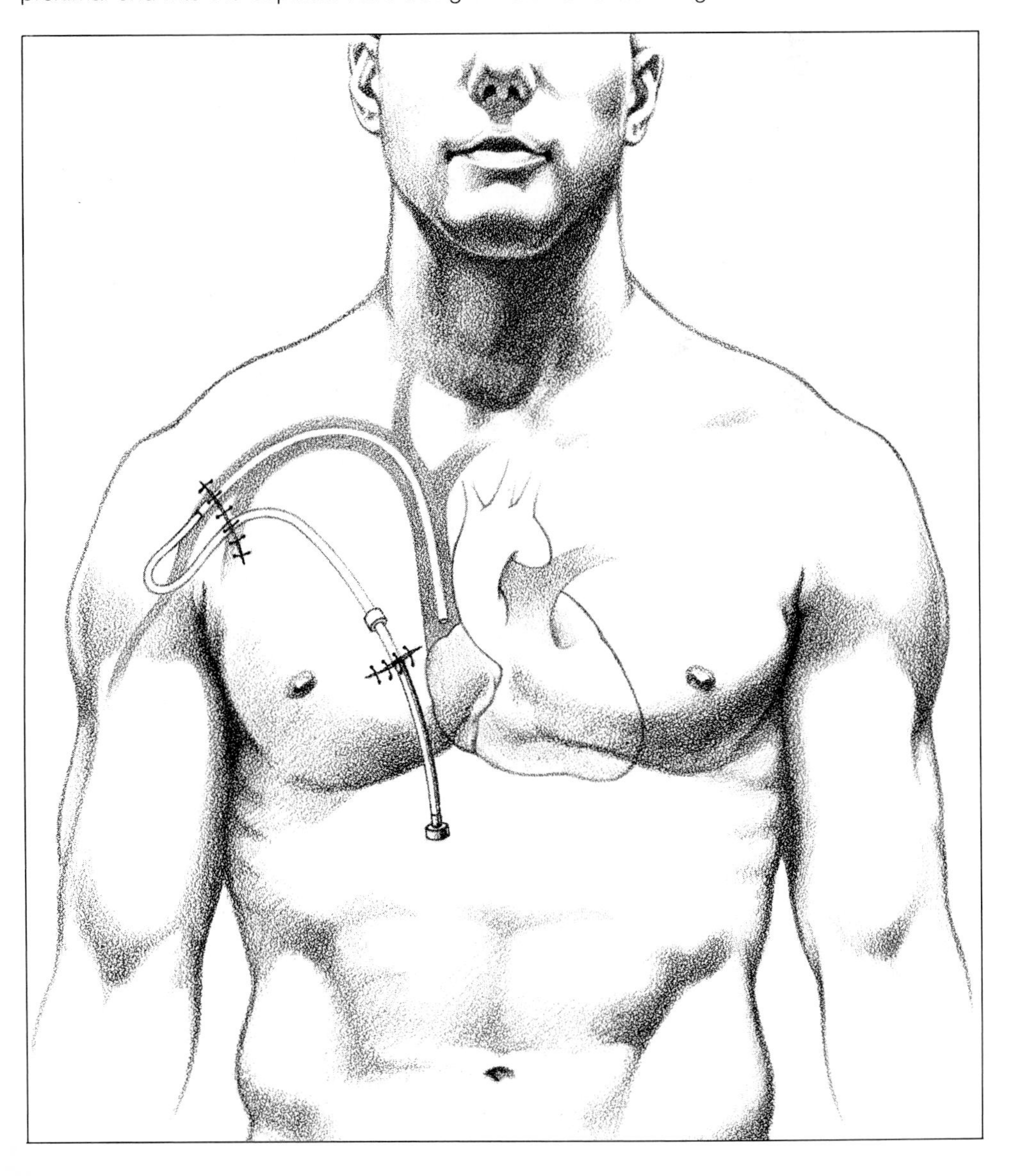

*Available in both the United States and Canada

Intravenous

Learning about the Hickman catheter continued

Alternate insertion sites

If for some reason the doctor can't use the patient's cephalic vein as an insertion site, he can choose from many other veins; for example, an internal or external jugular, common facial, or brachial vein. If the patient's superior vena cava is obstructed (as in superior vena cava syndrome, for example), the doctor can introduce the catheter into a femoral vein and feed it up the inferior vena cava to the right atrium, as illustrated at right. The catheter tunnel exits at the abdomen rather than the chest.

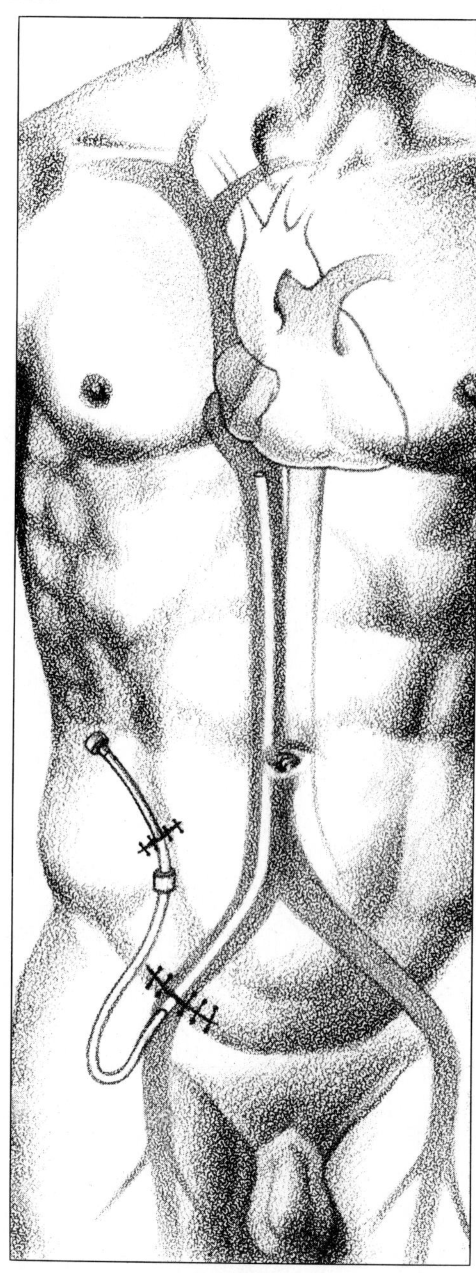

Care guidelines

If you're caring for a patient with a Hickman catheter in place, your responsibilities include the following:

- When your patient returns to his room after catheter insertion, remove the two pressure bandages and cleanse each site with hydrogen peroxide. Thoroughly rinse the sites with sterile normal saline solution or water. Then, apply antimicrobial ointment and tape sterile gauze pads over the incisions. *Important:* Use aseptic technique for dressing changes.
- Change the dressings daily (or more often if they become soiled), following the procedure described above. Examine the sites for redness, swelling, or discharge, and document your observations. Notify the doctor of any abnormalities.
- Discontinue dressing the deltopectoral incision after it heals (or as ordered), but continue dressing the catheter exit site for as long as the catheter's in place. After the incision heals, change the dressing every 3 days, or immediately if it becomes wet or soiled. *Remember:* Changing the dressing more often than necessary invites infection.
- If the patient's not receiving a continuous I.V. infusion, routinely flush the catheter with 6 to 8 ml of heparinized solution (100 units of heparin per 1 ml of normal saline solution) at least once a day to prevent clotting. While injecting the last 0.5 ml, reapply the clamp to the catheter. This measure ensures positive pressure in the catheter, preventing backflow.
- In addition, flush the catheter with heparinized solution after each use; for example, after medication injection or blood aspiration. This prevents sedimentation in the catheter that can cause catheter blockage. *Important:* If you're administering two drugs or other fluids at the same time, one after the other, take care to flush the line before and after giving the second fluid.
- Secure the catheter's distal end by wrapping it with a sterile gauze pad and taping it to the exit site dressing. Or, wrap tape around it and pin the tape tab to the patient's underclothing.
- If the patient's receiving a continuous I.V. infusion, heparinize the I.V. solution, as ordered. If you aspirate blood from the catheter, flush the catheter with normal saline solution before resuming the infusion.
- Replace the catheter cap every 2 weeks, or as needed. (Frequent punctures may weaken the cap or create nonsealing holes.)
- Protect the catheter from damage by using only smooth, toothless clamps or guarded hemostats. To avoid weakening the catheter, change the position of the clamp and protective tape once a day.

Patient teaching

Will your patient leave the hospital with a Hickman catheter in place? Begin patient teaching as soon as possible. You'll need at least 4 days to familiarize him and his family with care techniques they'll use at home. Begin by encouraging the patient to help with flushing and dressing changes; gradually, he should assume full responsibility. Stress the importance of performing routine care faithfully; failure to do so may result in an infection or other complication. (Teach him how to recognize the signs and symptoms of infection. Urge him to contact his doctor if he suspects an infection.) Beginning on page 89, we provide a home care aid to help reinforce your teaching.

Dealing with complications

Although the Hickman catheter minimizes the risk, complications *can* happen. An immunosuppressed patient, for example, may develop an infection despite the best nursing care.

But an infection doesn't necessarily mean the catheter must be removed. If the patient has no other complications, the doctor may treat the infection with the catheter in place. If so, collect specimens for culture and begin antibiotic therapy, as ordered. Catheter removal is indicated if subsequent cultures are positive or if the doctor suspects that the catheter is the infection source.

Air embolism is an unlikely complication, especially if you've taken appropriate precautions; for example, keeping a clamp on the catheter at all times and taping the catheter cap. If the cap does become dislodged and the catheter's unclamped, negative pressure generated by the central veins may pull air into the patient's vein. If this emergency occurs, follow these steps:

- Call for help.
- Place the patient on his left side. If the embolus has reached the heart, this position helps keep the air in the right atrium, near the superior vena cava.
- Attach a syringe to the catheter and aspirate blood. This maneuver may suck out the embolus.
- Keep the patient calm and still until help arrives.

Important: If your patient's receiving an infusion, thoroughly flush all infusion lines before use, and make sure all connections are secure. *Never* permit the I.V. container to run dry.

For more details on using a Hickman catheter, read the following photostories and the troubleshooting chart featured on page 88.

Collecting a blood specimen with a Hickman catheter

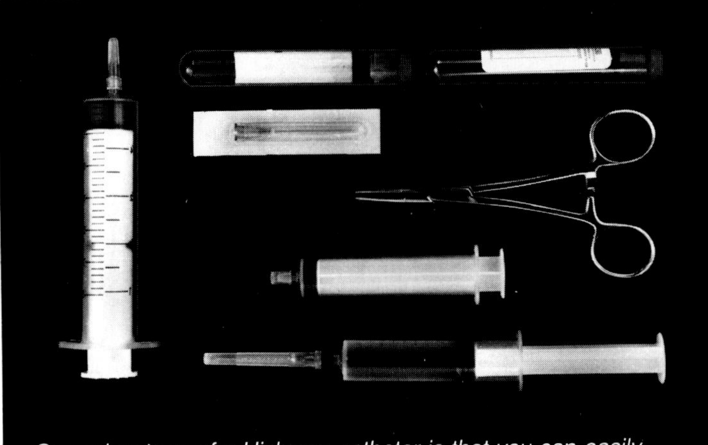

One advantage of a Hickman catheter is that you can easily collect blood specimens through it. Here's how.

First, find out which blood studies the doctor's ordered. Then, check your hospital lab manual to learn how many collection tubes you'll need, what size they should be, and what color tops they should have. We'll assume you need the equipment shown here: two red-top Vacutainer collection tubes, 30-ml syringe, large-gauge (19G) needle, empty 6-ml syringe, 6-ml syringe filled with heparinized solution, and guarded or toothless clamp. (If your patient will receive an I.V. infusion through the catheter immediately after specimen withdrawal, flush the catheter with 6 ml of normal saline solution.) Thoroughly wash your hands.

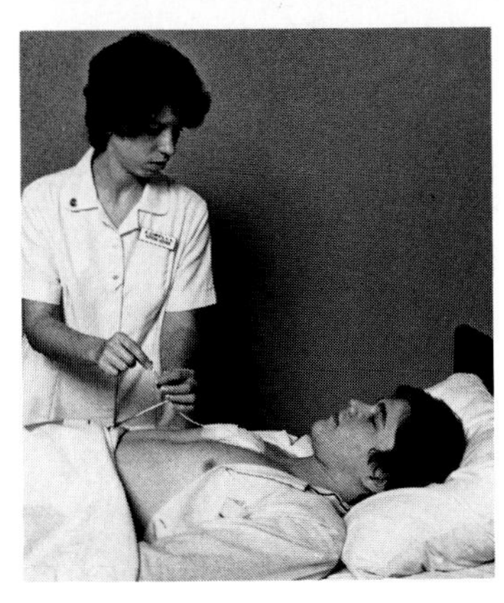

1 Explain the procedure to your patient. To minimize the risk of air embolism, caution him *not* to take deep breaths during the procedure. Then, clamp the catheter (if it's not already clamped) and remove the catheter's cap. (If the patient's receiving an infusion, stop the infusion pump, clamp the catheter, and disconnect the infusion line.)

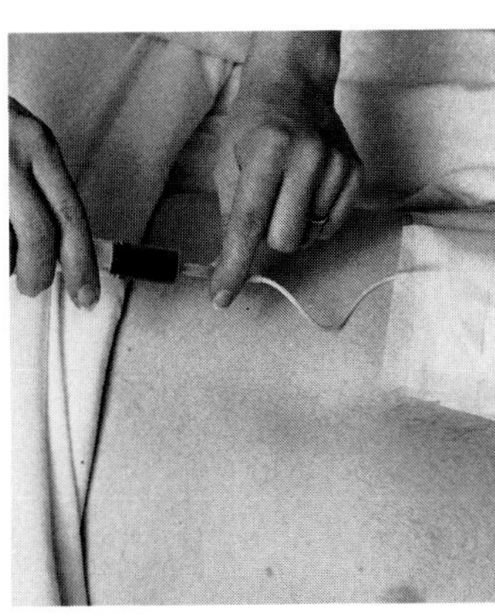

2 Connect the empty 6-ml syringe to the catheter, remove the clamp, and aspirate 6 ml of fluid (heparinized flush or I.V. solution and blood) from the catheter. Reclamp the catheter and remove the syringe. To ensure an undiluted specimen, discard this syringe, and prepare to aspirate a second specimen.

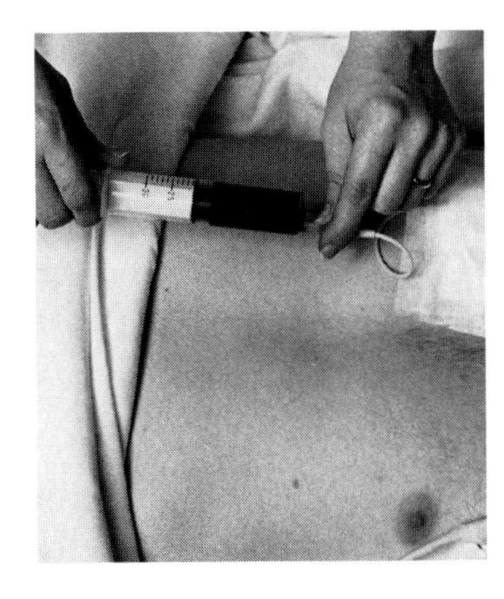

3 To do so, connect the 30-ml syringe to the catheter. Unclamp the catheter and aspirate the specimen, using a gentle, steady motion. After collecting the specimen, reclamp the catheter and remove the syringe.

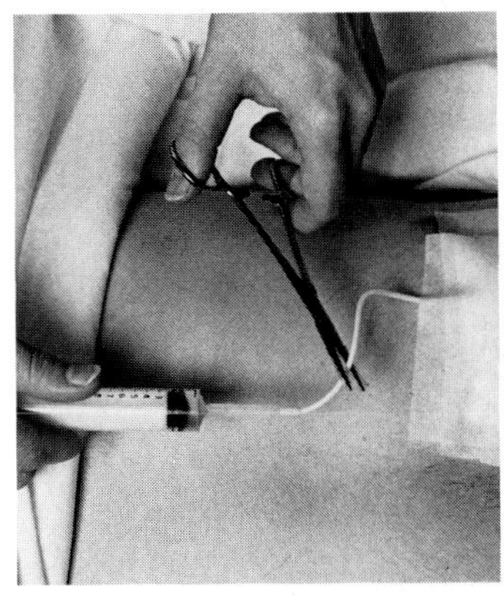

4 Next, remove the needle on the syringe filled with flush solution. Attach the syringe to the catheter, remove the clamp, and flush the catheter. To ensure positive pressure, reapply the clamp as you inject the last 0.5 ml of flush solution, as shown. This prevents backflow and blood clotting.

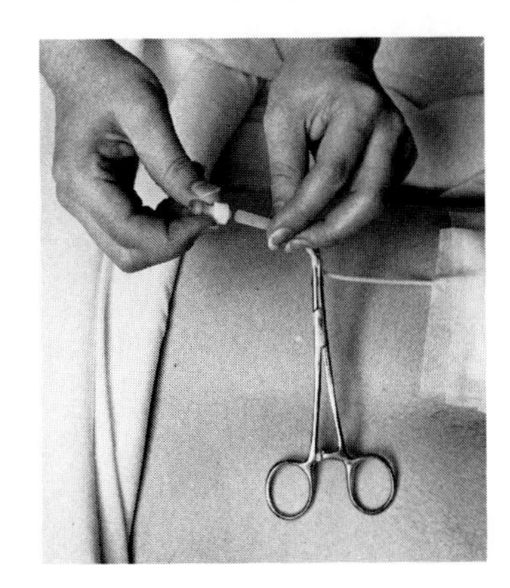

5 Replace the catheter's cap. Or, if your patient's receiving an infusion, reconnect the infusion line and remove the clamp. *Caution:* To prevent air embolism, make sure the entire infusion line is air-free and that all connections are secure. To prevent clotting in the catheter, ensure adequate I.V. flow rate with an infusion pump.

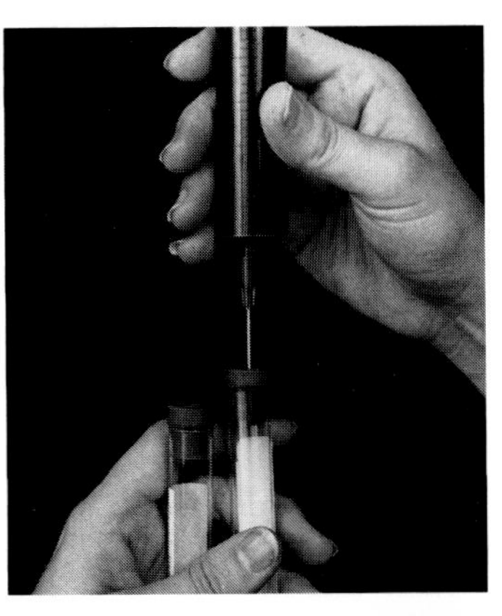

6 Using the 19G needle, transfer the specimen to labeled collection tubes, as shown here. Then, fill out the necessary lab slips, and send the specimens and slips to the lab at once.

If your patient's not receiving an infusion, tape the catheter securely to his chest, as illustrated in the home care aid beginning on page 89. Finally, document the procedure.

Intravenous

Troubleshooting Hickman catheter problems

When caring for a patient with a Hickman catheter in place, you may encounter one of the following problems. Study this chart to learn how to deal with it.

Clot or other blockage in catheter

Possible cause

- Failure to routinely flush catheter with heparinized solution
- Failure to flush catheter after a drug infusion or between infusions of incompatible drugs
- Switching off infusion pump (if one's in use) for an extended period or running an infusion too slowly

What to do

- Notify the doctor. *Important:* Don't attempt to irrigate a blocked catheter, unless directed by the doctor and hospital policy.
- Fill the catheter with no more than 2 ml of 1,000 units of heparin and temporarily apply *gentle* pressure; this may *loosen* the clot. *Important:* Don't apply too much pressure; you may rupture the catheter or cause a thromboembolism.
- Attempt to aspirate the clot with a 5- or 10-ml syringe.
- After aspirating the clot, flush the catheter with heparin.
- If you can't aspirate the clot, fill the catheter with 5,000 units of urokinase (Abbokinase, Breokinase), as ordered. Clamp the catheter and wait 15 to 30 minutes. (You may wait up to 4 hours for a stubborn clot to loosen.) Then, attempt to aspirate the clot. Repeat several times, if necessary.
- If precipitates from incompatible drugs have formed a solid plug in the catheter, the doctor may remove the catheter and clear it mechanically.

Difficulty aspirating blood but no difficulty giving infusions

Possible cause

- Catheter tip resting against atrium wall
- Fibrinous sheath grown around catheter tip, producing a ball-valve effect (especially likely if the patient has active cancer)

What to do

- Flush with heparinized solution. This may jar the tip free from the atrium wall.
- Use *less* pressure to aspirate blood. If the catheter's tip is jammed against the atrium wall, this may help free it.
- Ask the patient to change position, raise one or both arms, take a deep breath, or cough. These actions may also help free the catheter tip. *Note:* Unless contraindicated, you may also try lowering the patient's head and chest.
- If these steps don't work, notify the doctor. Prepare the patient for fluoroscopy to locate the catheter tip.
- If fluoroscopy indicates that the catheter's placed correctly, suspect a fibrinous sheath over the catheter tip. If ordered, inject 5,000 units of urokinase into the catheter and clamp the catheter. After 15 minutes, aspirate the urokinase. *Important:* During and after urokinase administration, monitor the patient for signs of anaphylaxis and bleeding disorders.
- If the catheter's still not patent, the doctor may have to remove the internal part of the catheter and clear it mechanically.

Tear in catheter's external portion

Possible cause

- Using clamps with teeth or prongs
- Failure to protect clamped portions of catheter with a strip of tape
- Accidental puncture with scissors or needle

What to do

- If the tear occurs more than 1½" (4 cm) from the chest wall, clamp the catheter close to the chest wall and insert a 14G indwelling I.V. catheter into the Hickman catheter. Remove the I.V. catheter's stylus, and tape the I.V. catheter securely to the Hickman catheter. Remove the clamp, flush with heparin, and cap the I.V. catheter. Then, reapply the clamp as close as possible to the chest wall. Notify the doctor and obtain a Hickman catheter repair kit. *Note:* You may insert a blunt needle instead of an I.V. catheter.
- If the tear is less than 1½" from the chest wall, clamp the catheter between the tear and the chest wall. Notify the doctor and prepare the patient for catheter replacement.

How to remove a Hickman catheter

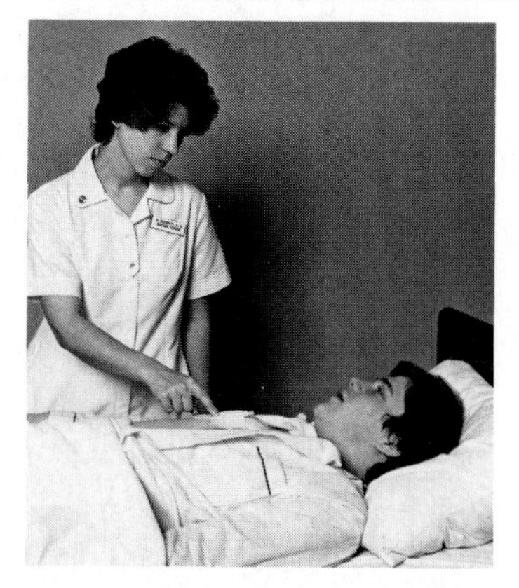

1 Is Hickman catheter removal a nursing responsibility in your hospital? If so, make sure you're familiar with the procedure by reviewing this photostory.

First, explain the procedure to your patient. Assure him that it's not painful, although he may feel a slight burning sensation. *Note:* If he's extremely anxious, give an antianxiety medication, as ordered.

Thoroughly wash and dry your hands.

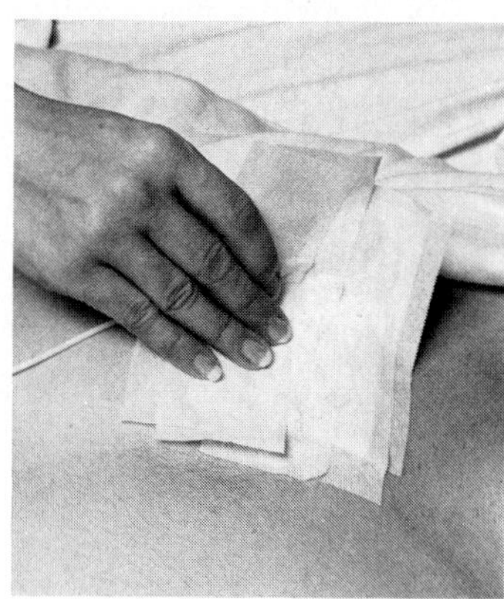

2 Now, remove the dressing over the exit site, as well as the gauze wrapping around the cap. Cleanse the site with hydrogen peroxide.

3 Wrap the catheter around your fingers, as shown, and stretch it with a firm, steady pressure. (Don't jerk it, or it may break.) After 2 or 3 minutes, the fibrous tissue around the catheter cuff will loosen, allowing the catheter to slide free. Pull it out with firm, constant pressure. Wrap it around your hand as it emerges.

If the catheter breaks, clamp it (if possible), apply pressure dressings, and notify the doctor, who'll remove it surgically.

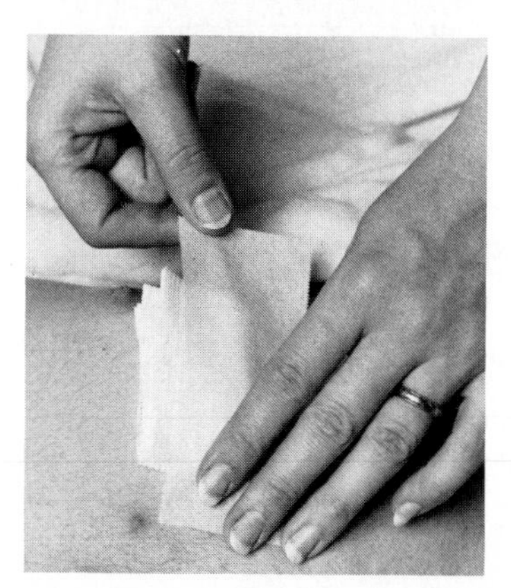

4 After catheter removal, some bleeding may occur at the exit site. Cleanse the site and apply a dressing. Chances are, you can remove the dressing in a day or two. Document the procedure. *Note:* The cuff may remain imbedded in the subcutaneous tunnel. If so, document this. The doctor probably won't remove the cuff unless an infection develops.

Home care

Caring for your Hickman catheter

Dear Patient:

Going home with a Hickman catheter in place? Make sure home care is trouble-free by following the simple—but important—instructions your nurse has given you. This home care aid will help you remember what you've learned. Keep these guidelines in mind:

- Routinely check the catheter for breaks, such as a nick or tear. If you see a break, immediately apply a clamp between the break and your chest and call the doctor.
- Whenever you change your dressing, carefully examine the skin around the catheter. Call the doctor at once if you see any sign of infection; for example, redness, soreness, swelling, or pus. Also call him if you develop a fever.
- Keep the dressing dry. When taking a shower, for instance, tape a plastic bag over the dressing to protect it. If the dressing gets wet, replace it immediately.
- Avoid wearing long necklaces that may become entangled in the catheter. Also, be careful when wearing shirts or tops that zip up in the front.
- If you have a baby, take precautions when holding him, so he doesn't pull or bump the catheter.

Flushing the catheter

To prevent blood clots from forming in the catheter, take care to flush the catheter at least once a day by injecting heparin solution into it. The following directions and illustrations will remind you what to do.

1

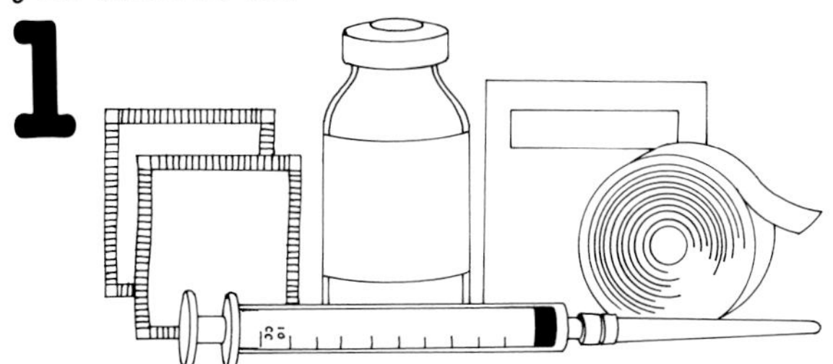

First, gather this equipment: bottle of heparin solution (as recommended by your doctor), disposable 10-ml syringe with needle (the needle's protected with a plastic needle guard), two povidone-iodine swabs, 4″ × 4″ gauze pad, and tape. *Remember:* To prevent infection, always use sterile equipment.

2

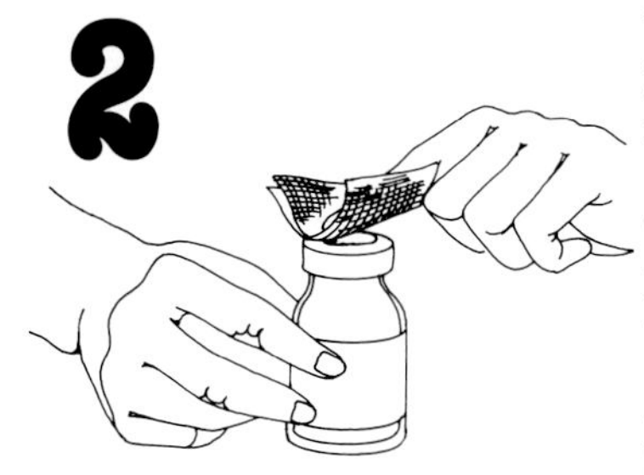

Wash and dry your hands. If necessary, remove the protective cap on the heparin solution bottle. Using a povidone-iodine swab, wipe the bottle top. (Don't touch the top after you've cleaned it.) Dispose of the swab.

3

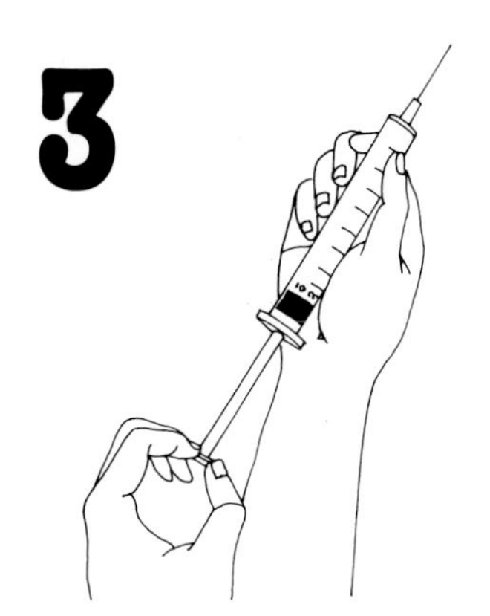

Remove the needle guard, and pull back the syringe plunger until the top of its rubber stopper meets the 10-ml line on the syringe, as shown here. By doing so, you draw air into the syringe. Then, insert the needle into the bottle top, and push down on the plunger to inject the air into the bottle.

4

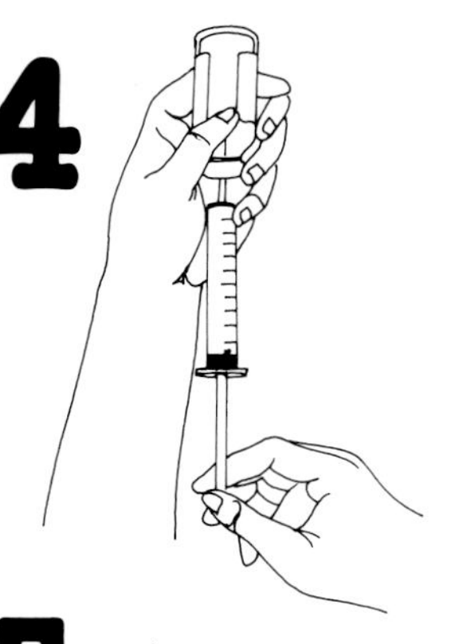

Turn the equipment upside down, as shown here, and pull back on the syringe plunger to fill the syringe with solution. Remove the needle from the bottle, and replace the needle guard to keep the needle clean until you're ready to use it.

5

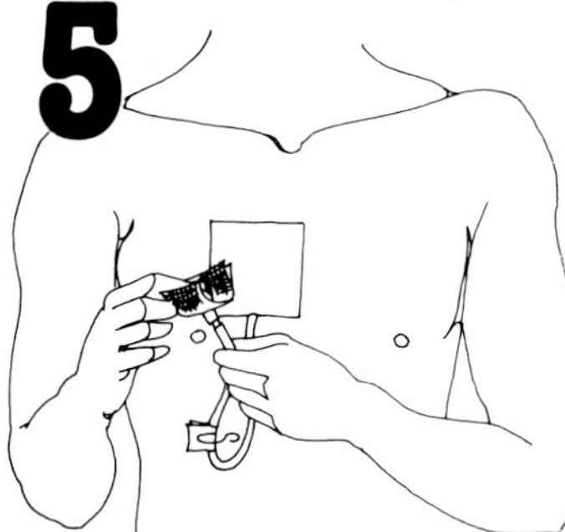

Now, remove and discard the gauze pad protecting your catheter cap. Using a clean povidone-iodine swab, wipe the top of the catheter cap. Discard the swab and wait for the cap to air-dry. (Don't let anything touch the catheter cap after you've cleaned it.)

Intravenous

Home care

Caring for your Hickman catheter continued

6

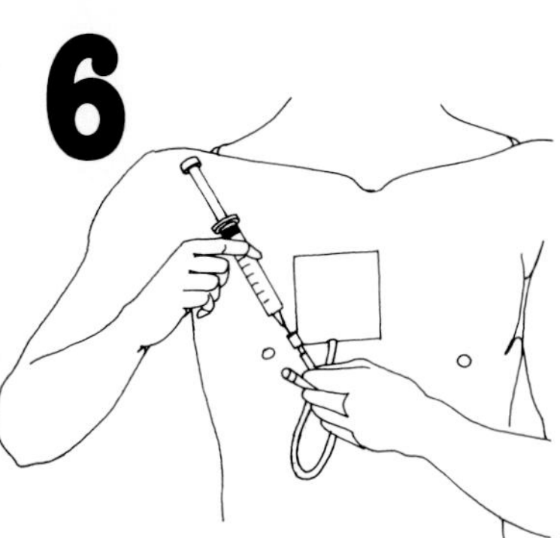

When the catheter cap's dry, remove your catheter's clamp. Then remove the needle guard and insert the needle into the cap, as shown. (Take care not to puncture the catheter with the needle.) Slowly and steadily press the syringe plunger until you've injected 8 ml of solution into the catheter. To prevent blood from backing up into the catheter, leave 2 ml of solution in the syringe. Withdraw the needle from the cap, replace the clamp, and discard the needle and syringe. *Remember:* Protect your catheter by applying a strip of tape under the clamp. Also, to avoid weakening the catheter, clamp it at a different place each time.

7

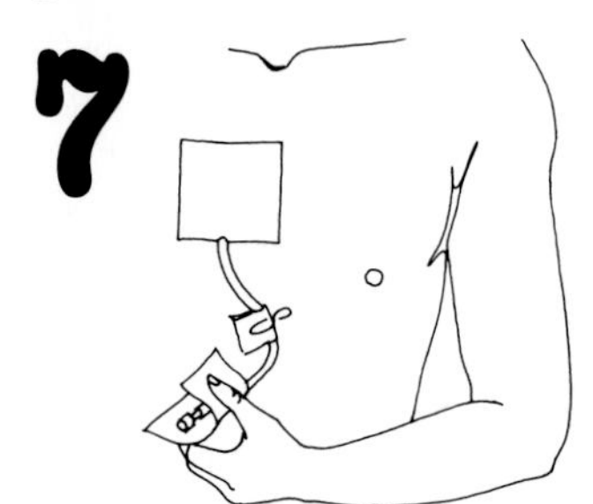

Now, prepare to reapply a gauze pad to your catheter cap to keep it clean. First, tear four strips of tape. Then, fold the sterile gauze pad around the cap, as shown here.

8

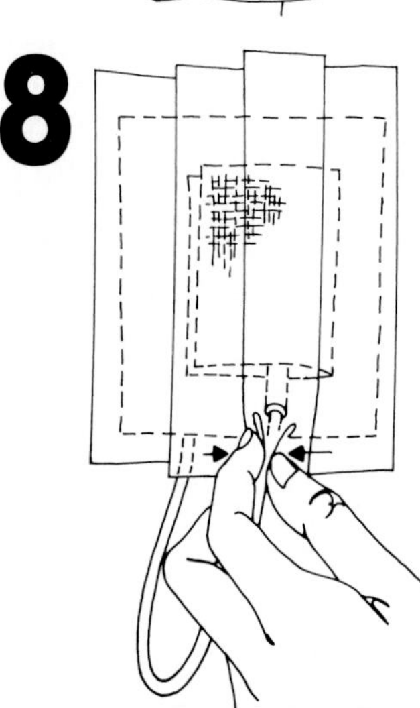

After wrapping the catheter cap, lay it against the dressing over the catheter exit site. Use the four strips of tape to secure the pad to the dressing. To keep the catheter cap from slipping out the bottom, pinch a strip of tape around it, as shown here.

Changing your dressing

At home, you'll change the dressing over the catheter's exit site every 3 days (or whenever it becomes wet or dirty). Follow the steps illustrated here.

1

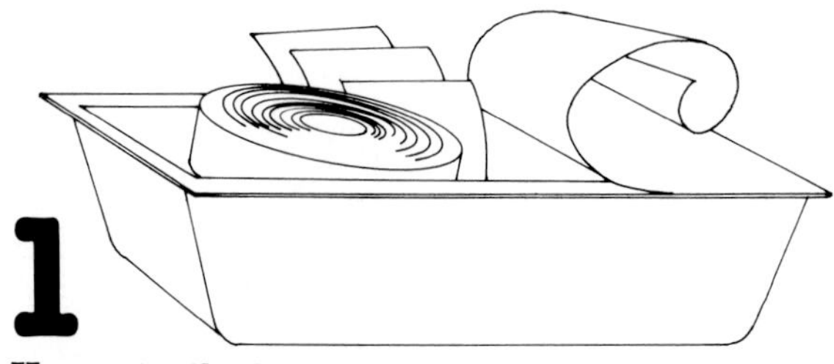

Use a sterile dressing change kit that includes gloves, four acetone-alcohol swabs, three povidone-iodine swabs, povidone-iodine ointment, gauze pads, tincture of benzoin, adhesive bandage, tape, and scissors.

2

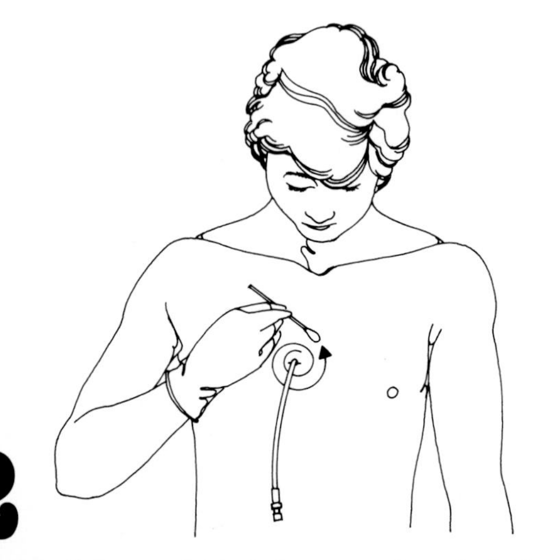

Thoroughly wash and dry your hands before beginning. Then, remove and discard the old dressing. Open the kit and put on the sterile gloves. (Keep them sterile by using the special technique the nurse showed you at the hospital.) Using an acetone-alcohol swab, cleanse the ointment and adhesive from the skin surrounding the catheter. To do so, begin near the catheter and work outward; then, dispose of the swab. Repeat this procedure as necessary, using a clean swab each time.

3 Now, cleanse your skin with a povidone-iodine swab, using the same motion. Discard the swab. Do this two more times, using a clean swab each time.

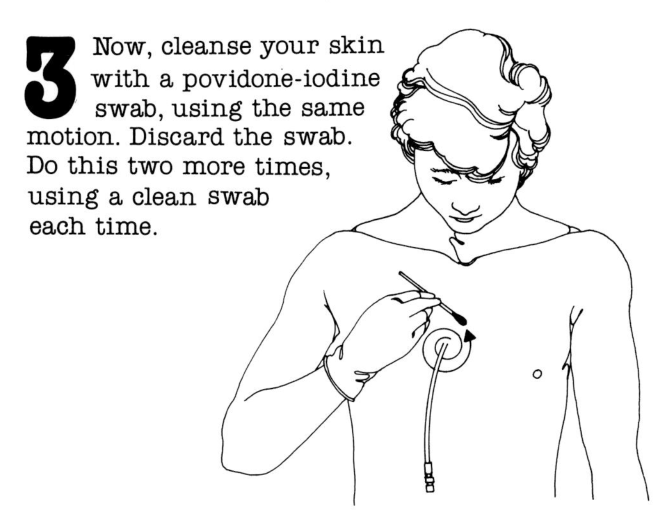

4 Squeeze povidone-iodine ointment onto a gauze pad, as shown here.

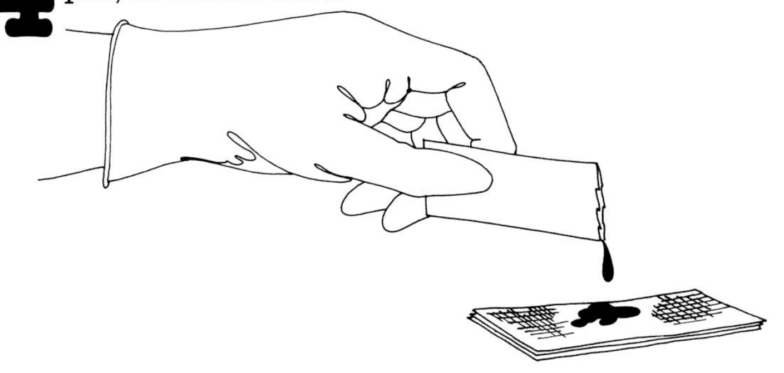

5 Using the sterile scissors, cut the adhesive bandage so it's large enough to overlap the gauze pad by ½″ (1.3 cm) on all sides.

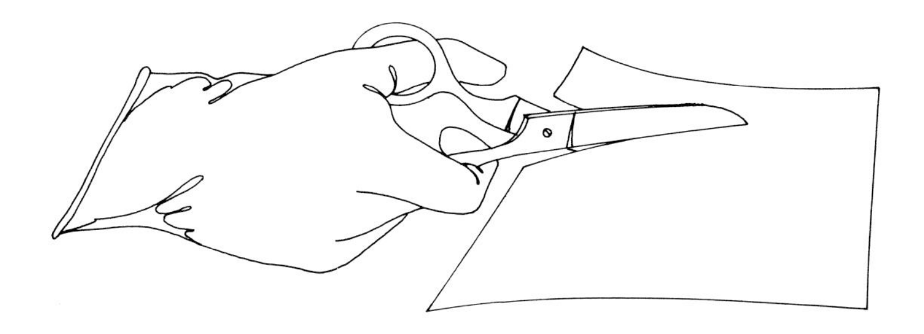

6 Now, put the gauze pad over the catheter exit site and hold it in place with one hand. Then, wipe tincture of benzoin on the skin alongside the gauze pad's edges. (This helps the adhesive bandage stick to your skin.) Let your skin air-dry for a few seconds.

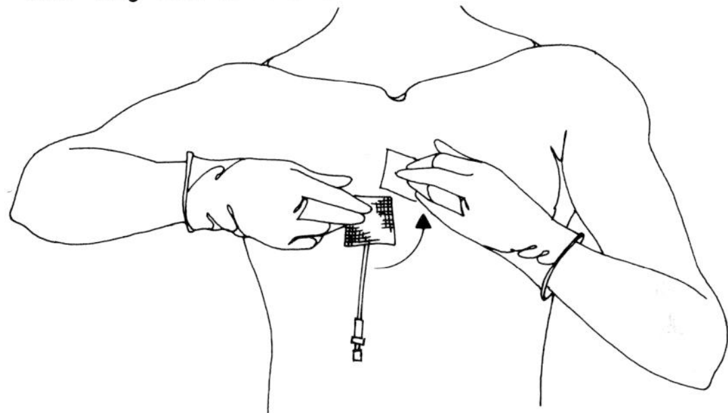

7 Next, peel off the adhesive bandage's backing. Apply the bandage over the gauze pad, so the bandage's edges stick to your skin.

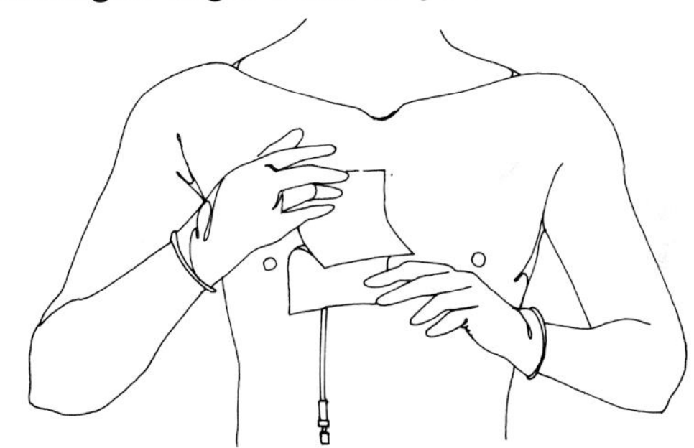

8 For extra security, tape the adhesive bandage's edges to your skin, as shown. Pinch the tape along the lower edge around the catheter.

Wrap the catheter cap in a sterile gauze pad and tape the cap on top of the dressing, as you'd do after flushing the catheter. Finally, remove your gloves, reapply the clamp, and dispose of all used equipment.

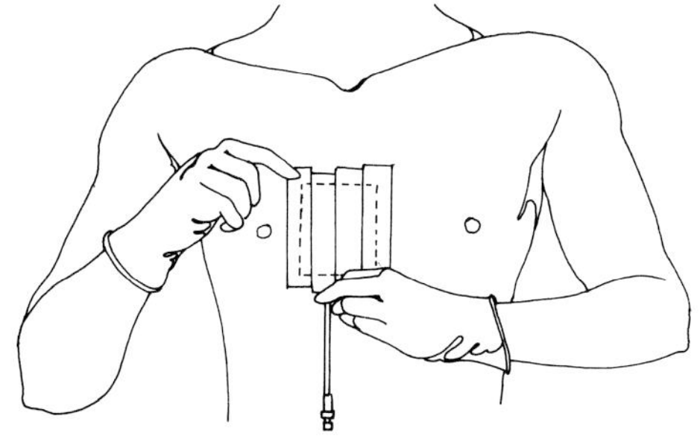

Intravenous

SPECIAL CONSIDERATIONS

When your patient needs TPN

Suppose your patient will be receiving home total parenteral nutrition (TPN) through his Hickman catheter. In addition to basic catheter care, you must teach him all he needs to know about giving himself TPN therapy.

At first, the prospect of TPN self-administration may seem overwhelming to him—after all, he has a lot to learn. This is why you'll begin active teaching long before he leaves the hospital. And because he'll probably need help when he returns home, you'll include his family in the teaching, too.

At first, let the patient and his family watch you as you perform the procedure. Explain everything you're doing and why as you go along. Encourage them to assume more responsibility as you continue to supervise them. For reminders of what to teach, see the checklist at right.

Before your patient leaves the hospital, give him a copy of the home care aid beginning on the next page; he can use it as a guide.

Infusion pump reminders

To give the patient freedom during the day, TPN therapy will probably be scheduled at night. An infusion pump ensures safe, accurate fluid delivery while he sleeps. Make sure you spend plenty of time teaching him how to operate his pump.

Because many types of pump exist, your instructions depend on the particular model the patient will use at home. No matter which pump he's using, take special care to familiarize him with its alarms. Remember, he may be startled the first few times he hears one. Reassure him that the problem is usually a minor one he can fix himself, but instruct him to attend to any alarm promptly. If a problem develops that he can't handle, stress that he should take precautions to keep his catheter patent (for example, by flushing it with heparinized solution and capping it) until help arrives.

Chances are, your patient's pump has the alarms listed below.

- *Volume delivered.* Show your patient how to set the pump to deliver the amount of TPN solution the doctor's ordered. Explain that the pump will alert him with an alarm when it's delivered the set amount. This safety feature prevents fluid overload and air embolism.
- *Air in the line.* This alarm's designed to signal that air is entering the catheter. Tell your patient if it sounds he should examine the pump tubing for a bubble, and teach him the procedure for clamping the catheter, disconnecting the pump tubing, and flushing the tubing.

If your patient discovers air in the tubing, tell him to double-check all connections to make sure they're secure. If he finds no air but the alarm continues to sound, suggest that he readjust the pump tubing where it passes through the air sensor.

- *Occlusion* (blocked line). Mostly, this alarm signals a minor problem; for example, the patient's rolled on the tubing while sleeping. Instruct him to check all the tubing, from the TPN container to the catheter, to make sure nothing's pressing on the tubing and that it's free of kinks. Also remind him to make sure the tubing's clamp is open.

If the line's still blocked, instruct your patient to clamp the catheter, disconnect it from the pump tubing, and flush TPN solution through the tubing. If the solution flows normally, the occlusion's probably in the catheter, not the tubing. Tell him to aspirate about 3 ml of blood from the catheter; if a clot's occluding the catheter, this may remove it. If he doesn't understand this technique (or if the catheter's still blocked after aspiration), tell him to clamp and cap the catheter and notify the doctor.

Note: Although most pumps can operate on battery power as well as electrical outlet power, caution your patient against using the battery except in an emergency. The pump's more reliable when it's plugged in.

Preparing for long-term care

Before your patient leaves the hospital, be sure to discuss home care arrangements—especially financial arrangements—with him and his family. Remember, long-term TPN therapy's expensive. If the patient's insurance doesn't cover the cost, refer him to the social service department.

Also, make sure he or a family member can pick up TPN solutions from the hospital pharmacy at least twice a week. If this is a problem, ask the social service department for assistance.

Finally, arrange for a visiting nurse to visit regularly.

Preparing your patient for home care: A checklist

When teaching your patient to administer total parenteral nutrition (TPN) solution through his Hickman catheter, take care to stress these important points:

☐ Take your temperature every day, just after getting up in the morning, and write it down. Also weigh yourself every morning, and write down your weight. (Wear similar clothing and use the same scale for each weighing.)

☐ Every morning, test a second-voided urine specimen for ketones and glucose. Keep a record of the result for your doctor.

☐ For convenience, try keeping your records on a small calendar; also jot down any problems you're having. These records help the doctor determine how you're doing.

☐ Don't forget to keep your appointments for regular blood testing (once a week or as directed by your doctor). If you can't regularly visit the doctor or clinic, a visiting nurse can help you at home. A weekly blood test helps the doctor decide if any changes need to be made in your TPN solution.

☐ Keep your TPN containers in the refrigerator. For your comfort during feeding, let a container warm to room temperature for about 1 hour before using it. *Note:* Don't freeze the solution.

☐ Store your TPN solution in a safe part of the refrigerator; for example, the top shelf, where nothing's likely to spill on it.

☐ Before using any TPN solution, hold it up to the light and make sure it looks clear. Don't use it if it looks cloudy or has an unusual color. (Some solutions look yellow, depending on the additives; make sure you know your solution's normal color.) Also, don't use it if the container is cracked, torn, or damaged. Finally, check the container's expiration date, to make sure the solution's fresh. Your pharmacist will probably mark on the container the date he mixed the solution. Use the solution within a week of this date, unless the pharmacist or doctor directs differently.

☐ Put all your supplies together in a box or basket, so you can easily find everything you need for each TPN administration. To keep your supplies clean, put them in a place where they won't get dusty or be disturbed. Also, place them out of children's reach.

☐ Never reuse any supplies, unless your doctor or nurse says it's O.K.

☐ Change your Hickman catheter's cap after each TPN administration.

Home care

Giving TPN through your Hickman catheter

Dear Patient:
At home, you'll use the Hickman catheter to feed yourself special I.V. fluid. These feedings are called TPN (total parenteral nutrition).

Your nurse has helped you learn how to give yourself TPN. Use this home care aid as a reminder of what you've learned. Carefully read this aid before you leave the hospital. If you have questions, be sure to ask your nurse. If you have questions or problems after you go home, contact ______________________.

Follow all the daily-care guidelines your nurse has taught you. By doing so, you reduce the risk of a complication, such as infection.

Now, here's how to prepare for a TPN feeding:

1 First, gather the infusion pump, pump tubing, filter, needle, tape, and TPN solution. Set up this equipment, according to the instructions for your pump. Then, use the tape to secure all tubing junctions, as shown here.

If you have long hair, tie it back. Make sure your catheter's clamp is secure. Then, thoroughly wash and dry your hands.

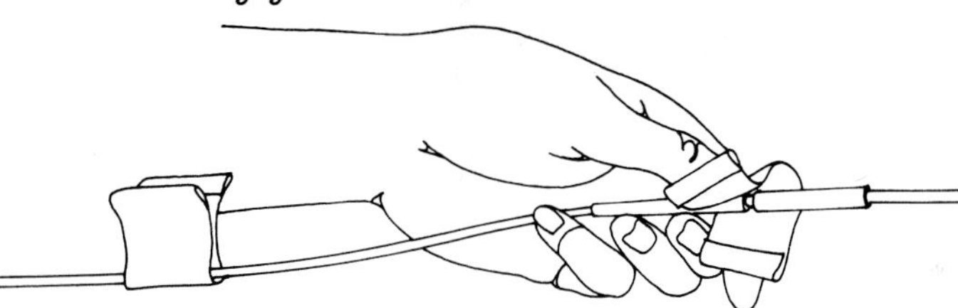

2

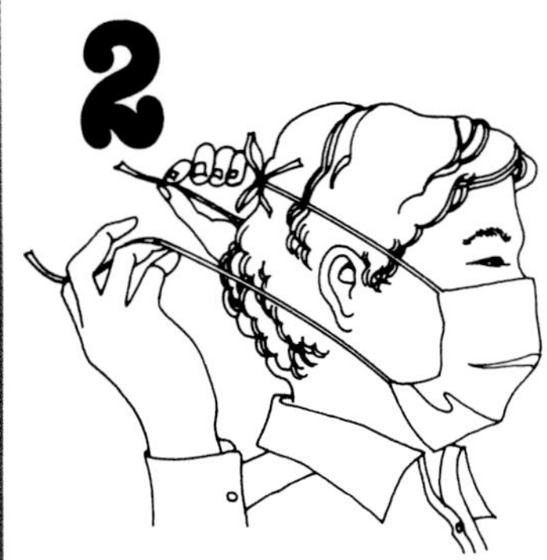

Chances are, the hospital or clinic has provided you with supplies for this procedure. For this home care aid, we'll assume you're using prepackaged supplies. If you're not, gather this equipment: two alcohol swabs, two povidone-iodine swabs, four sterile gauze pads, two pairs of sterile disposable gloves, face mask, sterile disposable towel, clean tape, empty plastic bag, scissors, a bottle of alcohol, and a clean cloth.

Put on the face mask.

3

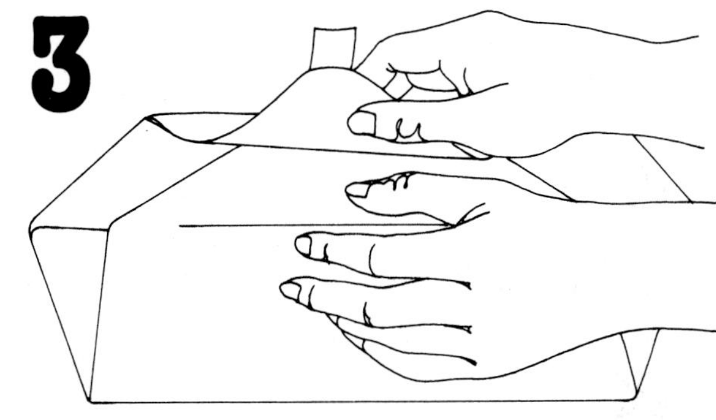

Using alcohol, wipe the table where you'll lay your supplies. Unbutton or take off your shirt, to expose the catheter. While the table dries, again wash and dry your hands.

Put the clean tape and scissors on the table, to one side. Tape the empty plastic bag to the table's edge to collect soiled equipment.

Among your prepackaged equipment, the sterile supplies are contained in a kit wrapped with sterile paper. Place the kit on the clean table and unwrap it. As you do, take care to touch only the *outside* of the paper. Remember, everything *inside* the paper is sterile. You'll find that the sterile gloves have been placed on top of your sterile equipment. *Important:* Don't let the sterile equipment touch *anything* that's not sterile; for example, your hands, the tape, or the scissors.

4

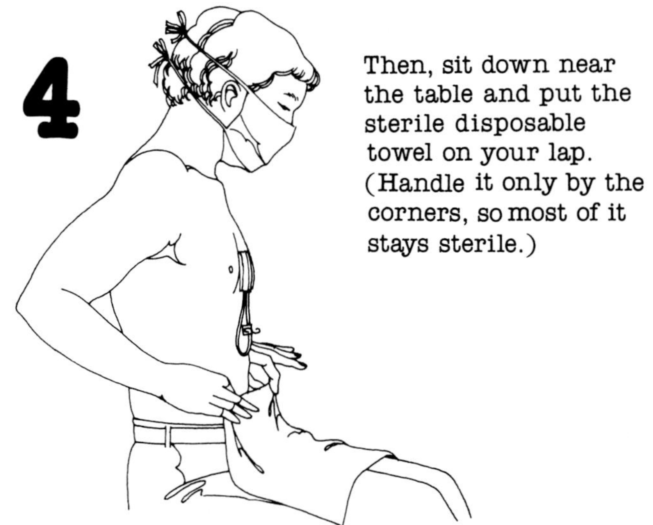

Then, sit down near the table and put the sterile disposable towel on your lap. (Handle it only by the corners, so most of it stays sterile.)

Intravenous

Home care

Giving TPN through your Hickman catheter continued

5 Free your catheter by removing the tape holding the catheter cap to the dressing. Discard the tape in the plastic bag. Also remove and discard the gauze pad and tape around the cap. Then, drop the capped catheter tip onto the sterile towel. *Note:* Once the catheter tip touches the towel, this part of the towel is no longer sterile.

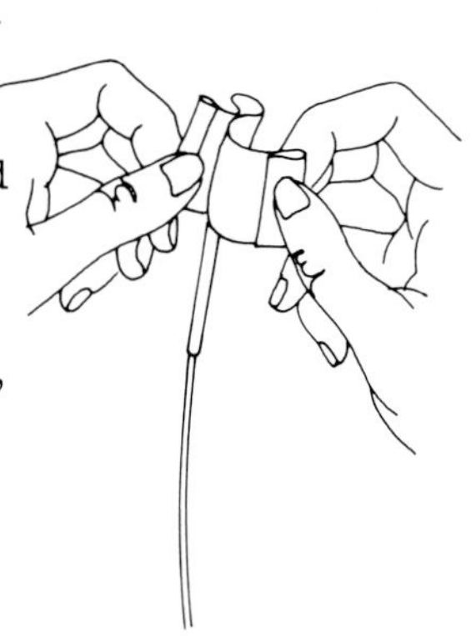

6 Put on a pair of sterile gloves, using the special technique your nurse has taught you. Then, put another sterile glove on your dominant hand. If you're right-handed, you now have two sterile gloves on your right hand and one sterile glove on your left hand. Now you can handle your sterile equipment without contaminating it. Unwrap the alcohol swabs, povidone-iodine swabs, and gauze pads. Spread them out *on the sterile paper,* so you can see and grasp everything.

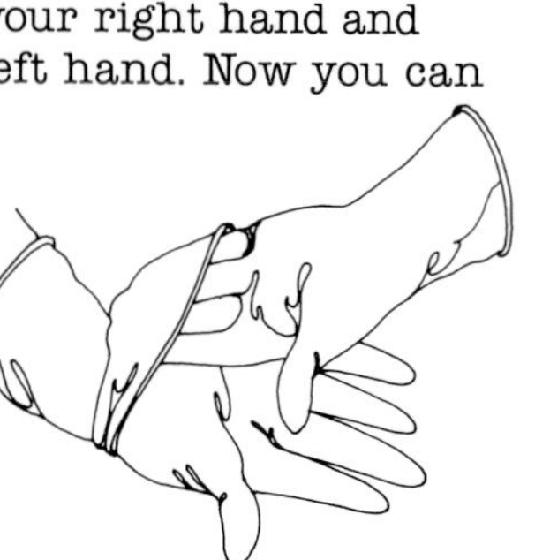

7 Grasp the catheter tip with your left hand, as shown here. (Your left hand is no longer sterile, because you've contaminated it by touching the catheter.) Using your right hand, pick up an alcohol swab and clean the catheter tip. To do so, first clean the junction between the catheter tip and the catheter cap (catheter-cap junction); then, clean above and below the junction. Discard the alcohol swab in the plastic bag.

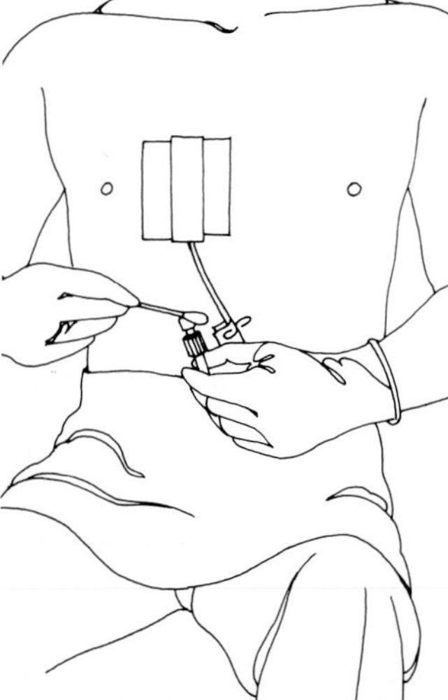

8 Repeat the procedure with a povidone-iodine swab, and discard the swab. Let the povidone-iodine dry for about 2 minutes, so it has time to work. While you wait, continue to hold the catheter in your left hand; don't drop it on the towel, because the towel is no longer sterile.

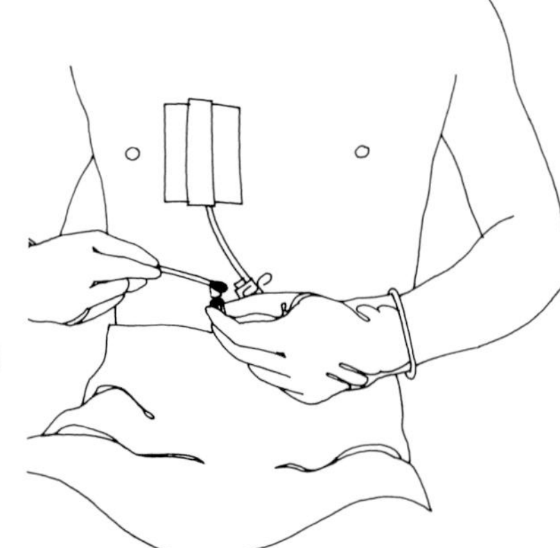

9 Then, pick up one dry gauze pad with your right (sterile) hand, and wipe the povidone-iodine from the catheter. Discard the gauze pad.

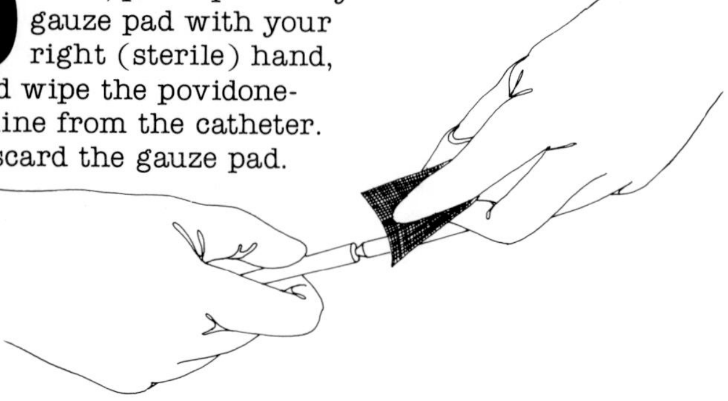

10 With your right hand, pick up a fresh gauze pad by a corner, so it falls open. Lay it on a dry part of the towel. Remember, this pad is sterile, so don't allow anything to contaminate it.

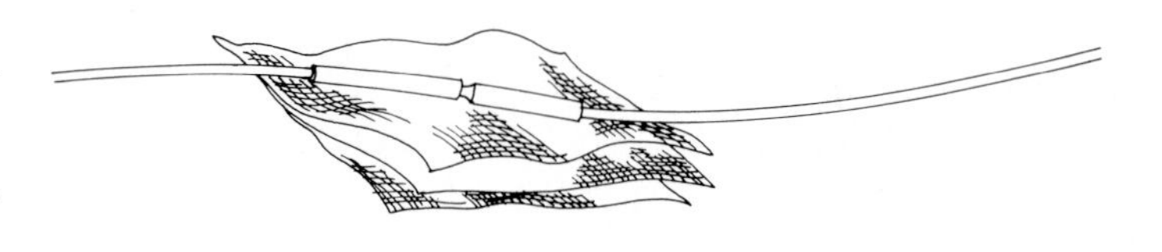

11 Using your right hand, unscrew the catheter cap and discard it in the plastic bag. (Your right hand is no longer sterile.) Then, still using your right hand, pick up the capped needle on the end of the infusion pump's tubing. Slip the cap between the second and third fingers of your left hand, and remove the needle from the tubing.

12 Connect the pump tubing to the catheter. Now, gently drop the junction between the catheter and pump tubing (catheter-tubing junction) into the center of the open sterile gauze pad, as shown.

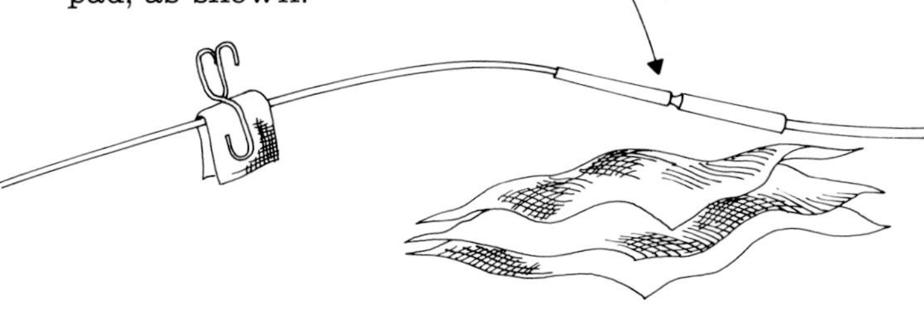

13 Check the pump setting for accuracy. Then, start the pump and immediately remove the clamp on your catheter. Place the clamp away from your sterile supplies.

Now, remove the outer glove from your right hand, and discard it in the plastic bag. Because you have another sterile glove underneath, your right hand is sterile again. Hold your right hand away from the catheter and sterile supplies, and rub your right hand's fingers together to remove any powder.

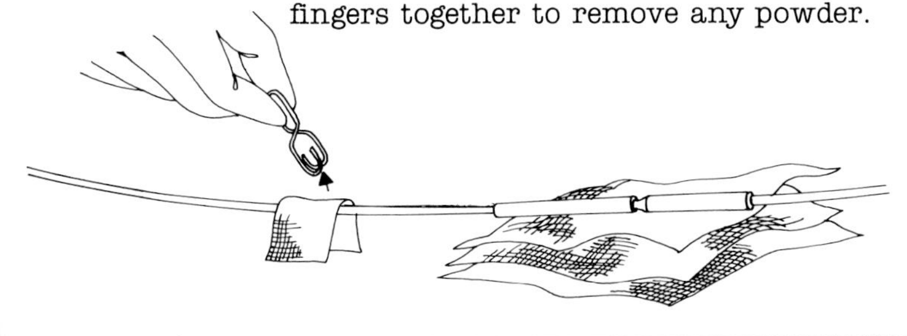

14 With your left hand, lift the catheter. Using your right (sterile) hand, clean the catheter-tubing junction with an alcohol swab. Repeat the procedure with a povidone-iodine swab. Wait at least 2 minutes; then, wipe the junction off with a sterile gauze pad.

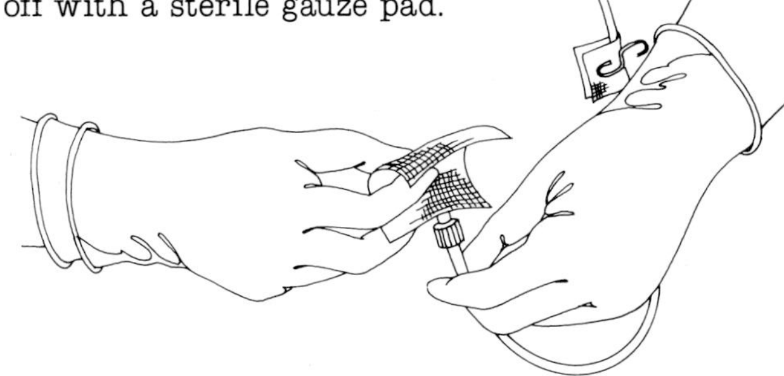

15 With your right hand, pick up another gauze pad by one corner, so it falls open. Drop it on a dry area of the towel. Gently drop the junction onto it.

Holding your hands away from the catheter-tubing junction and sterile supplies, remove your gloves. Rub your hands to remove any powder.

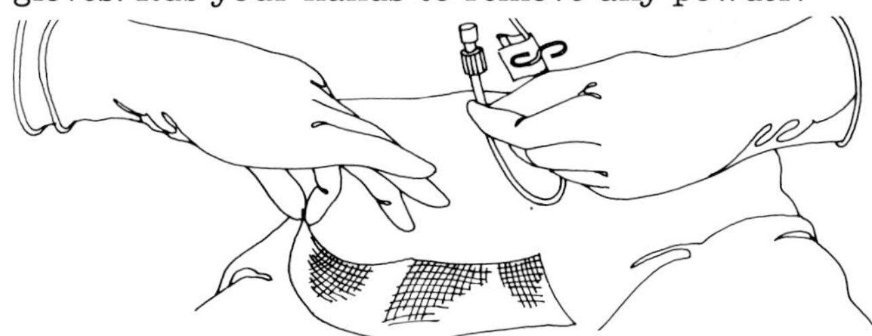

16 Cover and secure the junction with tape. (Don't touch the adhesive side of the tape or the junction with your hands.) Fold over the edges of the tape to make tabs for easier removal. Tape around the junction, and place another tabbed piece of tape lengthwise along the junction.

Remove your mask. Discard the mask, the towel, and the gauze pads in the plastic bag. Retape the catheter to the exit site dressing. Finally, make sure the tubing is free of kinks and all its connections are secure.

Intravenous

Learning about the heparin lock

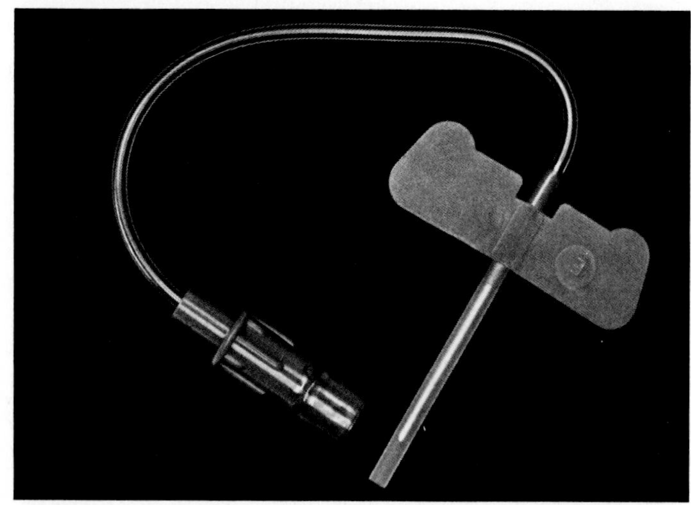

Consider this situation: Your patient, 27-year-old Roseanne Morrissey, needs intermittent I.V. antibiotic therapy. The relatively short length of time she's likely to need therapy doesn't justify implanting a long-term device, such as the Hickman catheter, and she doesn't need the continuous I.V. fluid infusion necessary to maintain a keep-vein-open (KVO) I.V. line.

In a situation like this, the doctor may order the insertion of an intermittent infusion reservoir, commonly called a *heparin lock.* As you see in the photo above, it consists of a small-gauge, winged-tip needle; short tubing (the reservoir); and an injection port.

By keeping the reservoir filled with dilute heparin solution, you keep the needle patent when not in use.

Nursing tip: You can easily make your own heparin lock by attaching a male adapter plug to any standard I.V. needle or catheter device.

The lock's advantages? Because the patient needn't cope with cumbersome I.V. equipment, he'll find it more convenient and comfortable than a KVO I.V. line. Equally important, the heparin lock reduces or eliminates risks associated with long-term I.V. therapy; for example, infiltration and fluid overload.

Besides using it to administer antibiotic therapy, you may use a heparin lock to:

- give a blood transfusion
- administer diuretics, steroids, and heparin
- provide access for I.V. cancer chemotherapy
- maintain an emergency I.V. route; for example, in a patient who recently suffered myocardial infarction.

Dealing with problems

When using a heparin lock, routinely monitor the site for:

- infiltration. Signs and symptoms include pain and absence of blood backflow during bolus administration. You'll have difficulty giving the drug, and a wheal may form under the skin during injection. If the patient's receiving an I.V. drip infusion, signs of infiltration include swollen, blanched, cool skin around the insertion site; leakage from the insertion site; and a sluggish I.V. flow rate.
- phlebitis from vein trauma or irritation by caustic drugs or the I.V. device itself. Signs and symptoms include a sore, hard, warm, cordlike vein; edema; and sluggish I.V. flow rate.
- hematoma.

If one of these problems develops, remove the heparin lock according to hospital policy. Insert another heparin lock at another site. Document the problem and your intervention.

Using a Tubex syringe set

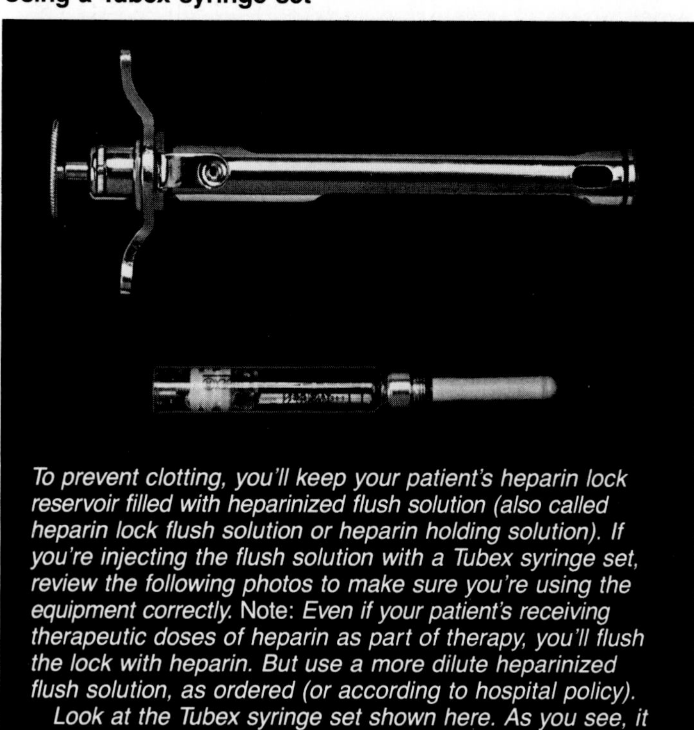

To prevent clotting, you'll keep your patient's heparin lock reservoir filled with heparinized flush solution (also called heparin lock flush solution or heparin holding solution). If you're injecting the flush solution with a Tubex syringe set, review the following photos to make sure you're using the equipment correctly. Note: *Even if your patient's receiving therapeutic doses of heparin as part of therapy, you'll flush the lock with heparin. But use a more dilute heparinized flush solution, as ordered (or according to hospital policy).*

Look at the Tubex syringe set shown here. As you see, it consists of a stainless steel syringe and a cartridge-needle unit (comprising a prefilled vial of heparinized flush solution, needle, and needle guard).

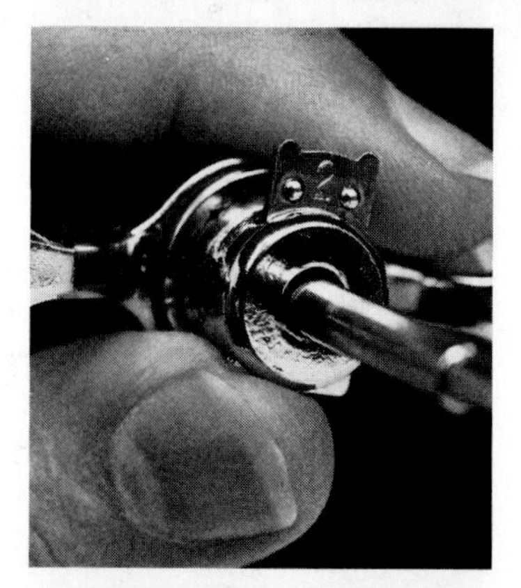

1 To assemble the set, first unlock the syringe (if the Tubex syringe you're using has a lock). Press the metal tab sideways, so the side marked with the number 2 protrudes. With the lock in this position, you can pull up the plunger as far as it'll go, as the nurse has done here.

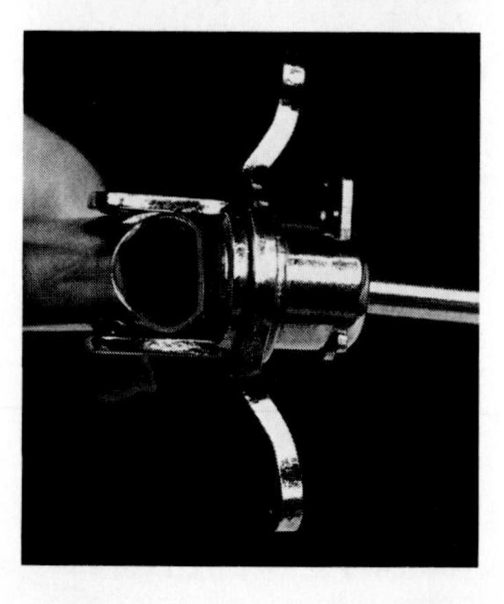

2 Holding the plunger with one hand, flip the syringe shaft to one side, as shown.

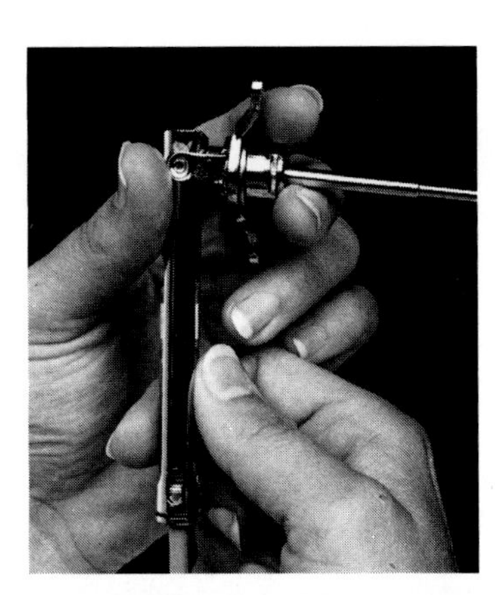

3 Now, slip the cartridge-needle unit into the shaft, so the needle points downward. Screw the needle hub into the base of the syringe shaft by spinning the cartridge. Flip up the plunger to straighten the equipment.

Next, slide the plunger toward the cartridge until it engages the screw protruding from the cartridge's rubber stopper.

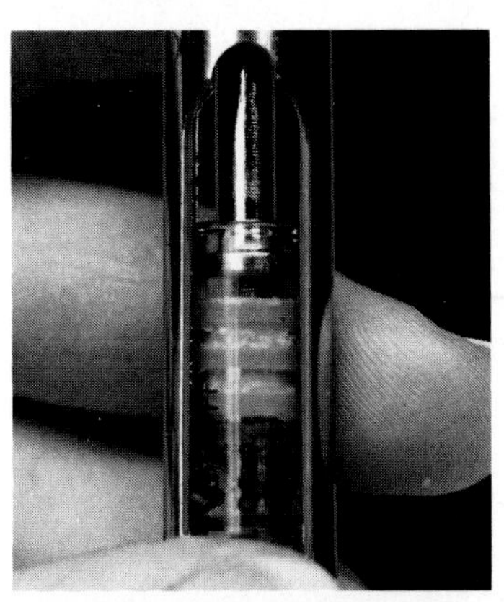

4 Screw the cartridge and plunger together. (Don't screw them together too tightly, or you'll have trouble disassembling the equipment.) Then, lock the plunger by adjusting the metal tab so the side marked with the number 1 is visible. This feature prevents you from accidentally pulling the stopper out of a 1-ml cartridge but doesn't prevent you from injecting the drug. (Locking the plunger isn't necessary for a 2-ml cartridge.)

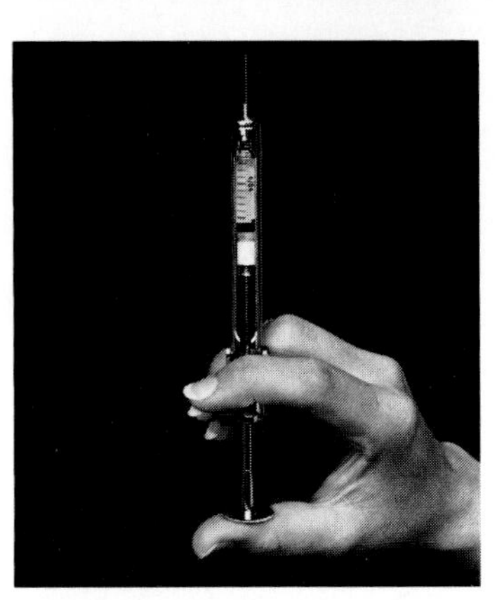

5 Pull off the needle guard and expel air from the cartridge, as shown. Inject the flush solution into the heparin lock port.

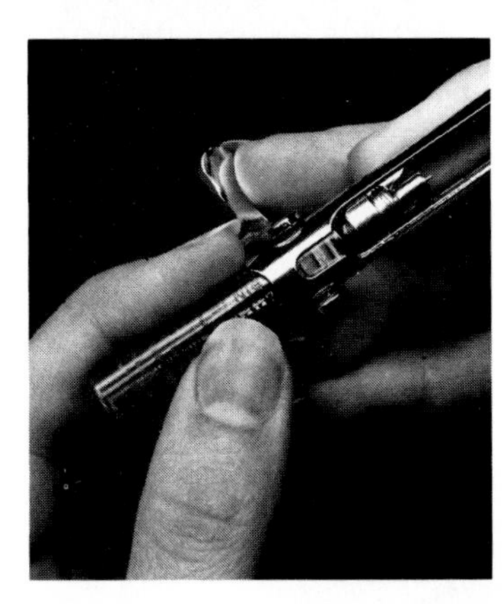

6 Then, cut off the needle and discard it.

To remove the empty cartridge, first unscrew the plunger from the cartridge stopper. Next, unscrew the needle hub from the base of the syringe shaft. Unlock the plunger, flip the syringe shaft to one side, and remove the cartridge, as shown. Discard the cartridge.

Now, read the following photostory to learn how to insert a heparin lock and fill its reservoir with flush solution.

How to insert a heparin lock

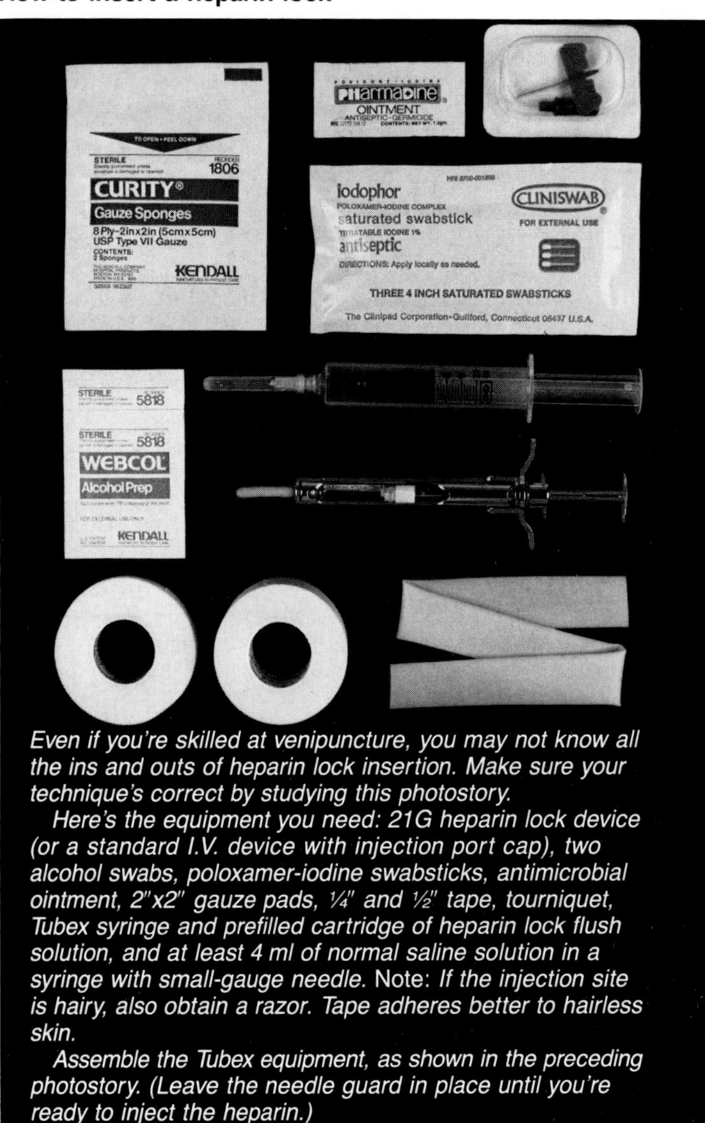

Even if you're skilled at venipuncture, you may not know all the ins and outs of heparin lock insertion. Make sure your technique's correct by studying this photostory.

Here's the equipment you need: 21G heparin lock device (or a standard I.V. device with injection port cap), two alcohol swabs, poloxamer-iodine swabsticks, antimicrobial ointment, 2"x2" gauze pads, ¼" and ½" tape, tourniquet, Tubex syringe and prefilled cartridge of heparin lock flush solution, and at least 4 ml of normal saline solution in a syringe with small-gauge needle. Note: *If the injection site is hairy, also obtain a razor. Tape adheres better to hairless skin.*

Assemble the Tubex equipment, as shown in the preceding photostory. (Leave the needle guard in place until you're ready to inject the heparin.)

Explain the procedure to your patient, and thoroughly wash and dry your hands. Important: *Before beginning, make sure your patient's not sensitive to iodine. If she is, cleanse her skin with 70% alcohol only.*

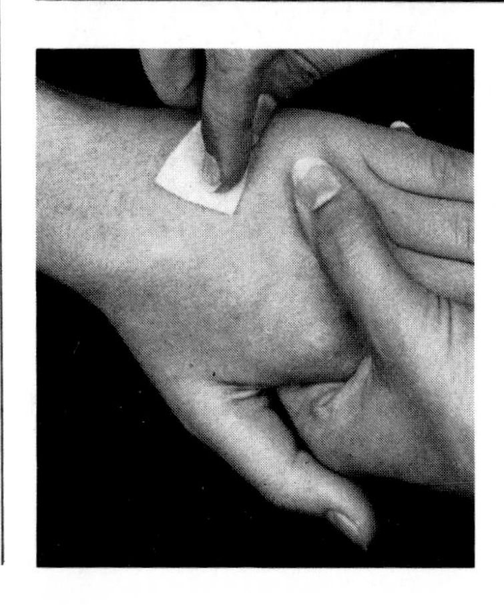

1 Select an appropriate vein for venipuncture. As a rule, you'll start with a distal vein, so you can later use veins farther up the arm, if necessary. But if your patient's receiving highly irritating drugs, choose a larger-volume vein; for example, a radial or ulnar vein.

If necessary, shave her skin near the proposed insertion site. Then, cleanse the site with an alcohol swab. Creating friction, work outward in a circular motion.

Intravenous

How to insert a heparin lock continued

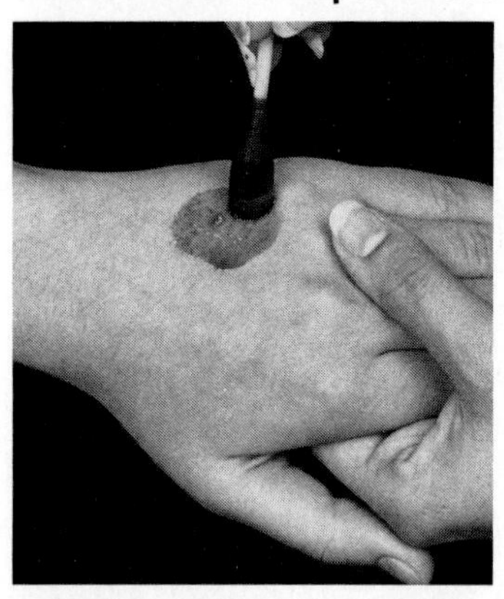

2 Repeat the procedure with a poloxamer-iodine swab-stick. Allow the patient's skin to air-dry for 30 seconds.

Apply the tourniquet to her arm.

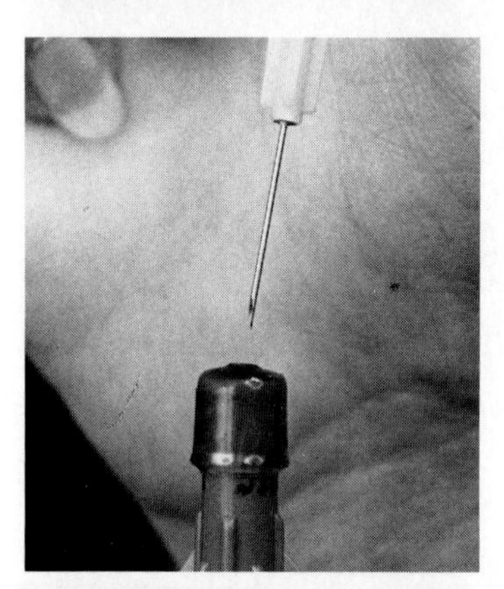

3 Using an alcohol swab, clean the heparin lock's injection port. Then, insert the needle connected to the syringe of normal saline solution, as shown here. *Note:* Whenever possible, use a small-gauge needle when injecting into the heparin lock, to minimize damage to the injection port. Also, take care not to insert the needle so far into the port that you perforate the reservoir.

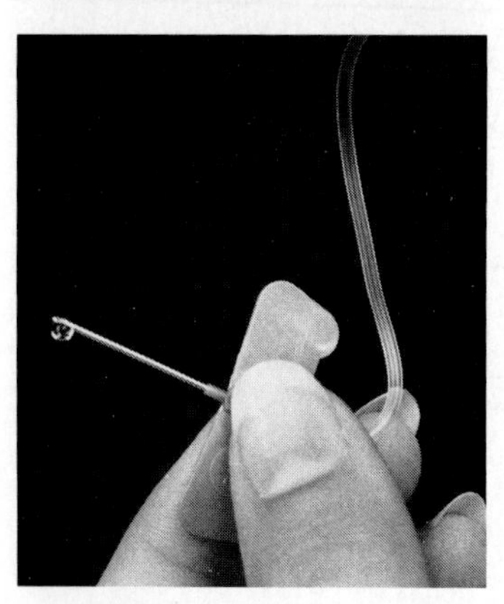

4 Flush air from the reservoir and needle by injecting about 1 ml of saline solution into the port. Leave the needle in the port.

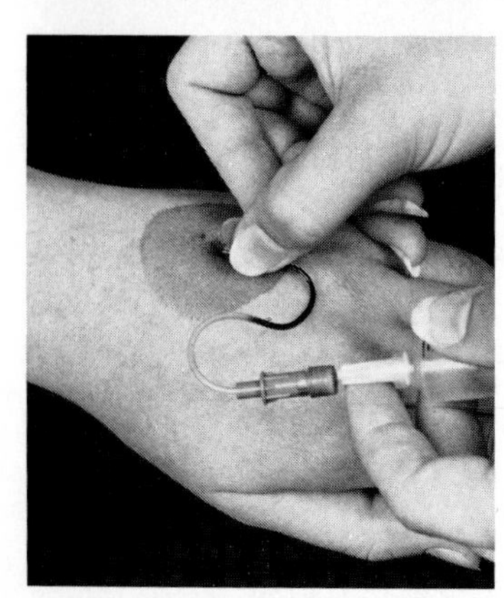

5 Perform venipuncture with the heparin lock needle. Watch for blood backflow, to confirm that the needle's placed properly.

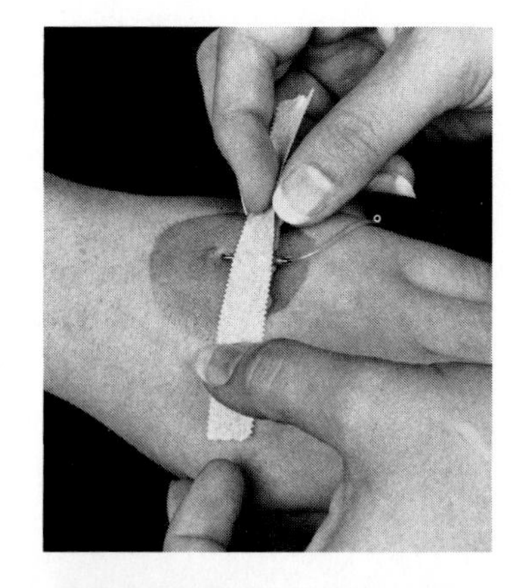

6 Place one piece of ¼" tape over the lock's wings to secure the needle. (Don't let the tape touch the venipuncture site.) Remove the tourniquet.

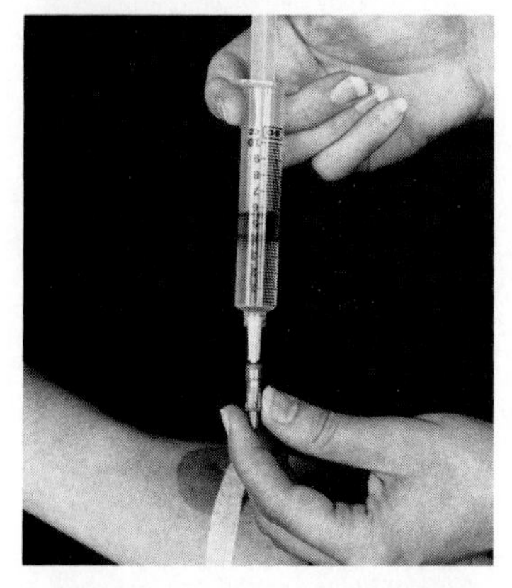

7 Clear blood from the lock by injecting 2 ml of saline solution, as shown here. Then, apply antimicrobial ointment to the site, cover it with a gauze pad, and secure the pad with ½" tape. Also coil and tape the reservoir, but take care to leave the injection port free. Then, lay the last piece of tape on the table and label it with the date and time of insertion, type and gauge of needle, and your initials. Place the tape over the insertion site.

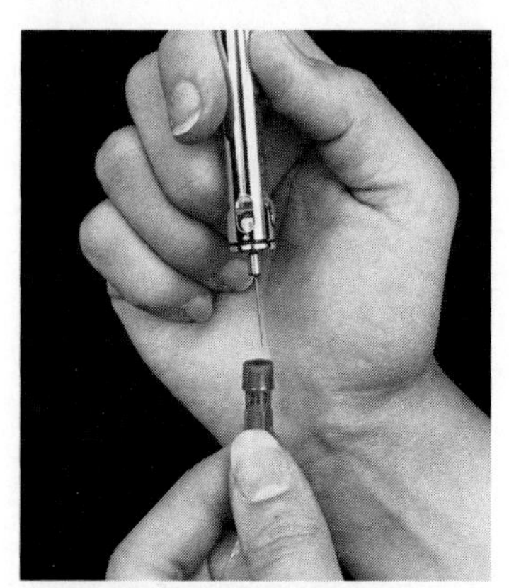

8 Remove the saline syringe's needle from the injection port. Then, remove the Tubex needle's guard and insert the needle into the port, as shown. Inject about 0.5 ml of heparinized flush solution into the reservoir.

Note: If you're using a standard I.V. device (such as a winged-tip needle) with a long reservoir, you'll need to inject slightly more than 1 ml to fill the reservoir.

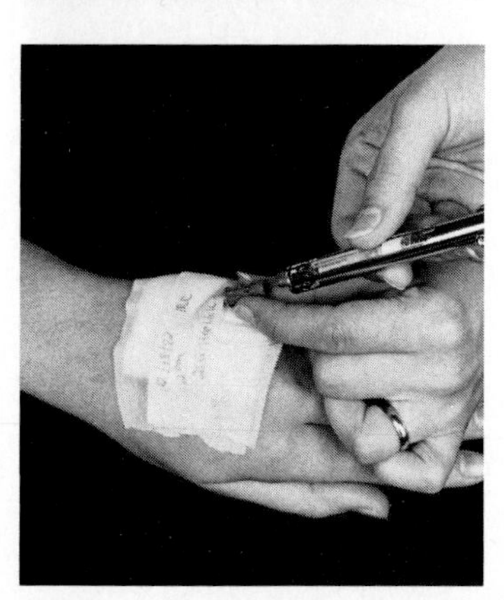

9 Remove the Tubex needle. Disassemble the Tubex equipment as shown in the preceding photostory, and dispose of all used equipment. Document the procedure.

Giving drugs through a heparin lock

You're preparing to administer two doses of drugs the doctor's ordered for your patient: 40 mg of furosemide (Lasix) I.V. bolus and 60 mg of gentamicin sulfate (Garamycin*) I.V. drip. If your patient has a heparin lock in place, do you know how to proceed? Read this photostory for guidance.*

Besides the ordered drugs and necessary I.V. equipment, you'll need 6 ml of normal saline solution in a syringe with a small-gauge needle, an alcohol swab, and 0.5 ml of heparinized flush solution drawn up in a tuberculin syringe. Note: *Of course, you can use heparinized flush solution prepackaged in a Tubex syringe set, as shown on pages 96 to 97. But we recommend that you use a tuberculin syringe in this situation, because it enables you to administer all drugs through the same small-gauge needle. This minimizes the number of times you perforate the injection port.*

Wash your hands and explain the procedure.

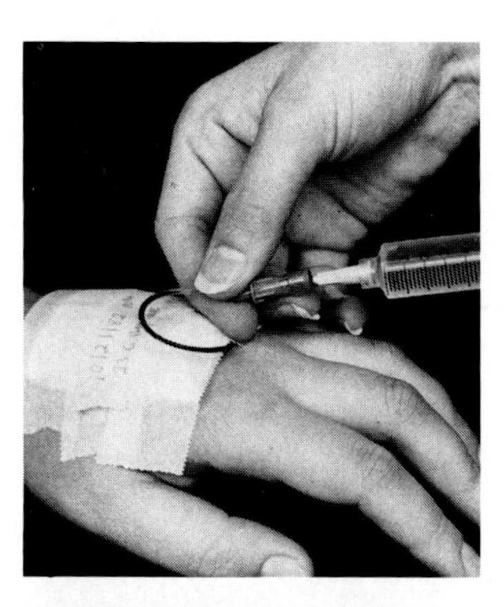

1 Clean the lock's injection port with the alcohol swab.

Insert the small-gauge needle connected to the saline solution syringe into the lock's injection port. Gently aspirate for blood backflow. If no blood appears in the reservoir, suspect that the needle is dislodged from the vein. Stop the procedure, remove the device, and insert a new heparin lock at a different location. *Note:* If the heparin lock is in a *small* vein, backflow may not occur.

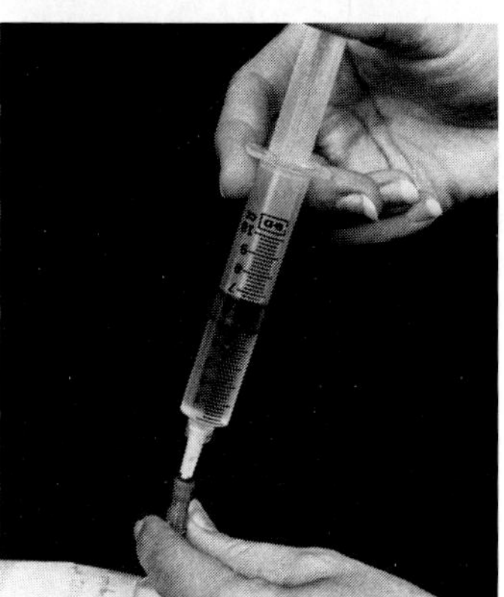

2 If blood backflow appears, inject 2 ml of saline solution into the reservoir, to flush out the heparinized flush solution. Inject the saline solution with a smooth, steady motion. *Note:* Stop the injection if the plunger's difficult to depress, if the patient complains of an intense burning sensation (a slight burning sensation is normal during heparin injection), or if you see a wheal forming under her skin. These signs and symptoms indicate infiltration.

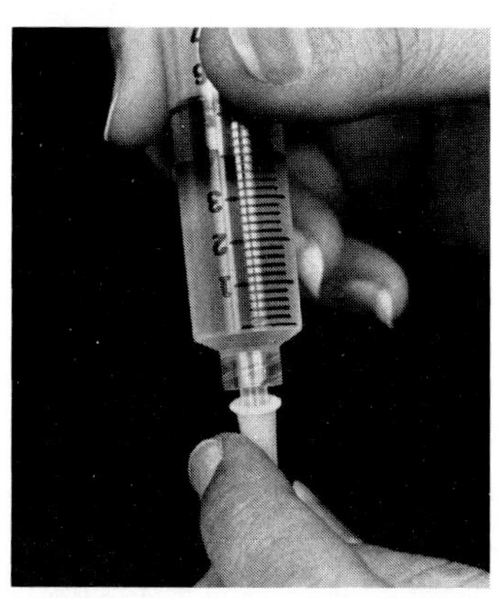

3 Now, leaving the syringe needle in place, detach the syringe barrel and cap it with the needle from the furosemide syringe. Then, attach the furosemide syringe to the needle, as shown. Administer the furosemide, as ordered.

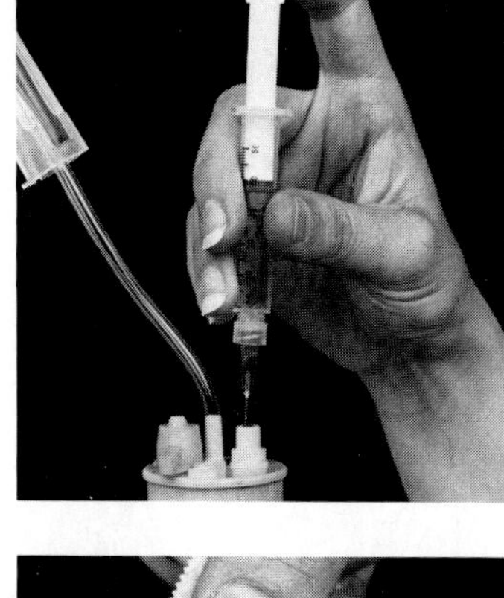

4 After giving the drug, detach its syringe from the needle. Uncap the saline solution syringe and reattach it to the needle. Flush the lock with 2 ml of saline solution. *Remember:* To prevent complications, always flush the lock between drug administrations.

Now, get ready to give the gentamicin sulfate. As shown here, prepare the I.V. solution and equipment, if you haven't done so already.

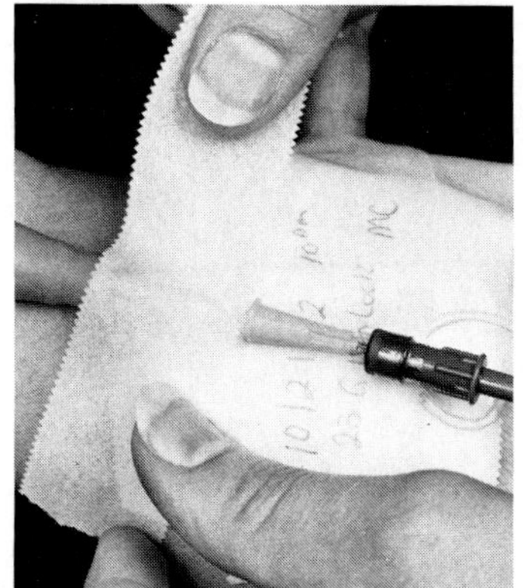

5 Then, remove the saline solution syringe from the needle in the port, cap the syringe, and attach the I.V. line to the needle. Infuse the drug, as ordered. *Important:* Because the gentamicin sulfate will infuse for about 30 minutes, tape the needle and tubing securely, as the nurse is doing here.

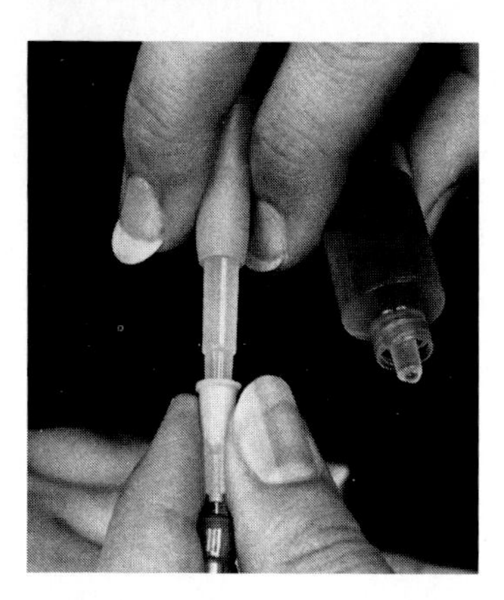

6 After the infusion's complete, close the I.V. flow clamp, detach the I.V. line from the needle, and reattach the saline solution syringe. Again flush the heparin lock with 2 ml of saline solution. Then, remove the saline solution syringe.

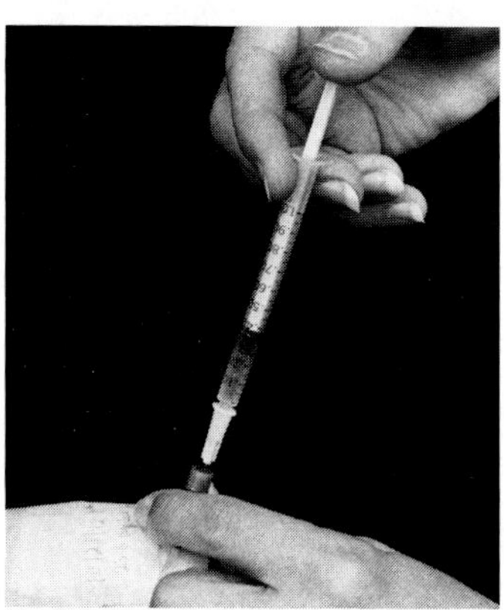

7 Now, attach the tuberculin syringe containing heparinized flush solution to the needle. Inject 0.5 ml of heparinized solution into the reservoir, to maintain patency.

Finally, remove the needle and syringe. Properly dispose of all used equipment. Document the procedure.

*Available in both the United States and Canada

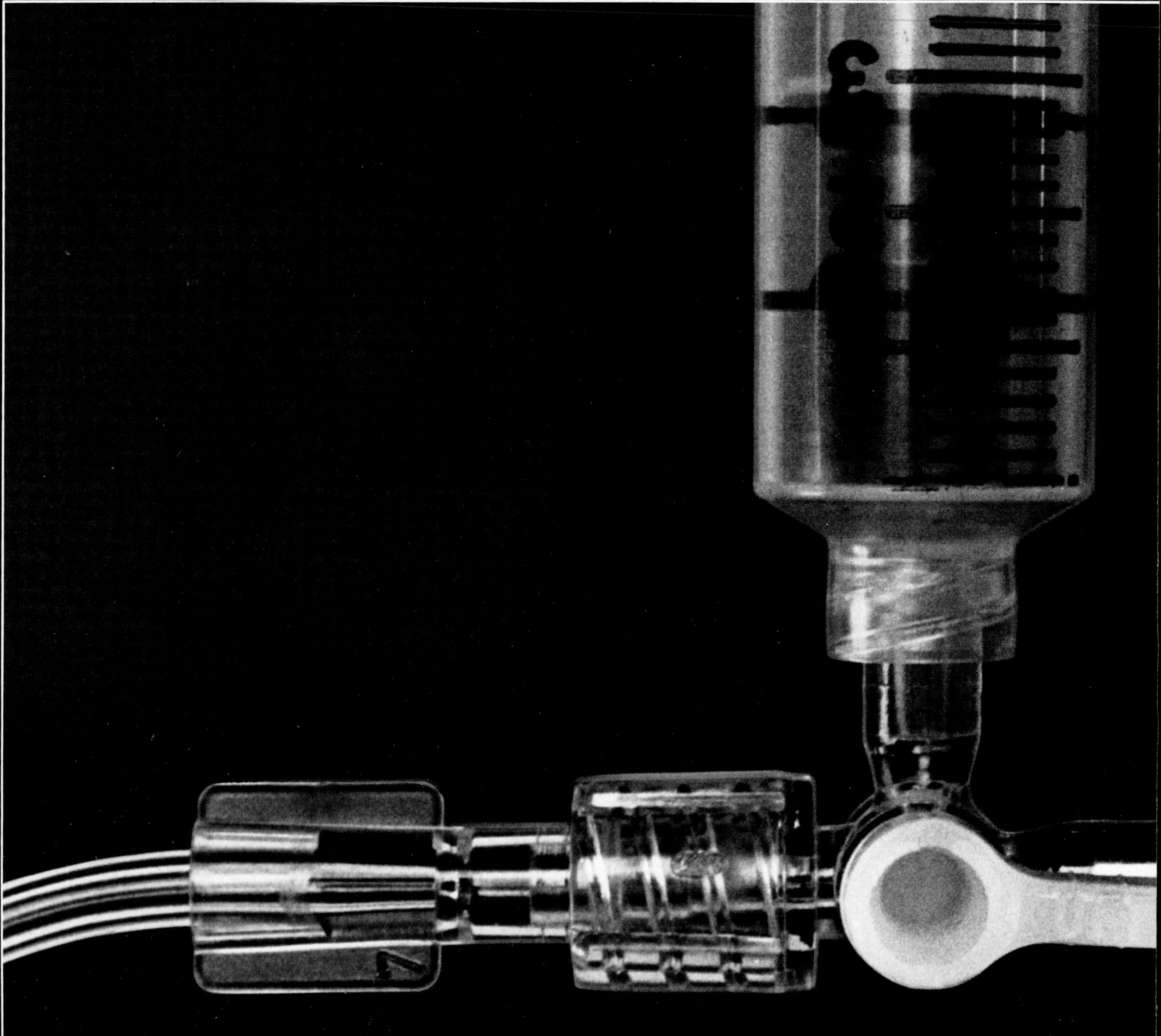

Dealing with Special Problems

Trauma

Kidney disease

Radiation therapy

DIC

Coma

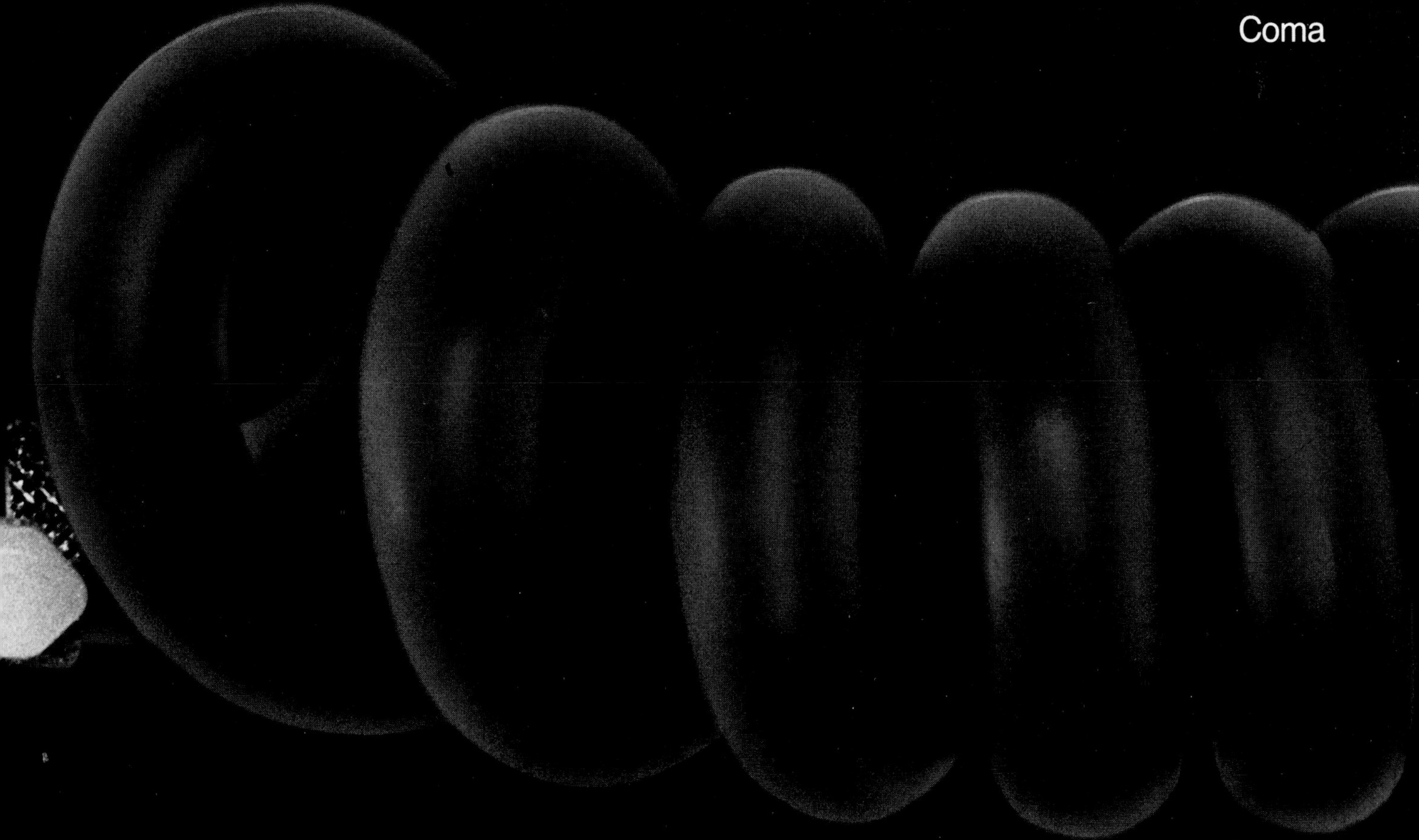

Trauma

Caring for a patient with traumatic injuries? His successful recovery may depend on your expertise.

In the following pages, we don't try to discuss everything you need to know when caring for a trauma patient. But we do familiarize you with a few special procedures that can help your patient recover completely. For example, you'll learn how to:

- monitor your patient for early signs of compartment syndrome.
- assist with peritoneal lavage and interpret the results.
- set up and use autotransfusion equipment.
- prepare your patient for hyperbaric oxygen therapy.

In addition, we acquaint you with equipment that enables you to perform wound irrigation with maximum efficiency.

Sound like important information? Read on.

Learning about compartment syndrome

Imagine this: You're on duty in the emergency department (ED) when 16-year-old Robert Delgano arrives with several deep dog bites on his right leg. Because his leg's swollen, you've elevated it above heart level and applied ice packs. Every 10 minutes you assess his right leg and foot for pulse rate, capillary refill, color, sensation, and warmth. You're relieved to note that all these indicators are nearly normal. You assure Robert that his leg, although painful now, will heal quickly and completely.

Or will it? You're giving care by the book, but you may be surprised to learn that it may not be enough to forestall a potential crippler called *muscle compartment syndrome*—compartment syndrome for short. In fact, traditional nursing measures for controlling edema—ice and elevation—may contribute to the problem.

What's compartment syndrome?

To understand compartment syndrome, you must recall some basic anatomic principles. As you know, muscle groups are contained in a compartment of tough, inelastic fascia. (In the illustration at right, the thigh's muscle compartments are distinguished by different shadings.) The entry and exit points for these muscle compartments are large enough to accommodate only major blood vessels, nerves, and tendons, with little room to spare. Edema *within* the compartment compresses these structures, leading to ischemia of muscle and nerve tissue.

Normally, compartmental pressure is below 20 mm Hg. If pressure rises above 40 mm Hg, circulation becomes impossible. If compartmental pressure remains above 40 mm Hg for longer than a few hours, nerve and muscle damage is irreversible.

Be alert for compartment syndrome if your patient suffers from burns, fractures, crushing injuries, gunshot wounds, animal bites, or idiopathic infection. Vascular or orthopedic procedures performed on an arm or leg also predispose a patient to this syndrome, as does pressure from a cast or dressing.

Early detection

Now that you understand the problem, how can you cope with it? Clearly, early detection of compartment syndrome is vital. Unfortunately, clinical signs don't appear until compartmental pressure's at least 30 mm Hg for several hours. By then, some permanent damage may have occurred. The only reliable way to assess compartmental pressure—before it's too late—is by taking direct pressure readings.

To do so, you may use pressure transducer equipment like that used for hemodynamic monitoring. Or, you can use a saline or mercury manometer. To use any of these systems, the doctor inserts a needle or catheter into the affected compartment. You'll be responsible for monitoring pressure readings and reporting readings higher than 30 mm Hg (or as ordered). In the following pages, we show you how to monitor compartmental pressure.

Important: If you're using a saline manometer, don't forget the conversion factor. To convert centimeters of water (cm H_2O) into mm Hg, divide cm H_2O by 1.36. For example:

$$22 \text{ cm } H_2O \div 1.36 = 16.17 \text{ mm Hg.}$$

Cross section of muscle compartments at midthigh

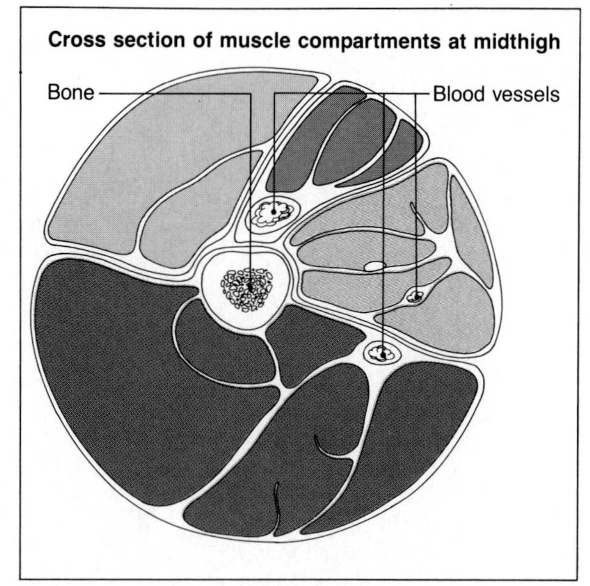

If monitoring reveals elevated compartmental pressure, the doctor will perform a fasciotomy. For more information on this procedure, see page 105.

Nursing care

Whether or not you're using a monitoring system, don't neglect regular nursing assessment and continuing care. What's the best way to proceed? Think back to Robert Delgano. By elevating his leg above heart level you hoped to control local edema. At the same time, you reduced blood supply to the compartment, increasing ischemia. You can modify this traditional nursing technique by placing Robert's leg *level* with the heart or only slightly above heart level.

For similar reasons, don't pack the leg in ice; the resulting vasoconstriction further reduces tissue perfusion. Instead, keep the leg *cool;* don't let its temperature fall below 32° F. (0° C.).

Closely monitor your patient's systemic blood pressure. A systemic blood pressure drop below the affected compartment's pressure reduces compartmental blood perfusion and increases ischemia. *Important:* Take blood pressure readings on the *unaffected* arm or leg.

As part of your assessment, compare the injured leg with the unaffected leg, and note differences in size and muscle hardness. Check the skin distal to the affected compartment for coolness, pallor, and poor capillary refill. Also assess for absent or weak pulse and for sensory changes in or between digits. Other signs and symptoms of compartment syndrome include:

- restlessness
- increasing, severe pain out of proportion to the injury; pain may be poorly localized and unrelievable by narcotics
- muscle weakness (especially in the absence of nerve injury)
- cool, white, or swollen fingers or toes
- referred pain to the affected compartment during passive movement of fingers or toes.

Using a mercury manometer to measure compartmental pressure

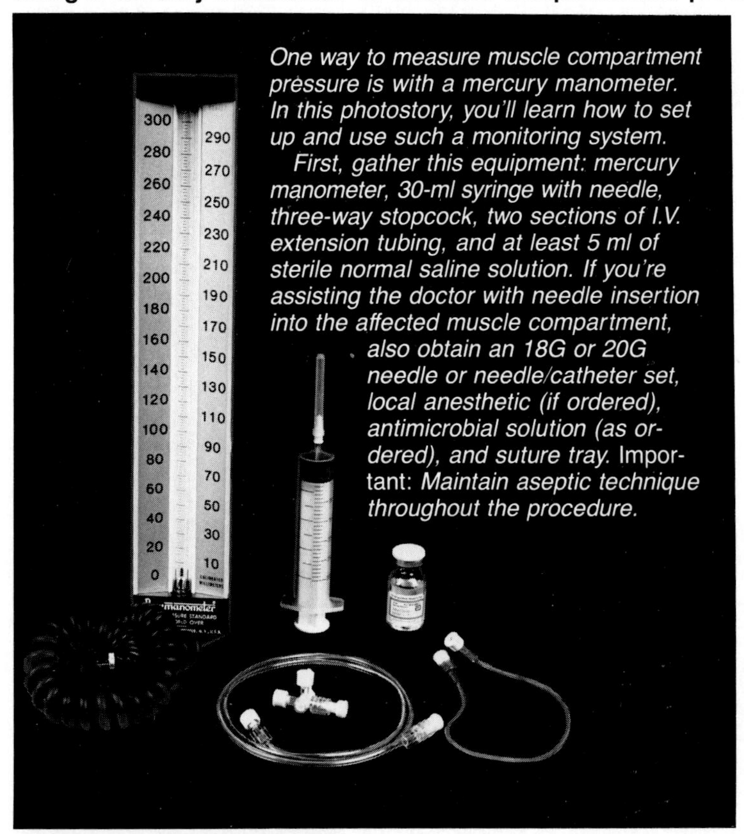

One way to measure muscle compartment pressure is with a mercury manometer. In this photostory, you'll learn how to set up and use such a monitoring system.

First, gather this equipment: mercury manometer, 30-ml syringe with needle, three-way stopcock, two sections of I.V. extension tubing, and at least 5 ml of sterile normal saline solution. If you're assisting the doctor with needle insertion into the affected muscle compartment, also obtain an 18G or 20G needle or needle/catheter set, local anesthetic (if ordered), antimicrobial solution (as ordered), and suture tray. Important: *Maintain aseptic technique throughout the procedure.*

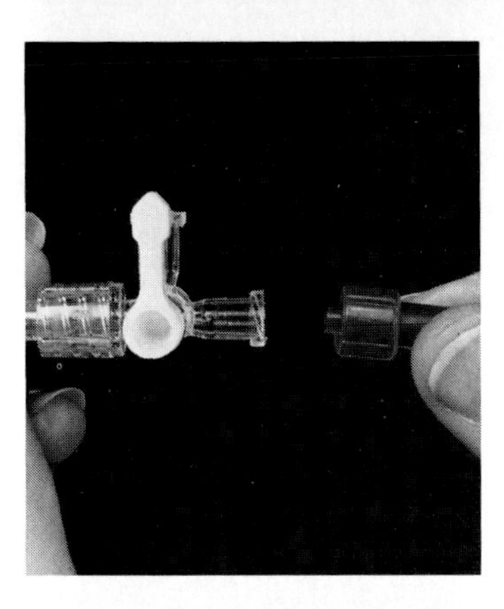

1 To assemble the monitoring equipment, first attach extension tubing to each side of the stopcock, as shown, leaving the top port free. Then, attach one end of extension tubing to the mercury manometer.

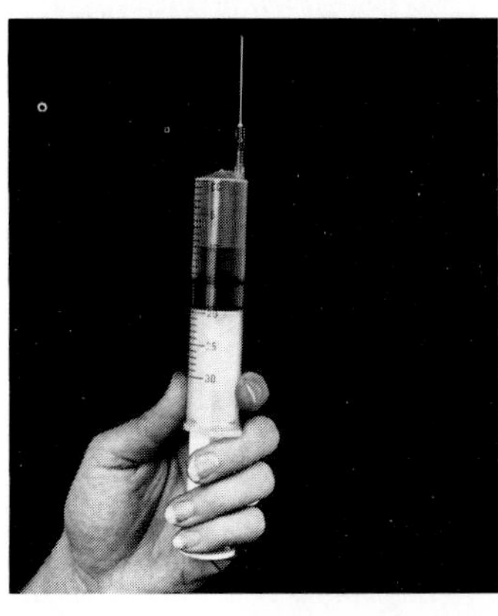

2 Draw up about 5 ml of saline solution; then, draw up about 15 cc of air into the syringe. Remove the needle and insert the syringe tip into the stopcock's top port.

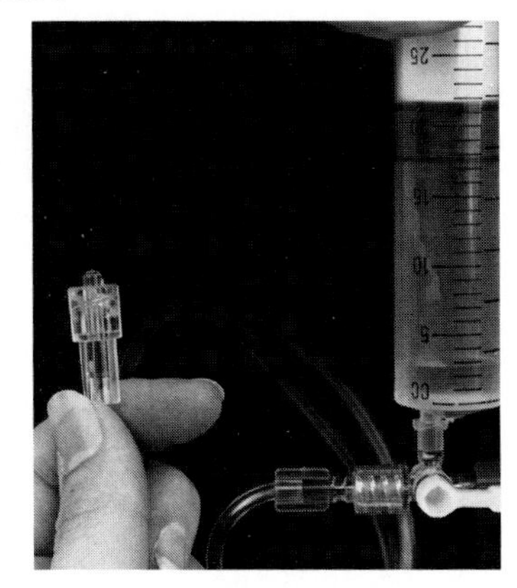

3 Now, turn the stopcock so the line's open between the syringe and the unattached portion of tubing. Remove the tubing's cap, invert the syringe and depress the plunger until solution fills about half the tubing's distal end and air fills the proximal end. Cap the tubing, and close the stopcock.

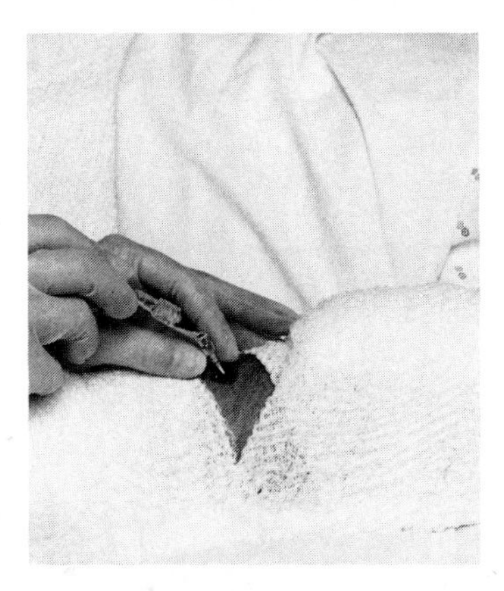

4 After the doctor inserts a needle into the patient's affected compartment, he connects the unattached tubing to the needle hub. Now, you're ready to take a compartmental pressure reading.

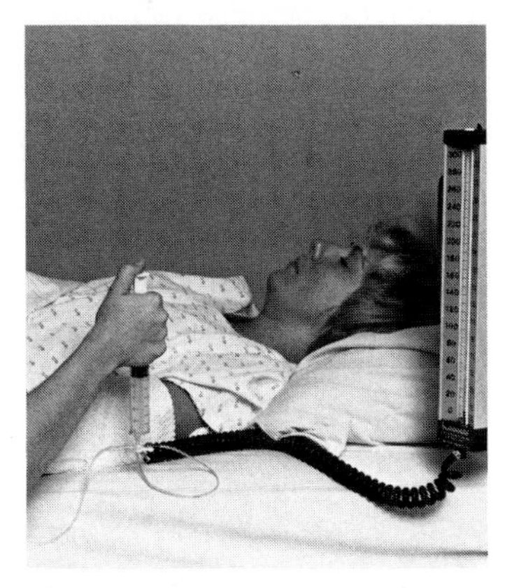

5 To do so, first position the patient's affected arm or leg so it's approximately level with her heart. Then, position the manometer so its zero point is level with the compartment. (For accuracy, use a leveling arm.) Open the stopcock between the syringe and the patient.

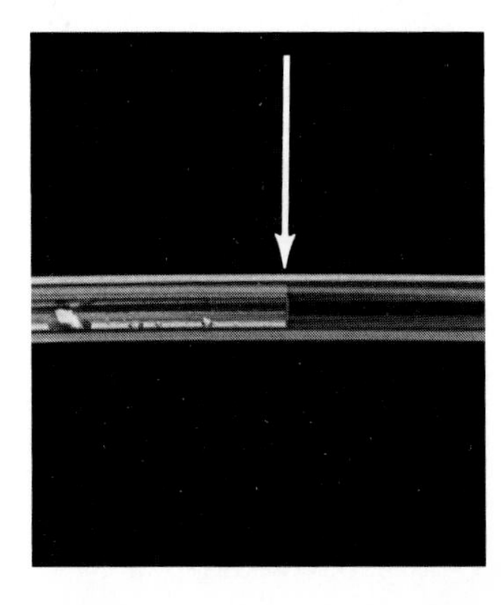

6 Using slow but steady pressure, depress the syringe plunger. Watch the air/saline meniscus in the tubing (see arrow). When it flattens, stop depressing the plunger and reposition the stopcock so the line is open between patient and manometer. Document the pressure reading shown on the manometer.

Trauma

Monitoring compartment syndrome with a pressure transducer

Do you need to take continuous muscle compartment pressure readings for your patient? If so, use a pressure transducer setup like the one shown below.

With this system, a syringe pump infuses sterile normal saline solution into the affected compartment at a rate of 0.03 ml/hour. A transducer measures the pressure necessary to maintain this rate; a monitor displays the pressure reading. This accurate system can alert you to small but significant pressure changes almost immediately.

To use this system, the doctor inserts an 18G or 20G I.V. catheter (or needle) into the muscle compartment and secures it with sutures or tape. He may leave the catheter in place for up to 72 hours. You'll change the dressing daily, or according to hospital policy. *Important:* During each dressing change, carefully inspect the site for signs of infection.

To ensure accurate pressure readings, remember the following points. (For more information, see the NURSING PHOTOBOOK USING MONITORS.)

- Use small-bore, high-pressure I.V. tubing.
- When assembling equipment, take care to avoid trapping air between the transducer and transducer dome.
- Eliminate air bubbles from the transducer dome and *all* tubing and stopcocks.
- Limit the total length of pressure tubing to less than 8′ (2.4 m).
- Before balancing and calibrating the equipment, position the patient's affected compartment at heart level. Then, position the transducer so its *balancing port* is level with the affected compartment throughout monitoring. *Remember:* If the patient changes position, you must reposition the transducer and rebalance and recalibrate the equipment.
- Repeat balancing and calibration procedures at least once every 8 hours. To confirm the equipment's accuracy, test it periodically with a mercury sphygmomanometer.
- When redressing the catheter site, don't apply the tape tightly. Pressure at the catheter site will distort readings.
- If clots obstruct the catheter, flush them with saline solution. Notify the doctor if clots continue to form; he may slightly increase the flow rate.

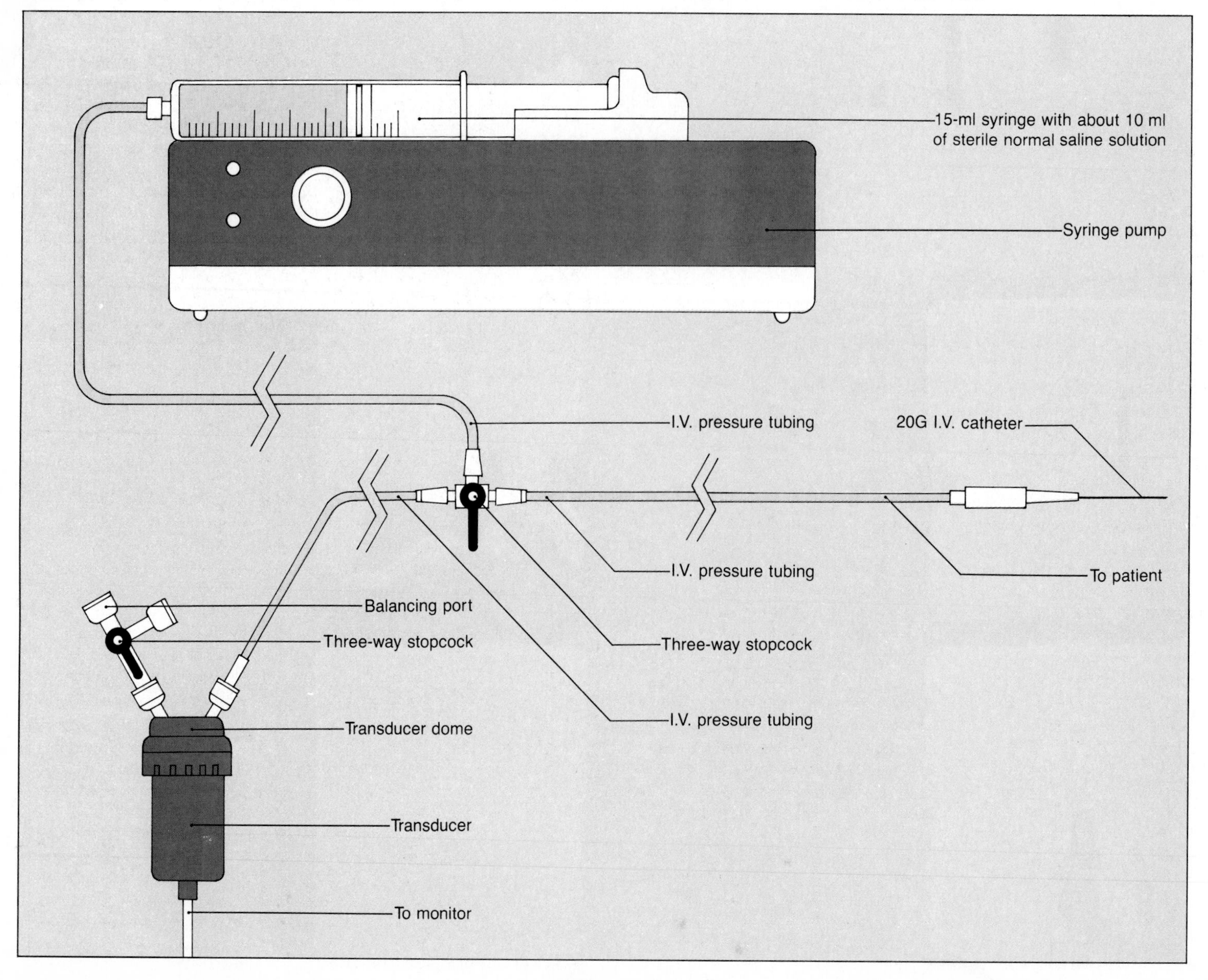

Monitoring compartment syndrome with calipers

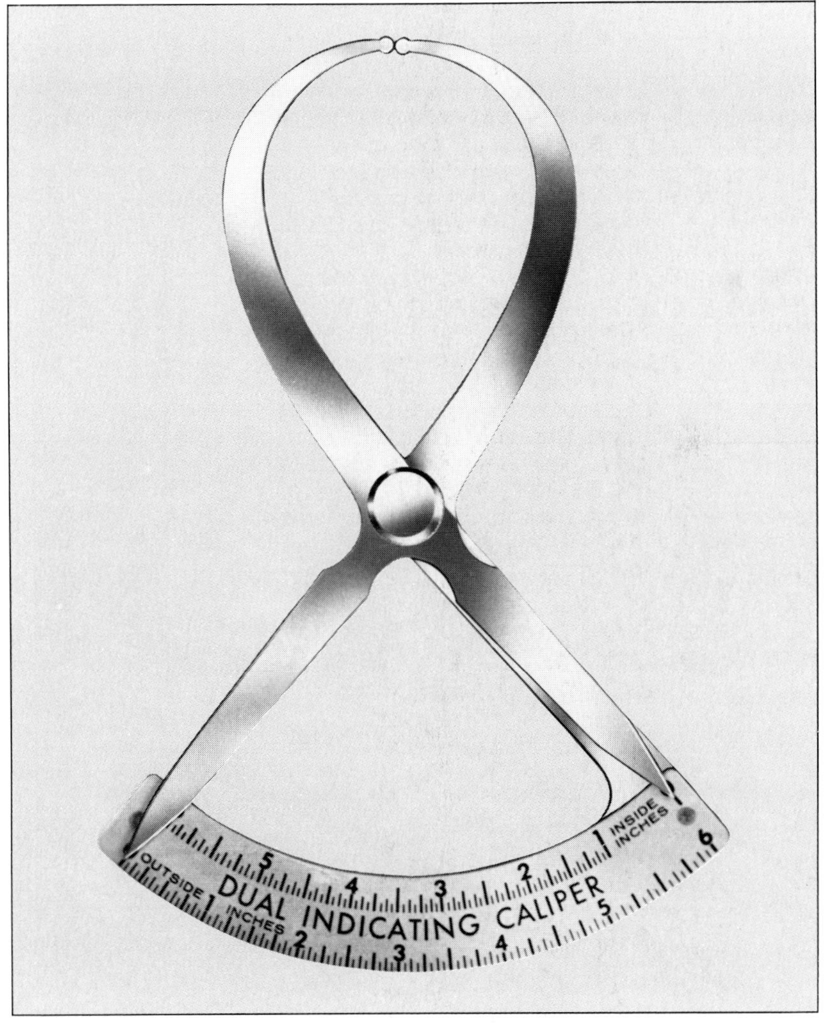

Invasive monitoring is the most accurate way to assess compartment syndrome. But suppose your hospital or clinic isn't equipped for invasive monitoring? The next best assessment technique is serial extremity measurements taken with calipers, such as the Dual Indicating Calipers featured here. By using calipers instead of a tape measure, you avoid having to ask the patient to lift a painful extremity for each measurement.

Let's say you're monitoring your patient's injured left arm for compartment syndrome with calipers. Take these steps:

- Using an indelible marker, put a dot on the medial aspect of his left arm, several inches above the injury.
- Mark another dot at a parallel site on his arm's lateral aspect.
- Mark a second pair of dots 1" (2.5 cm) distal to the first pair. Repeat this procedure until you have a series of dots 1" apart extending the length of the patient's arm.
- Open the calipers and place the jaws' tips on the proximal pair of dots. Gently close the jaws so they rest lightly on the dots. (Don't force the jaws closed, or you're likely to get an inaccurate reading.)
- Read the measurement on the calipers' *outside* scale.
- Repeat the measurement procedure for each pair of dots.
- Document all measurements. Repeat the procedure every 15 to 30 minutes, and note any trend toward increasing diameter.

Note: To assess trends in two planes, mark pairs of dots on the ventral and dorsal aspects of the patient's affected arm and record serial measurements from these points, too.

SPECIAL CONSIDERATIONS

When your patient needs a fasciotomy

Let's say you're using a mercury manometer to monitor your patient for signs of compartment syndrome. For 2 hours you've recorded pressure measurements between 40 and 45 mm Hg. The doctor probably won't wait any longer before surgically relieving pressure with a fasciotomy. By doing so now—before clinical signs and symptoms appear—he may prevent muscle necrosis, acidosis, nerve damage, and blood vessel compromise, which, in turn, can cause irreversible muscle contracture and paralysis.

To perform the procedure, the doctor makes an incision through the skin covering the medial aspect of the affected compartment; then, he incises the fascia. To prevent tearing, both incisions are the same length—from 4" to 6" (10 to 15 cm). Chances are, he'll also make an identical incision along the compartment's lateral aspect, too. These incisions allow the compartment to swell freely, relieving pressure inside the compartment.

After the procedure, the doctor may ask you to keep the incisions wet by applying dressings soaked with sterile saline solution or water. Or, he may order a petrolatum-saturated gauze dressing to be applied instead. Secure the dressing by *loosely* wrapping the arm or leg with a bulky dressing like Kling or Kerlix.

Note: Under unusual circumstances, the doctor may leave the incisions open to air; for example, if the patient has an infection (such as gas gangrene) caused by an anaerobic organism.

After swelling subsides (probably within a few days), the doctor sutures the incisions or closes them with skin grafts.

Providing nursing care

When caring for a patient who's recovering from a fasciotomy, follow these guidelines:

- Change the dressing every 4 hours, or as ordered. Maintain strict aseptic technique; infection spreads quickly in long fascial incisions. During each dressing change, observe and document the amount, color, and odor of drainage and the wound's appearance. *Note:* Serosanguinous drainage is normal.
- Protect bed linens from drainage by placing a sterile barrier under the arm or leg.
- Don't ask the patient to hold up his arm or leg during dressing changes. Instead, ask a co-worker to support it while you work. Remember, after surgery, the arm or leg will be painful.
- If infection develops, irrigate the incisions with antibiotic solution, as ordered.
- Provide continuing emotional support for the patient. Keep in mind that these large, open wounds may upset him. Inform him that although the incisions will probably leave scars, scarring can be minimized with plastic surgery. Give him more information if he wishes.

Trauma

Peritoneal lavage: Learning the basics

Your patient was brought to the emergency department after the car she was driving skidded into a ditch. The doctor suspects internal abdominal injuries. To confirm his suspicions, he decides to perform peritoneal lavage. To refresh your knowledge of this diagnostic procedure, read what follows and study the illustration at right.

Understanding the procedure

To perform peritoneal lavage, the doctor makes a small incision at midline, about 1" to 2" (2.5 to 5 cm) below the umbilicus. (Under certain circumstances, he'll choose another site; for example, if the patient has a scar at this spot.) Then, he inserts a cannula through the peritoneum and into the abdominal cavity. After aspirating a peritoneal fluid specimen, he introduces about 1,000 ml of lavage solution and allows it to spread throughout the abdominal cavity. Finally, he drains the fluid and examines it for blood, bile, and other signs of internal injury. After the procedure, you'll send fluid specimens to the lab for more detailed analysis. *Note:* If the patient's a child or a small adult, the doctor introduces less lavage fluid, according to this formula: 20 ml of fluid per kilogram of body weight, up to 1,000 ml.

Possible complications of peritoneal lavage include perforation of the bladder, intestine, or a major blood vessel or organ.

Your role

In the following photostory, you'll learn how to assist with peritoneal lavage. Besides the guidelines shown there, keep these points in mind:

- Explain the procedure to your patient and her family (if present) and answer their questions. Prepare the patient to experience some discomfort during needle insertion, but assure her that she'll receive a local anesthetic to minimize pain. Tell her the procedure takes from 30 minutes to 1 hour.
- Make sure the patient's signed a consent form. If for any reason she can't, make sure a responsible family member has done so.
- Take baseline vital signs and abdominal girth measurements. *Important:* Notify the doctor if the patient's vital signs are unstable.
- Document the patient's pain symptoms.
- Ask the patient to urinate before the procedure begins. This reduces the risk of bladder perforation during the procedure. If she can't urinate, prepare to catheterize her.
- During the procedure, check vital signs every 15 minutes. Compare your readings with the baseline measurements, and observe for dizziness, pallor, perspiration, and increasing anxiety.
- After the procedure, check vital signs every 15 minutes until stable and then every 30 minutes for 2 hours, hourly for 4 hours, and every 4 hours for the next 24 hours.
- Periodically ask the patient if she has more or less pain now than before the procedure or if the pain is different in any way. Document her responses.
- Check the dressing over the incision site whenever you monitor vital signs. Reinforce the dressing or apply a pressure dressing, if necessary.
- Periodically measure the patient's abdominal girth, and compare this measurement with the baseline measurement.
- Monitor urinary output for hematuria, which suggests bladder perforation.

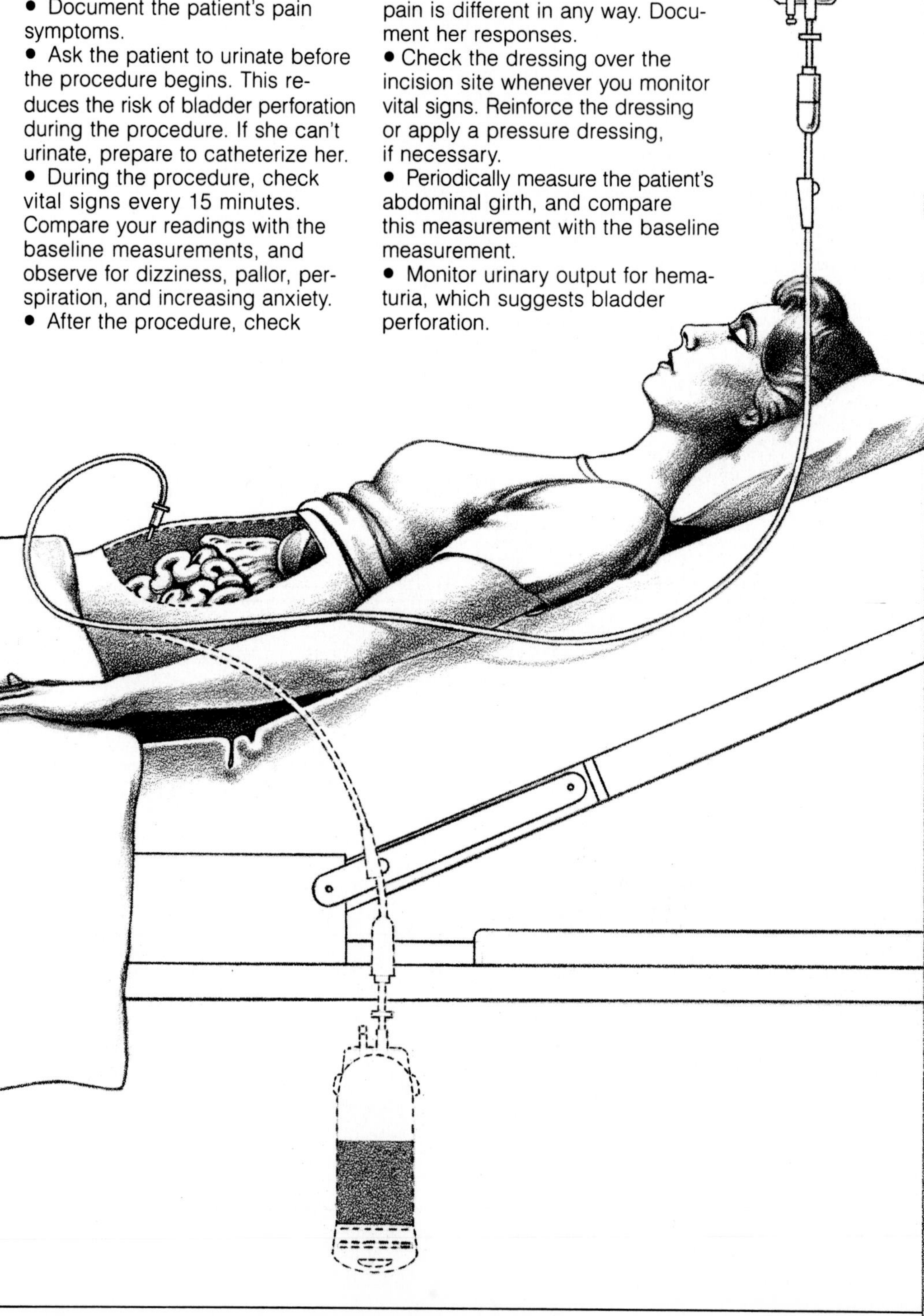

Assisting with peritoneal lavage

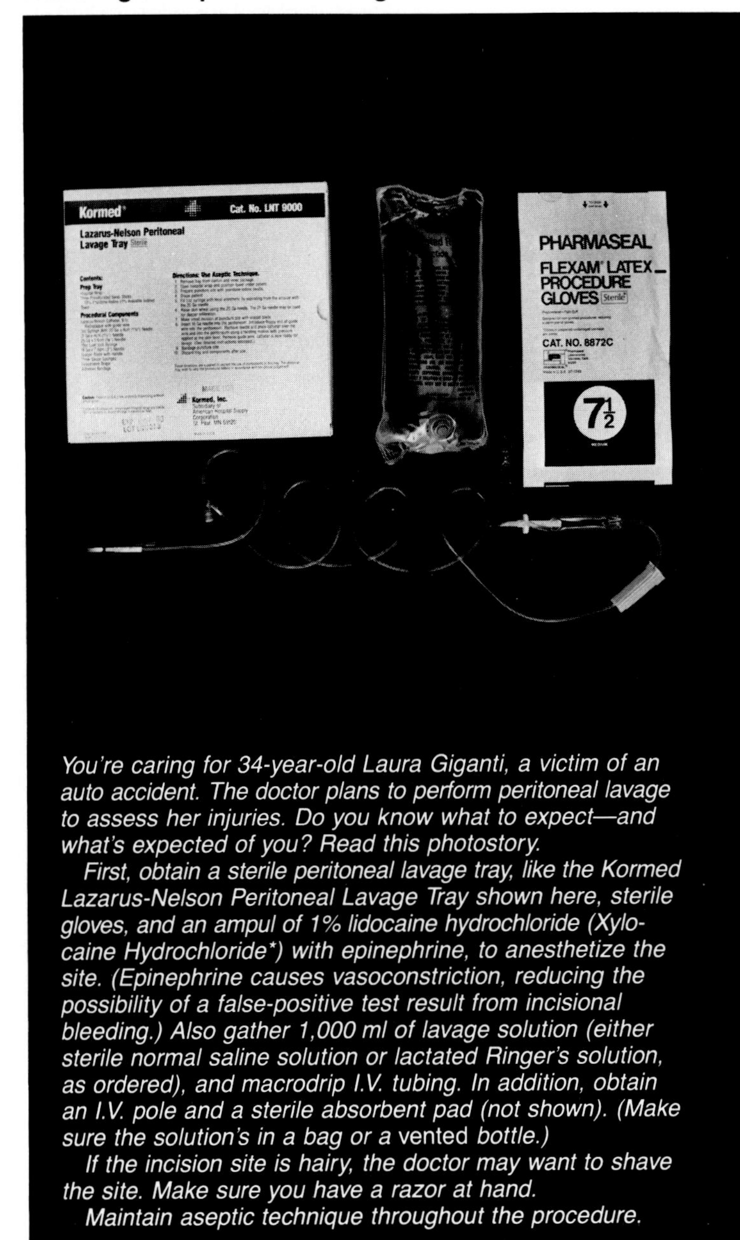

You're caring for 34-year-old Laura Giganti, a victim of an auto accident. The doctor plans to perform peritoneal lavage to assess her injuries. Do you know what to expect—and what's expected of you? Read this photostory.

First, obtain a sterile peritoneal lavage tray, like the Kormed Lazarus-Nelson Peritoneal Lavage Tray shown here, sterile gloves, and an ampul of 1% lidocaine hydrochloride (Xylocaine Hydrochloride) with epinephrine, to anesthetize the site. (Epinephrine causes vasoconstriction, reducing the possibility of a false-positive test result from incisional bleeding.) Also gather 1,000 ml of lavage solution (either sterile normal saline solution or lactated Ringer's solution, as ordered), and macrodrip I.V. tubing. In addition, obtain an I.V. pole and a sterile absorbent pad (not shown). (Make sure the solution's in a bag or a vented bottle.)*

If the incision site is hairy, the doctor may want to shave the site. Make sure you have a razor at hand.

Maintain aseptic technique throughout the procedure.

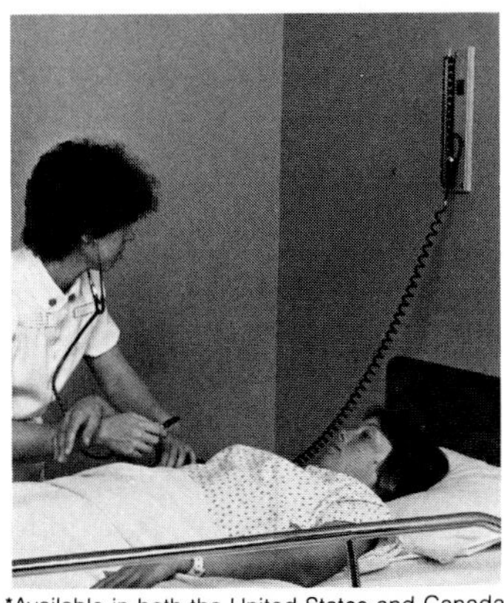

1 Explain the procedure to your patient, and answer her questions. Document baseline vital signs measurements, abdominal girth, and pain symptoms. Then, provide her with a bedpan, and ask her to urinate.

Meanwhile, the doctor dons sterile gloves.

*Available in both the United States and Canada

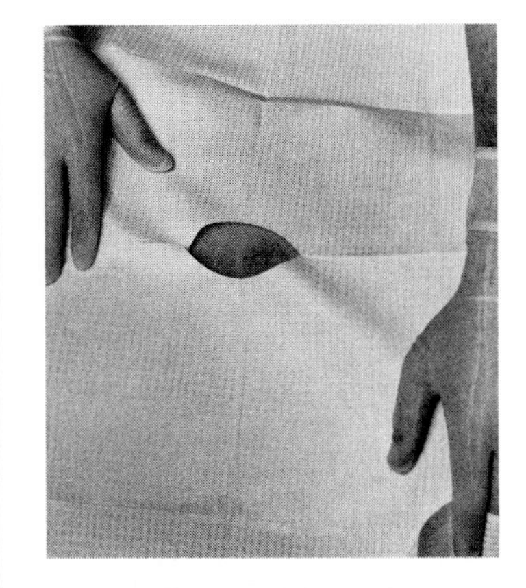

2 Place the patient in supine position. Cover her as necessary to prevent chilling. Observing aseptic technique, open the sterile tray and position its sterile towel under her to catch drainage.

Prep the surgical area with the tray's three povidone-iodine swabs, if ordered. (The doctor may prefer to do this himself.) Then, the doctor drapes the patient with the fenestrated drape, so the proposed incision site's visible.

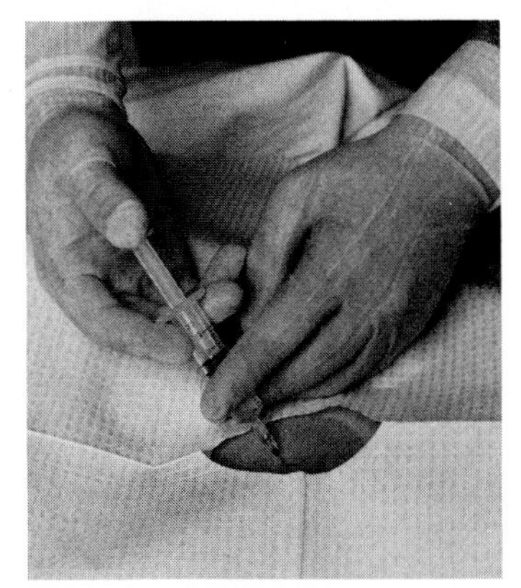

3 Snap off the ampul's neck and invert the ampul so the doctor can draw up the appropriate amount of local anesthetic (between 1 and 3 ml). Now, the doctor anesthetizes the site.

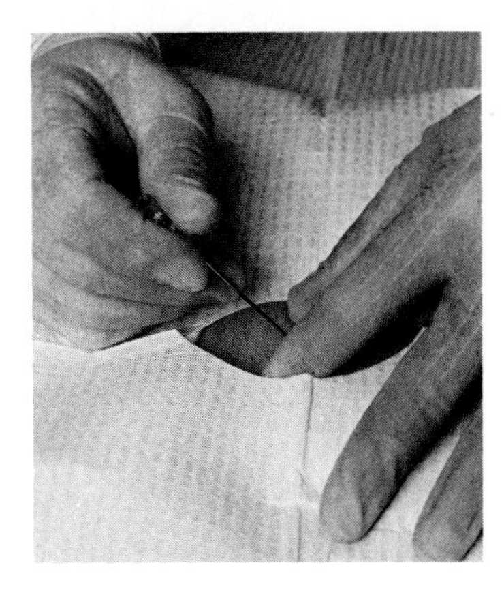

4 Next, he makes a 3-mm vertical incision with the scalpel blade. Then, he inserts the 18G needle through the incision into the abdominal cavity. You may hear a popping sound as the needle punctures the peritoneum. *Important:* Provide support for the patient, because the puncture may be painful. Tell her to tense her abdomen, as if having a bowel movement, during this part of the procedure.

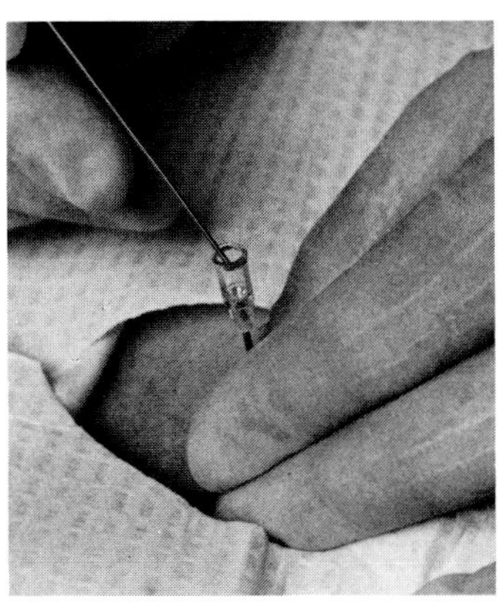

5 Now the doctor inserts the floppy end of the guide wire through the needle and into the peritoneum. If he's placed the needle correctly, the wire will fall freely into the cavity. When about half the wire's inside the cavity, he carefully removes the needle, leaving the wire in place.

Trauma

Assisting with peritoneal lavage continued

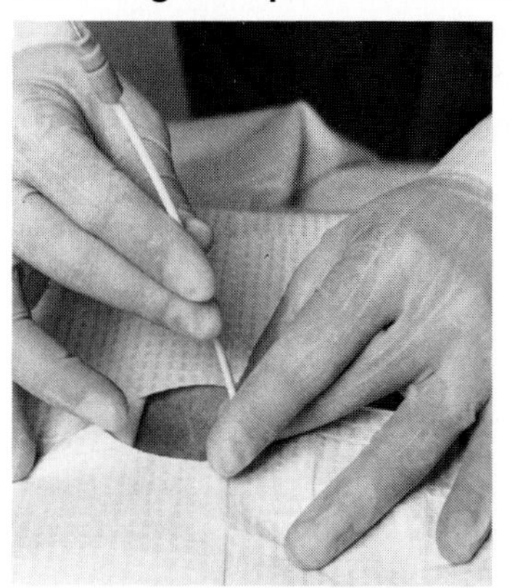

6 Next, he places the catheter over the wire, as shown, and inserts the catheter into the peritoneum. He uses a twisting motion to force the catheter through the fascia. The wire's stiff end still protrudes from the catheter. When the catheter's in place, the doctor removes the wire. *Note:* If the catheter touches the rectum, the patient may feel an urge to defecate.

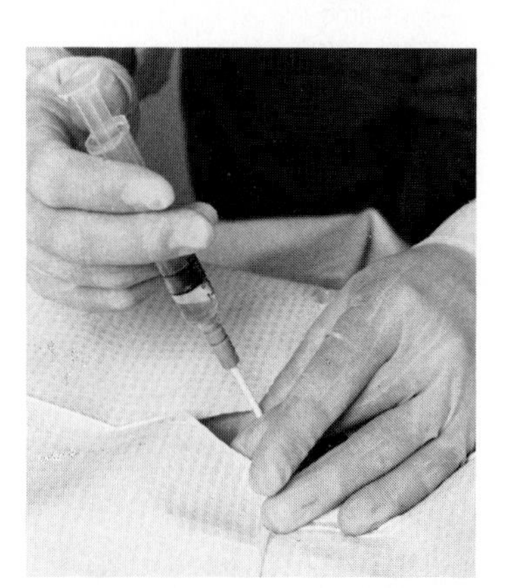

7 Using a 10-ml syringe, the doctor aspirates a specimen. If he recovers less than 10 ml of free-flowing blood or peritoneal fluid, he considers the specimen nondiagnostic and prepares for lavage.

Important: If he aspirates more than 10 ml of blood, he may have lacerated a blood vessel during needle insertion. Prepare the patient for emergency surgery. Be sure the patient or a family member signs a consent form, if possible.

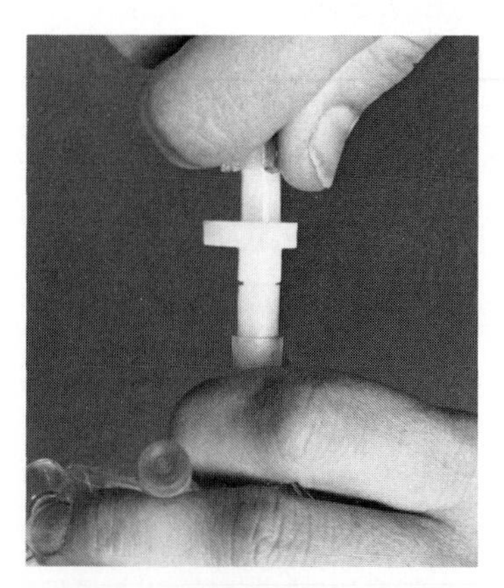

8 Spike the I.V. container, hang it on the I.V. pole, and prime the tubing. Then, close the I.V. tubing's clamp. The doctor now attaches the I.V. tubing to the peritoneal catheter, fully opens the clamp, and allows I.V. solution to run into the abdominal cavity.

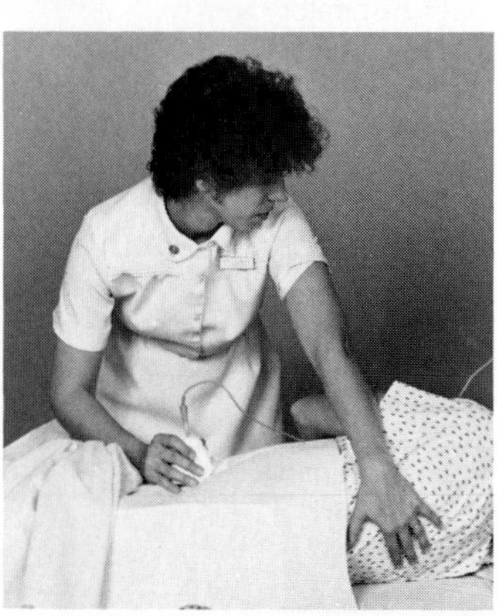

9 To help mix the I.V. solution and peritoneal fluids, turn or roll the patient from side to side. While you do, take care to support the catheter by wrapping it in a sterile pad and holding it, as shown here. (Explain this step to your patient before beginning.) *Caution:* This step is contraindicated if the patient has hypotension or a suspected spinal injury.

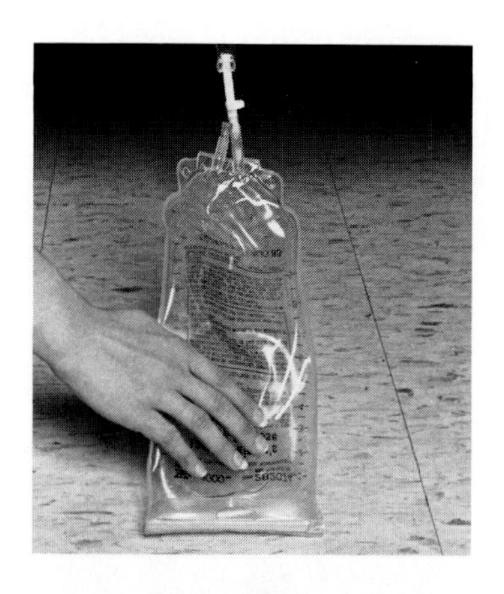

10 After about 10 minutes, place the I.V. container on the floor. The mixture of lavage solution and peritoneal fluid will now siphon into the container. *Note:* If your patient becomes hypovolemic or shows signs of shock, slow the drainage rate by raising the I.V. container. If necessary, stop drainage by clamping the tubing.

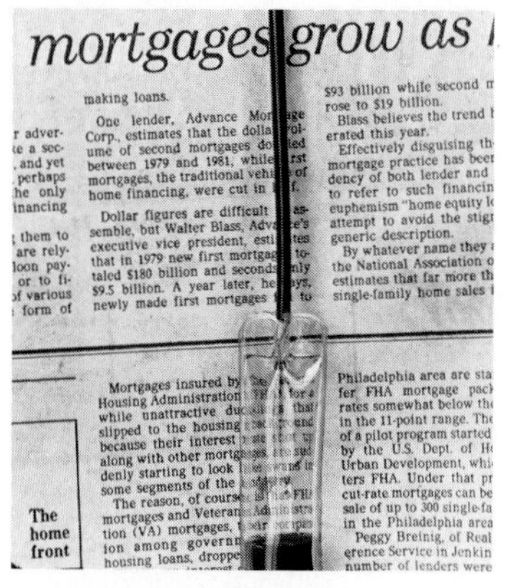

11 Because blood is present, the doctor checks to see if he can read newspaper print through the fluid in the I.V. tubing. If he can't, the test is strongly positive; if he can, the test is weakly positive. (If the fluid is clear, the test is negative.) *Note:* If the test is strongly positive, as shown here, prepare the patient for emergency surgery.

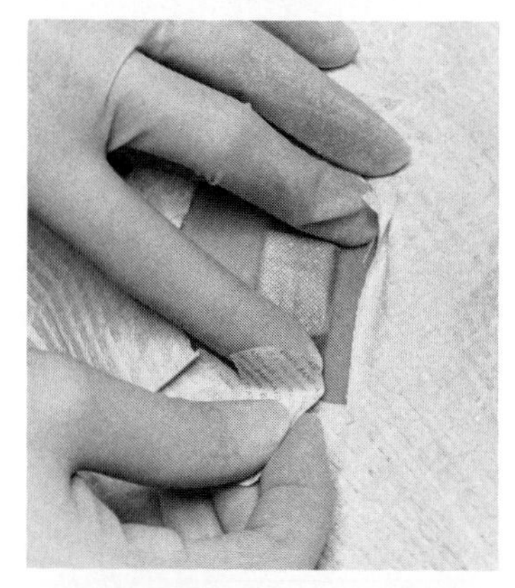

12 When lavage is complete, the doctor removes the catheter. Apply an adhesive bandage strip over the incision and help the patient into a comfortable position. *Note:* The doctor may close the incision with one or two sutures or cover it with a butterfly adhesive strip.

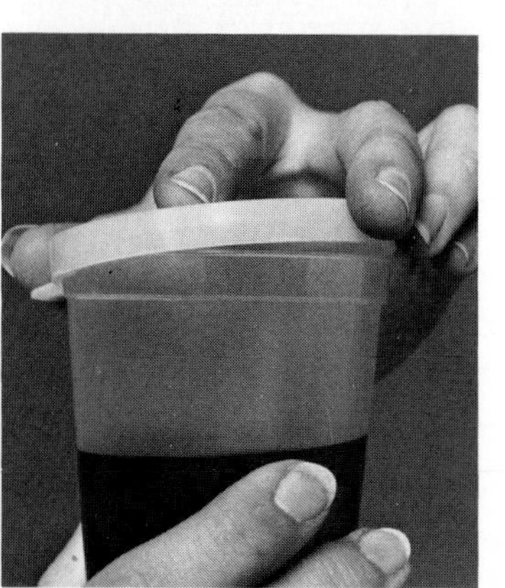

13 According to hospital policy, transfer the lavage specimen to a specimen container and label it properly. (Take care to specify that the specimen is peritoneal lavage fluid.) Also label the undiluted specimen fluid the doctor aspirated initially. Fill out the appropriate lab slips, and immediately send the specimens to the lab.

Document the procedure, including the lavage fluid's appearance.

Peritoneal fluid: Assessing its appearance

You needn't wait for a lab analysis for a clue to your patient's condition; your own observations during peritoneal lavage can tell you a lot. Normally, peritoneal fluid (if present) is clear or slightly yellow. Review the following to learn possible reasons for abnormal appearance.

Red (bloody)
Trauma, intra-abdominal tumor, acute hemorrhagic pancreatitis

Green (bile-stained)
Ruptured gallbladder, acute pancreatitis, perforated intestine, or perforated duodenal ulcer

Cloudy or turbid
Peritonitis from ruptured bowel, primary bacterial infection, pancreatitis, strangulated or infarcted intestine, appendicitis, ruptured appendix

Milky
Escaping chyle from a damaged thoracic duct, escaping barium sulfate from stomach or intestinal perforation after upper or lower gastrointestinal tests

Recognizing normal lab values

When you receive the results of your patient's peritoneal fluid analysis, can you correctly interpret the findings? The following chart will help you recognize normal values. *Important:* Keep in mind that these values apply to an *undiluted* specimen. Values measured per volume will be smaller if the specimen was diluted with lavage solution.

General qualities
Sterile, odorless, clear to pale yellow color; scant amount (less than 50 ml)

Red blood cells (RBCs)
None

White blood cells (WBCs)
Less than 300/μl

Protein
0.3 to 4.1 g/dl (albumin, 50% to 70%; globulin, 30% to 45%; fibrinogen, 0.3% to 4.5%)

Glucose
70 to 100 mg/dl

Amylase
138 to 404 units/liter

Ammonia
Less than 50 μg/dl

Alkaline phosphatase
Males over age 18: 90 to 239 units/liter
Females over age 45: 87 to 250 units/liter
Females under age 45: 76 to 196 units/liter

Cytology
No malignant cells present in specimen

Bacteria
None

Fungi
None

INDICATIONS/CONTRAINDICATIONS

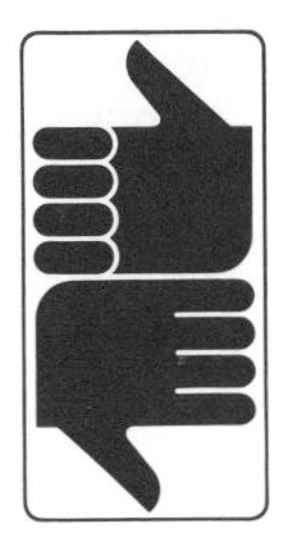

Autotransfusion: Pros and cons

With the development of less complex, safer equipment and techniques, autotransfusion—the collection and transfusion of a patient's own blood rather than donor blood—is becoming widely accepted as therapy for emergency trauma patients. If you wonder why, read the information below. Then, study the following pages for details.

Pros

- Provides compatible blood immediately. Autotransfusion avoids time-consuming typing and cross matching procedures.
- Eliminates the risk of transfusion reaction or the transmission of such diseases as hepatitis, cytomegalovirus, and malaria
- Supplies blood as close as possible to circulating blood. Blood that's transfused soon after collection has normal pH and normal levels of 2,3-diphosphoglycerate (2,3-DPG), which permits adequate oxygen delivery to tissues. It also has normal levels of all clotting factors, except fibrinogen. (Keep in mind that stored blood that's close to the 21-day shelf limit has many lysed red cells, platelet microaggregates, low platelet activity, diminished clotting factor levels, and biochemical anomalies.)
- Eliminates danger of overtransfusion
- Avoids transfusion hypothermia, because recently collected blood is warm
- May be used with patients who refuse donor blood for religious reasons
- Significantly reduces blood transfusion costs
- Conserves stored blood supplies

Cons

- May cause bacteremia from transfusion of contaminated blood (especially blood aspirated from the abdominal cavity)
- Increases risk of air embolism (especially if blood is transfused under pressure) and particulate embolism
- Increases risk of coagulopathies, especially after autotransfusion of 4,000 ml or more of blood
- Increases risk of respiratory and kidney insufficiency (unless damaged white cells and the lysosomal enzymes they release are removed from the blood before it's transfused)
- May encourage dissemination of aspirated cancer cells.

Note: None of these disadvantages is a contraindication in a life-threatening emergency. Air embolism is a significant risk only with certain older types of equipment, such as the Bentley ATS-100. Risk of bacteremia from contaminated blood is significantly reduced by concurrent administration of a broad-spectrum antibiotic.

Trauma

Learning about autotransfusion

Your patient in the emergency department is hemorrhaging from extensive internal injuries. Is autotransfusion indicated?

Chances are, the answer's *yes*. Generally, autotransfusion's indicated whenever 2 or 3 units of pooled blood is recoverable from a body cavity. Blood recovered from the abdominal cavity is less desirable than blood from the thoracic cavity, because it may be contaminated with bile, feces, and other abdominal contents. But when a patient's in danger of bleeding to death, the benefits of transfusing possibly contaminated blood from the abdominal cavity outweigh the dangers.

Autotransfusion consists of these steps:

- collection of shed blood with specially designed suction and collection equipment
- anticoagulation of collected blood (if necessary)
- processing to eliminate undesirable blood components and products (this step may be skipped in an emergency, when blood's needed quickly)
- transfusion of filtered blood.

Comparing equipment

Equipment used to treat traumatic injuries must be simple and easy to use; otherwise, risk of error during an emergency is high. In addition, such equipment should minimize blood cell damage during collection, reduce the risk of air embolism during transfusion, and contain a filtering system to screen out microclots and contaminants.

The Receptal ATS Trauma, made by Sorenson Research Company, meets these requirements. A special suction regulator limits the power of ordinary room suction to about 10 mm Hg, minimizing blood cell damage. Because the unit mounts on an I.V. pole, you can take it wherever it's needed. For details on operating this equipment, read the following photostory.

The more complex Haemonetics Cell Saver is a much larger, free-standing unit that employs a centrifuge to spin off blood components, debris, and contaminants, leaving only red blood cells. Then, it washes and packs the cells and returns them, suspended in normal saline solution, to the patient. In an emergency, this

Getting acquainted with the Receptal ATS Trauma

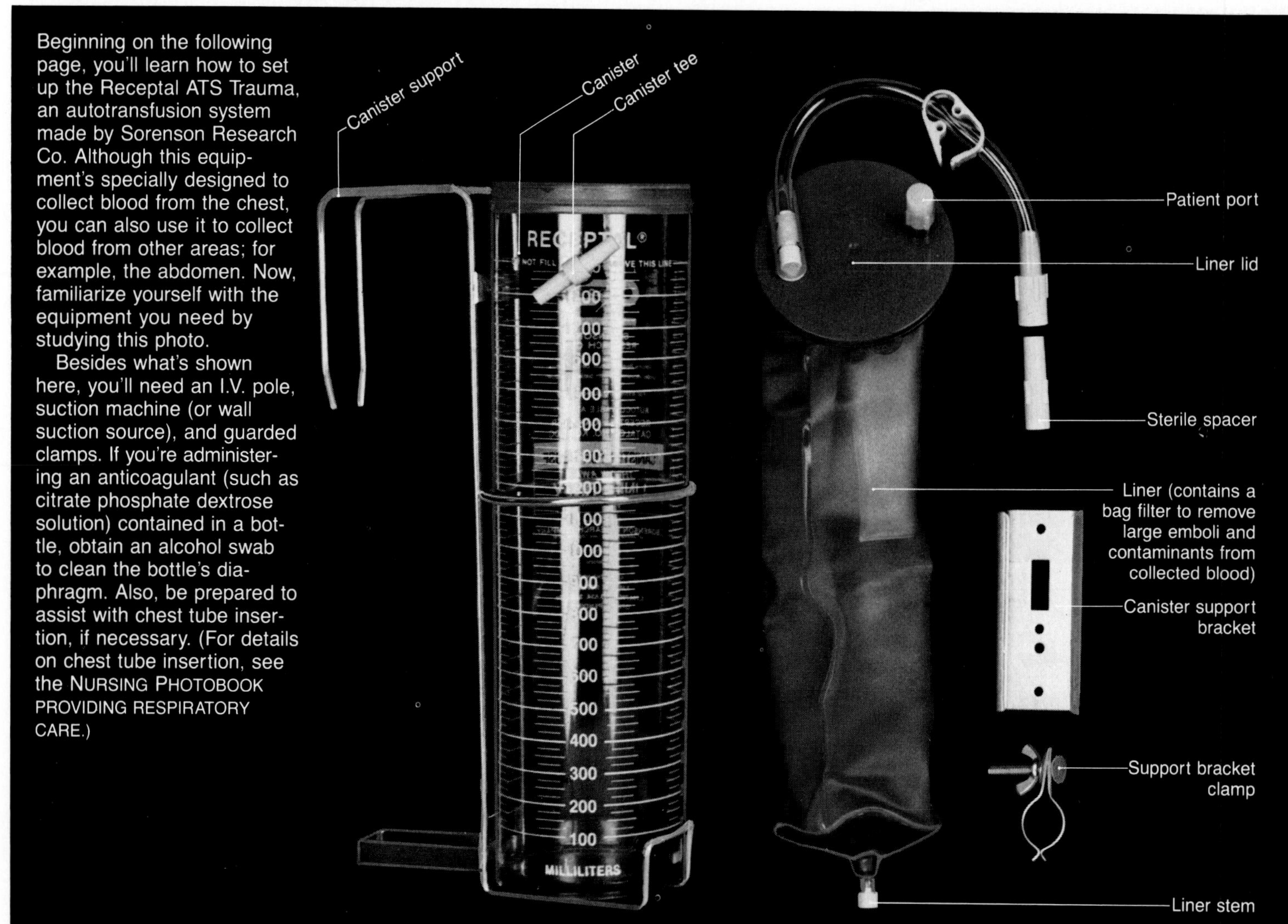

Beginning on the following page, you'll learn how to set up the Receptal ATS Trauma, an autotransfusion system made by Sorenson Research Co. Although this equipment's specially designed to collect blood from the chest, you can also use it to collect blood from other areas; for example, the abdomen. Now, familiarize yourself with the equipment you need by studying this photo.

Besides what's shown here, you'll need an I.V. pole, suction machine (or wall suction source), and guarded clamps. If you're administering an anticoagulant (such as citrate phosphate dextrose solution) contained in a bottle, obtain an alcohol swab to clean the bottle's diaphragm. Also, be prepared to assist with chest tube insertion, if necessary. (For details on chest tube insertion, see the NURSING PHOTOBOOK PROVIDING RESPIRATORY CARE.)

equipment is less useful than the Receptal, because it delays blood return to the patient while processing occurs. Also, it's more expensive and requires a specially trained operator.

Note: Autotransfusion equipment formerly made by the Bentley Corporation (for example, the Bentley ATS-100 and ATS-200) has been discontinued because of recurring problems with pump-induced hemolysis and air embolism caused by operator error.

Anticoagulation problems

As a rule, collected blood must be anticoagulated before it's transfused. (An exception is blood collected after some types of chest injury, because blood that contacts the lungs or pericardium anticoagulates naturally.) Using a systemic anticoagulant, such as heparin, can be disastrous for a patient who's already bleeding massively. To avoid the added risk of systemic anticoagulation, anticoagulate shed blood with citrate phosphate dextrose (CPD). Because the body quickly metabolizes CPD, anticoagulation is limited to the blood in the autotransfusion system. *Note:* To avoid citrate toxicosis and heart failure, the doctor will probably order calcium to be given with any large transfusion.

Other indications for autotransfusion

Autotransfusion has a place in nonemergency surgery, too. Blood may be obtained:

- *preoperatively.* If a patient's scheduled for surgery that may produce considerable blood loss (such as vascular surgery), he may donate his blood for storage and later use (if necessary) during surgery.
- *immediately before surgery.* After anesthetizing the patient but before beginning surgery, the doctor withdraws 1 to 2 units of blood and replaces the volume with crystalloid or colloid. Now, fresh, warm, compatible blood is available for immediate use. This method's widely used for cardiac bypass surgery.
- *postoperatively.* Blood shed during surgery is collected and replaced postoperatively in the recovery room or surgical ICU.

Note: Autotransfusion is contraindicated if the patient has a previously diagnosed coagulation disorder and during cancer surgery.

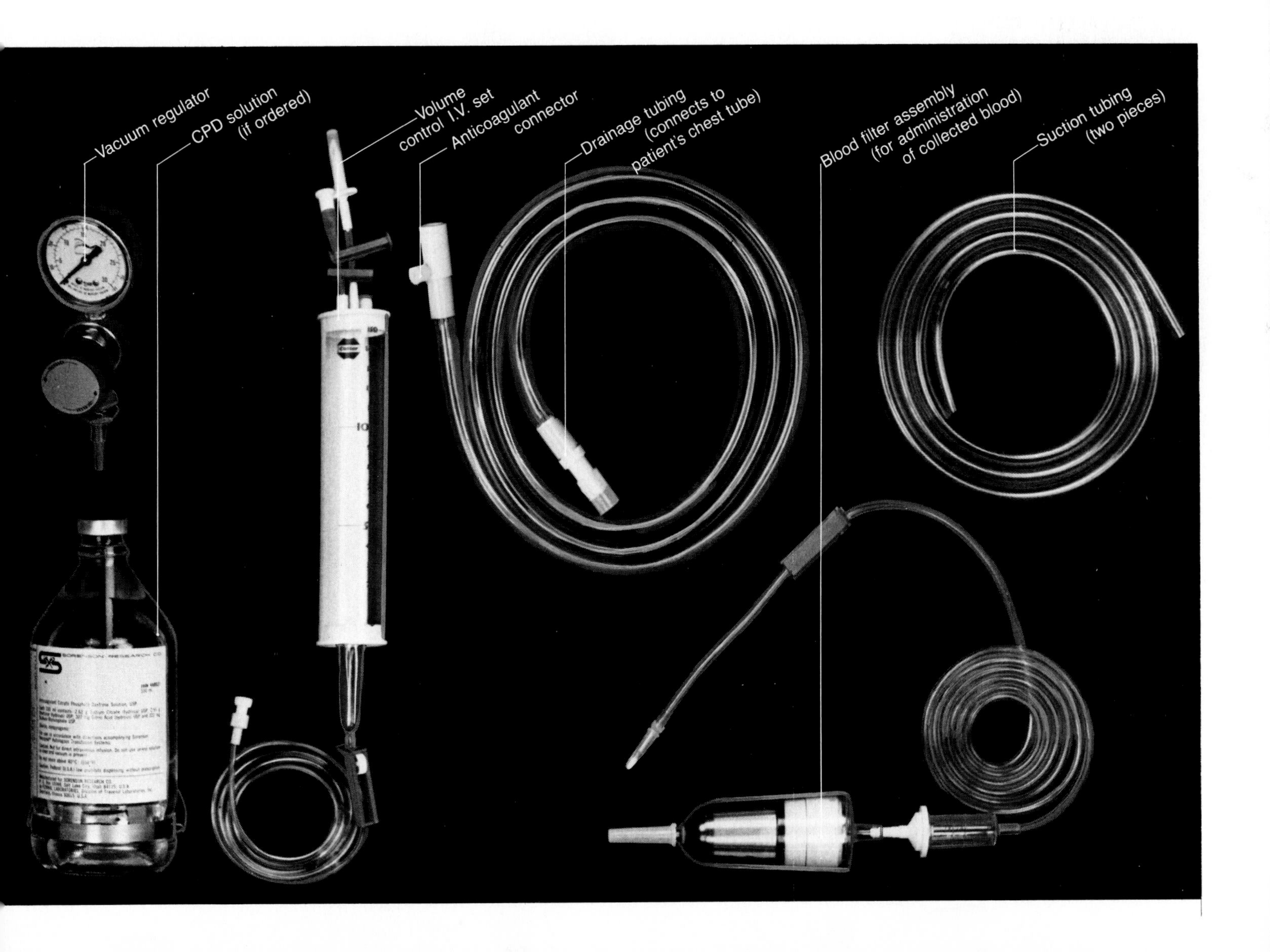

Trauma

Performing autotransfusion

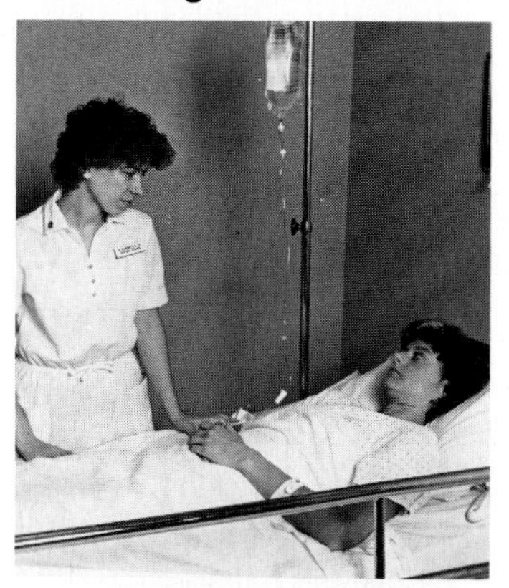

1 Your patient suffered traumatic chest injuries during a car accident. Because she's developed a large hemothorax, the doctor's ordered chest drainage and autotransfusion. To assist, first gather the equipment you need (see preceding page). Then, thoroughly wash and dry your hands. Maintain strict aseptic technique throughout the procedure.

Explain the procedure to your patient.

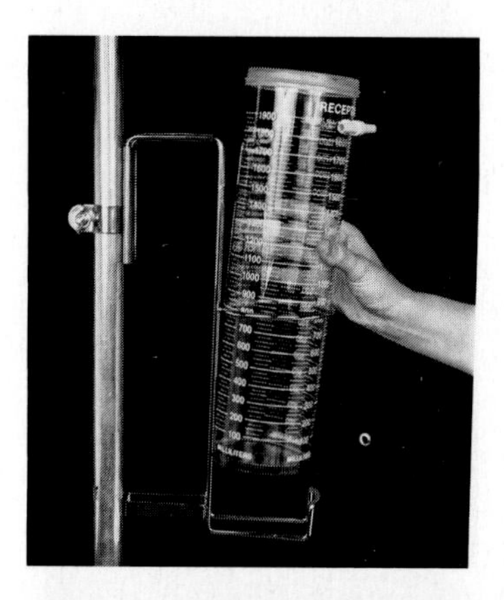

2 To assemble the autotransfusion equipment, first slip the support bracket in place on the canister support. Then, using the bracket clamp, attach the canister support to an I.V. pole. Insert the canister, as shown. *Note:* For convenience, you may permanently mount the canister support on a wall; for example, for use in an operating or emergency room.

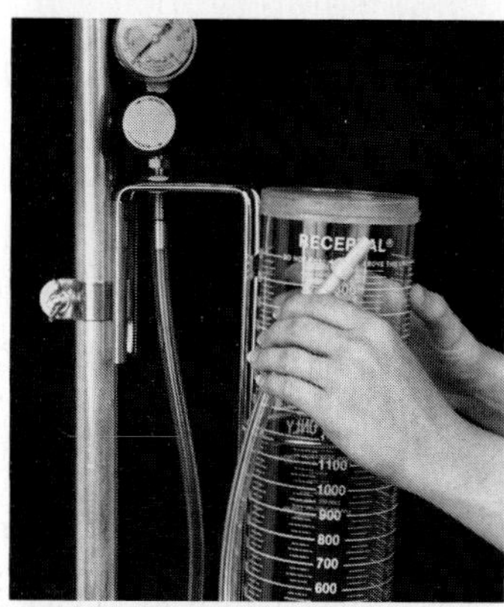

3 Mount the vacuum regulator on the canister support, as shown. Then, use suction tubing to connect the regulator with the canister tee, as the nurse is doing here.

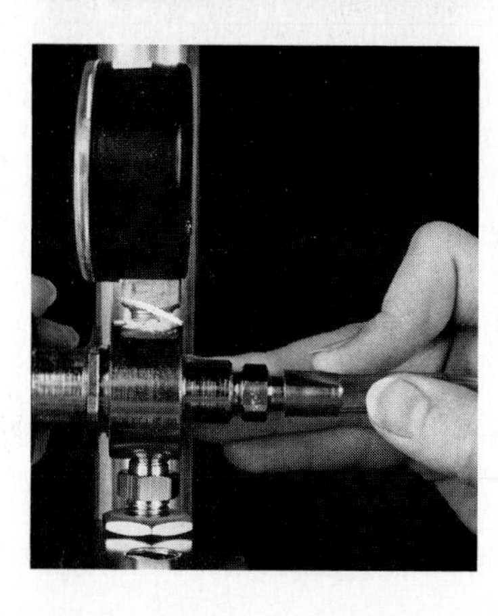

4 With another piece of suction tubing, connect the vacuum regulator with the suction source (suction machine or wall suction outlet). *Note:* Instead of mounting the vacuum regulator on an I.V. pole, you can insert it directly into a wall suction outlet. Depending on the outlet's size, you may need an adapter.

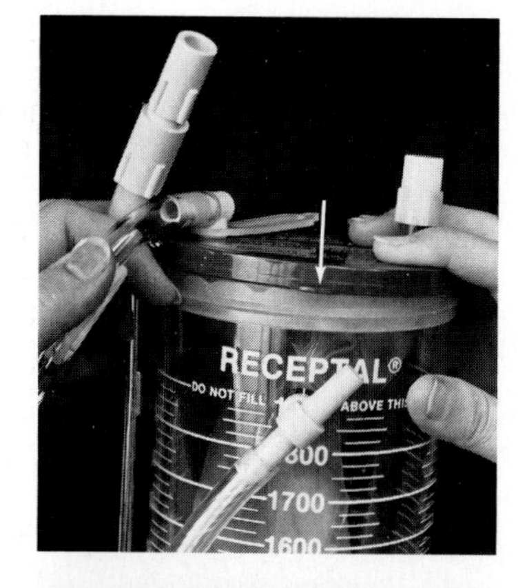

5 Remove the sterile liner assembly from its plastic wrapping. Unfold the liner and extend it to its full length.

Caution: Don't contaminate the sterile spacer attached to the liner lid's tubing.

Insert the liner in the canister, as shown. Line up the lid's thumb tab (see arrow) with the canister tee; then, firmly press the lid in place.

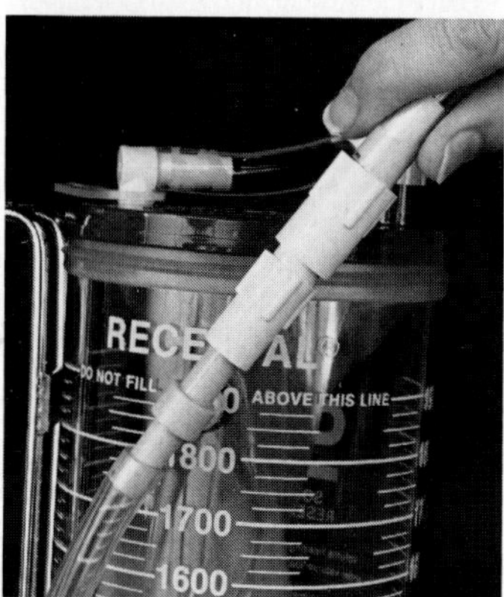

6 Grasp the sterile spacer and connect the lid's tubing with the canister tee. Turn on the vacuum machine. Then, using a guarded clamp, occlude the tubing between the regulator and the vacuum machine. Adjust the vacuum to between 10 and 30 mm Hg, as ordered.

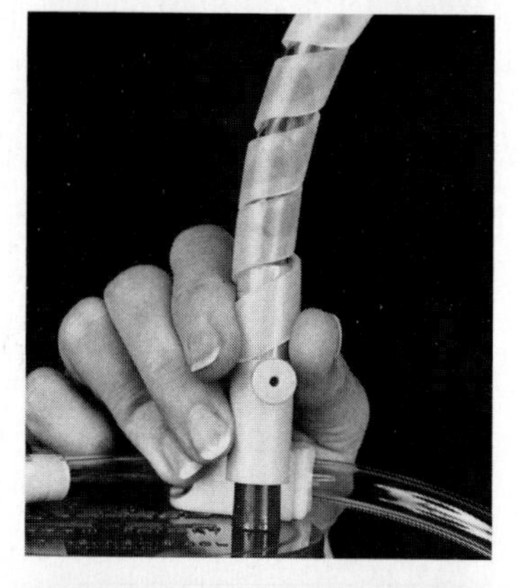

7 After the doctor's inserted the chest tube, remove the sterile drainage tubing from its package. Uncap the male end and insert it into the patient's chest tube. Then, uncap the patient port on the liner lid and attach the drainage tubing's other end to it, as shown.

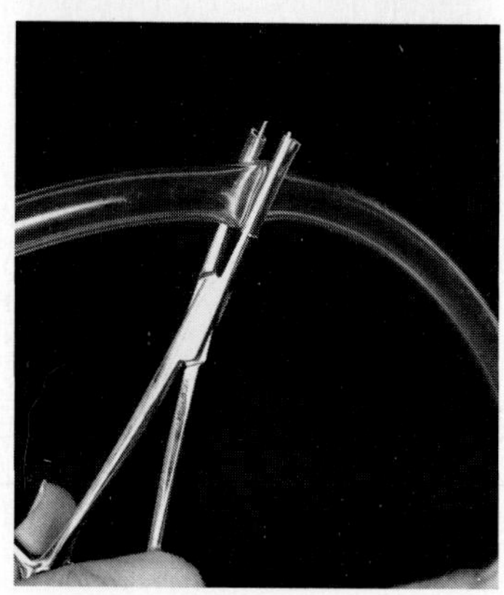

8 Unclamp the suction tubing between the regulator and the canister. Now, blood collection begins.

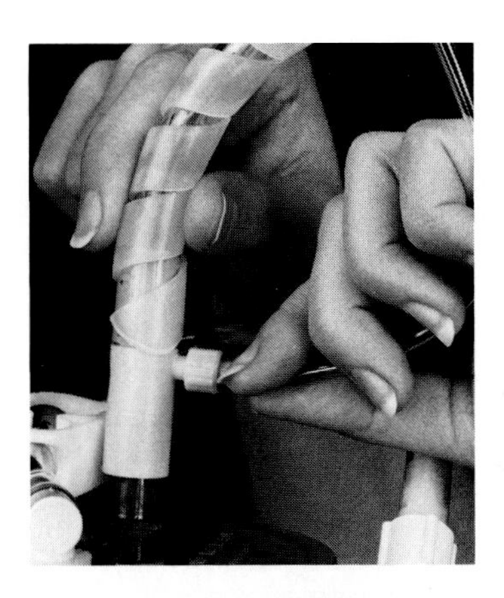

9 If the doctor's ordered anticoagulation with citrate phosphate dextrose (CPD), spike and hang the I.V. container; then, flush the line and close the flow clamp. *Important:* Always deliver CPD with a volume control I.V. set.

Now, remove the cap from the anticoagulant connector and attach the I.V. tubing, as shown. *Note:* If you're not using anticoagulant, leave the anticoagulant connector's cap in place.

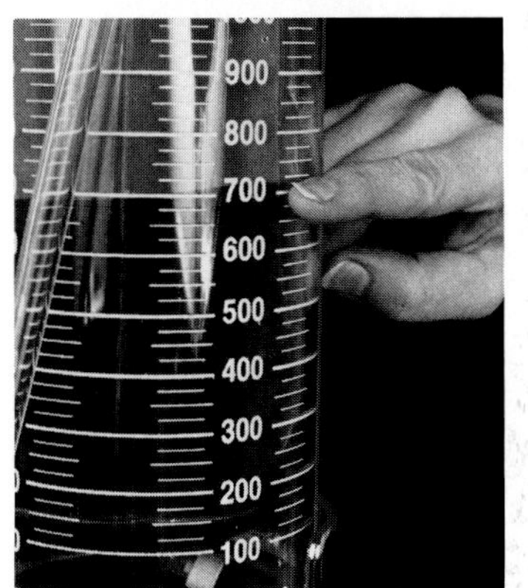

10 Start the CPD infusion, regulating flow rate as ordered. (The recommended mix for CPD is between 25 and 60 ml per 500 ml of blood. To help you set the correct flow rate, Sorenson supplies a handy blood-to-CPD ratio guide.)

Carefully monitor the liner's blood level, as the nurse is doing here. Don't permit the liner to overflow.

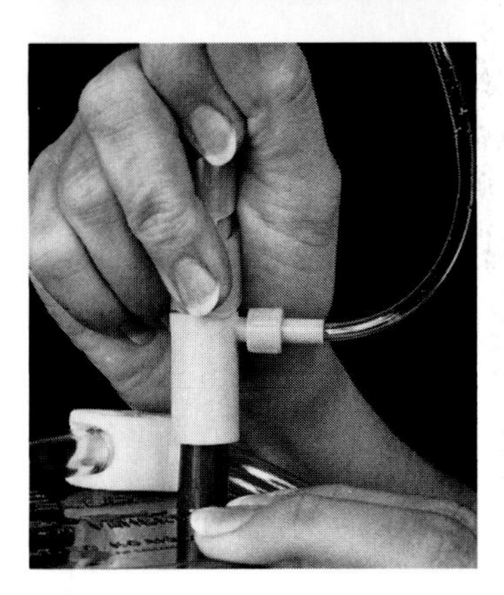

11 Prepare to transfuse the collected blood by clamping the patient tubing close to the canister. *Caution:* Always clamp the patient's line before turning off the suction or disconnecting any part of the suction line. Otherwise, pneumothorax may result.

Then, stop the CPD infusion and disconnect the patient line (which includes the anticoagulant connector) from the liner lid's patient port.

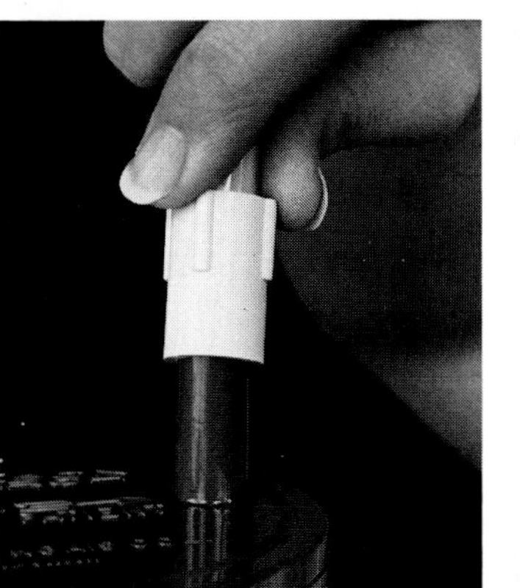

12 Disconnect the sterile spacer from the lid tubing and discard it. Immediately connect the lid tubing to the patient port, as shown here. Secure the connection by giving the tubing a hard push and twist.

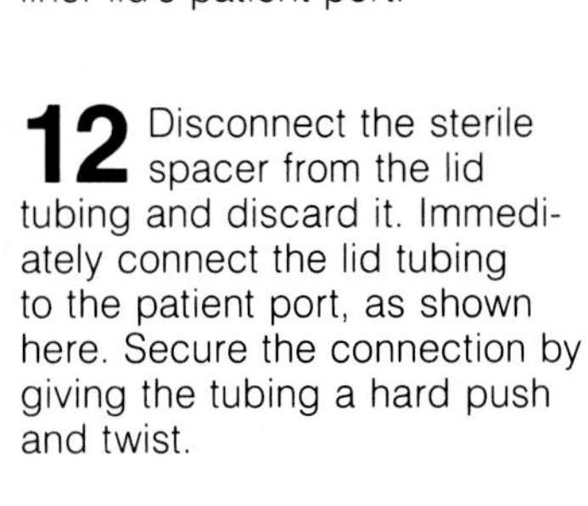

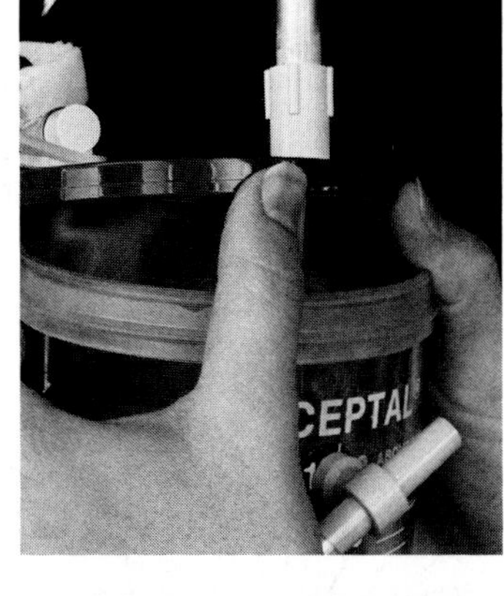

13 Remove the liner by pressing against the lid's thumb tab. If you plan to continue blood collection, replace the liner with a sterile one. Reconnect the patient and vacuum lines, as already shown.

Nursing tip: As an alternative, consider preparing a second canister and lining beforehand. To continue blood collection, simply connect the tubing to the second set of equipment.

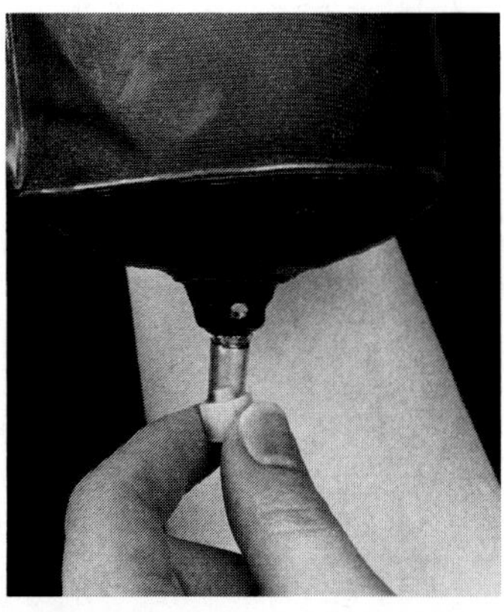

14 Now, grasp the capped stem on the filled liner bag and pull it out, as shown.

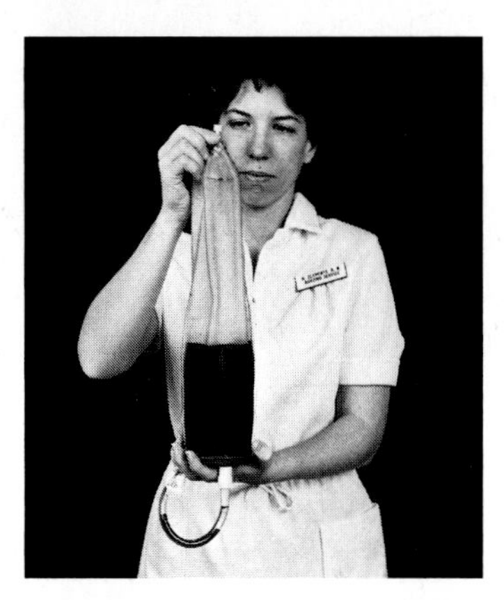

15 Invert the liner, so the capped stem points up.

16 Remove the filter assembly from its package. (We're featuring the Sorenson-Swank Blood Filter. Other types may require a set-up procedure that's slightly different from the one shown here.)

Remove the protective caps from the filter spike and the liner's stem. Insert the spike into the stem, as shown.

Trauma

Performing autotransfusion continued

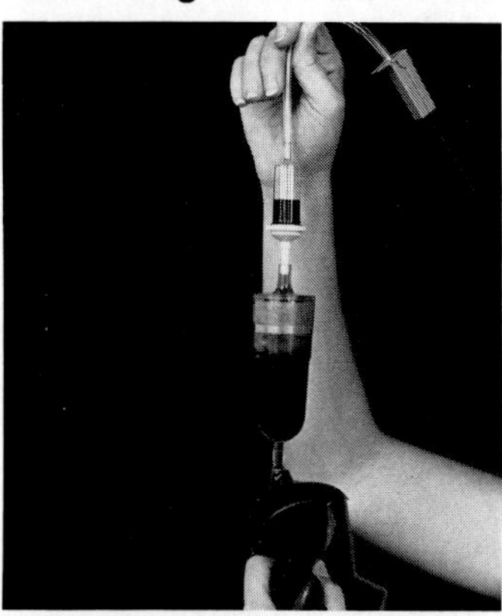

17 Open the filter assembly's flow clamp and gently squeeze all air out of the liner. Continue gentle squeezing until the filter's saturated with blood and the drip chamber is half full.

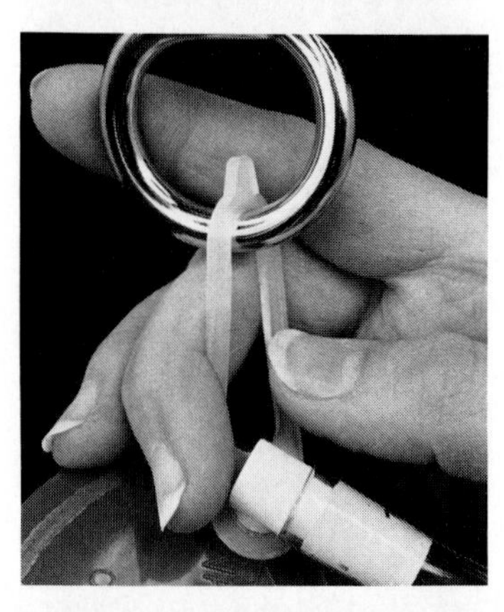

18 Close the clamp. Invert and hang the liner on the I.V. pole, using the liner lid's plastic hanger tab.

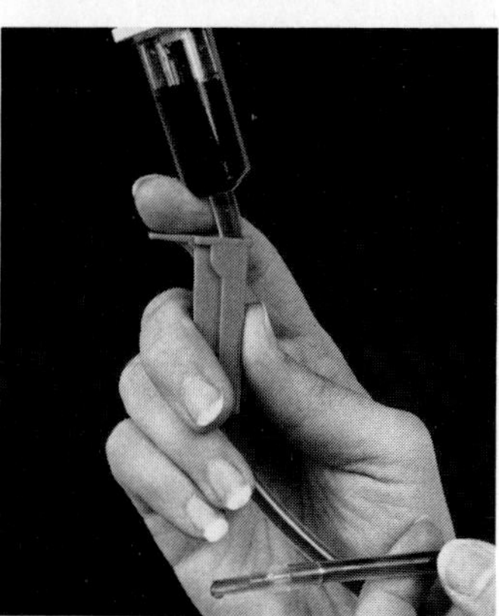

19 Open the clamp and flush air out of the rest of the tubing. Close the clamp.

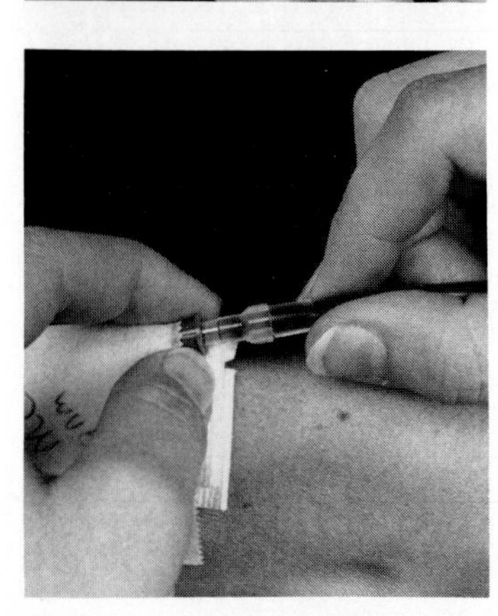

20 Connect the filter tubing to the patient's I.V. catheter or needle, and begin the infusion at the ordered rate. Use gravity or hand pressure; the liner lid may rupture a pressure bag. *Note:* For details on giving a blood transfusion, see the NURSING PHOTOBOOK MANAGING I.V. THERAPY.

After the procedure, document everything, including the amount of blood transfused.

Using the Irrijet Irrigation and Wound-cleansing System

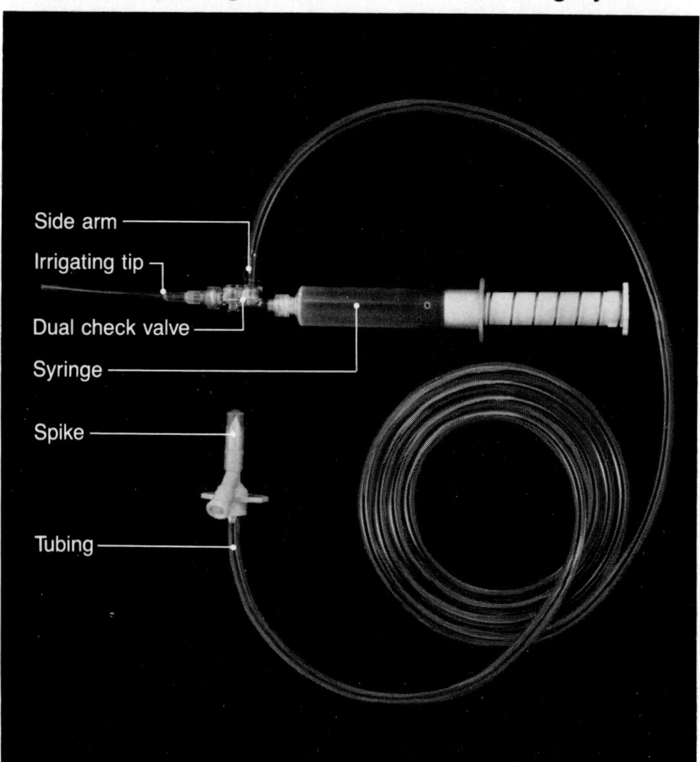

Burt Shoemaker, a 37-year-old television producer, has an infected laceration on his right arm. To expel debris from the wound, the doctor's ordered irrigation with sterile normal saline solution every 4 hours.

Wound irrigation, as you know, necessitates aseptic technique. Gathering and assembling sterile equipment every 4 hours can be time-consuming. The Irrijet Irrigation and Wound-cleansing System, by Ackrad Laboratories, offers an efficient alternative.

Look at the photo above. As you see, the Irrijet consists of a syringe with spring-action piston plunger; dual check valve; 6′(1.8-m) tubing with spike; and short, flexible irrigating tip. (The manufacturer supplies five individually wrapped sterile tips with each syringe.) The only additional equipment you need is an I.V. container of the ordered irrigating solution and an I.V. pole. (If your container's a bottle, you'll also need an alcohol swab to clean the diaphragm.)

The Irrijet tubing connects a hanging I.V. container to the check valve's side arm. The check valve permits you to alternately aspirate irrigating solution from the container and eject it into the wound without retrograde contamination.

For thorough cleansing, place the flexible tip within the wound while irrigating. When irrigation's complete, dispose of the tip and attach a sterile one. (To maintain sterility between treatments, leave the tip in its wrapper until you're ready to use it.) When you've used all five tips, dispose of all the equipment and continue treatment with new equipment, as ordered.

INDICATIONS/CONTRAINDICATIONS

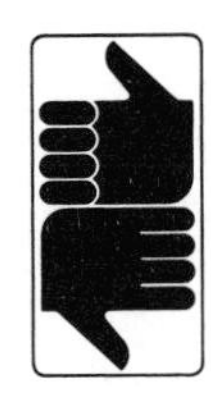

When to use hyperbaric oxygen therapy

As primary treatment, hyperbaric oxygen therapy's indicated for:
- anaerobic infection, such as gas gangrene
- anemia caused by hemorrhage
- carbon monoxide poisoning
- cyanide poisoning
- decompression sickness
- air embolism.

As secondary treatment, it's indicated for:
- smoke inhalation
- cerebral edema
- spinal cord injury
- osteomyelitis
- maintaining skin graft integrity.

For some patients, it may be helpful in treating:
- cerebrovascular accident
- bone fracture
- frostbite
- meningitis
- myocardial infarction
- sickle cell crisis.

Hyperbaric oxygen therapy's contraindicated in:
- untreated pneumothorax
- emphysema with carbon dioxide retention
- untreated metastatic cancer
- epilepsy
- upper respiratory tract infection
- history of thoracic or ear surgery
- pregnancy (especially in the first trimester).

Note: None of the above is an absolute contraindication for a primary life-threatening condition that's best treated by hyperbaric oxygen therapy; for example, gas gangrene or decompression sickness.

Treating gas gangrene with hyperbaric oxygen therapy

Three days ago, Henry Wolcott was admitted to your unit after suffering traumatic leg injuries in a farming accident. When you detected signs of developing ischemia (cool skin, pallor, edema, absent pulses) in his right leg, you immediately notified the doctor. The diagnosis? Gas gangrene. As part of Mr. Wolcott's treatment, the doctor orders hyperbaric oxygen (HBO) therapy. To understand why, first review what you know about gas gangrene.

Gas gangrene is caused by *Clostridium perfringens,* an anaerobic organism that's commonly found in soil. A patient who's suffered a traumatic injury that has broken the skin is vulnerable to *C. perfringens* wound contamination—especially if his injury occurred outdoors.

As you know, anaerobic organisms thrive in oxygen-free environments. Once a contaminated wound closes—either from surgical repair or normal tissue growth—these organisms are likely to multiply and spread along fascial layers, causing a potentially deadly infection.

HBO therapy helps your patient by destroying the organisms' anaerobic environment. Administered in a sealed chamber, HBO therapy delivers pure (100%) oxygen at high pressure, increasing the amount of oxygen reaching the tissues. This, in turn, inhibits or halts multiplication of anaerobic organisms.

How HBO therapy works

You'll recall that a person normally breathes an air mixture that's about 21% oxygen. Oxygen bonds to the hemoglobin on red blood cells (RBCs), which then transport the oxygen throughout the body.

If the patient's heart and lungs function normally, increasing the oxygen content of the air he breathes to 100% forces the RBCs to carry the greatest amount of oxygen possible. Of course, once the RBCs are working at maximum capacity, they can't carry more oxygen. By increasing atmospheric pressure also, you encourage unbonded oxygen to dissolve in plasma, further increasing the blood's oxygen content. The increased pressure then permits the oxygen molecules to diffuse into tissues harboring anaerobic organisms. Doubling normal atmospheric pressure provides up to 15 times more oxygen to the tissues.

Learning about chamber types

Two types of hyperbaric pressure chamber exist: monoplace and multiplace. The versatile, cost-effective monoplace chamber accommodates the patient only. During treatment, the patient lies on a stretcher that slides into the chamber. Pressurized pure oxygen is then piped into the chamber.

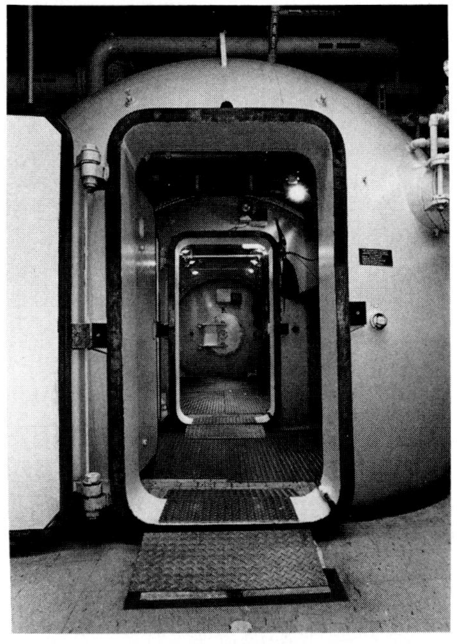

Although the monoplace chamber doesn't allow you direct access to your patient, it can support even a critically ill patient through use of special attachments and support systems. Most models are also equipped with communication systems, which enable the patient to speak with health-care professionals or listen to music during therapy.

Depending on its size, a multiplace chamber (see photo) can accommodate several health-care professionals and one or more patients. One advantage is obvious: Treatment necessitating hands-on care—cardiopulmonary resuscitation, for example—can be given within the chamber. A large multiplace chamber can even be used as an operating room. For a patient like Mr. Wolcott, who needs surgery to excise necrotic tissue, this is another important advantage. By performing surgery in the chamber, the doctor can give Mr. Wolcott the benefits of HBO therapy during surgery.

In a multiplace chamber, the patient receives pure oxygen through a face mask, hood, head tent, or endotracheal tube. Atmospheric pressure is raised by pumping compressed air into the chamber.

Even if you don't perform HBO therapy yourself, you'll prepare your patient beforehand and care for him afterward. Make sure you understand your role by reading the information on the following page.

Trauma

Hyperbaric oxygen therapy: Your role

Let's say your patient's anticipating his first hyperbaric oxygen (HBO) treatment. What are your responsibilities?

First, consider the medications he's taking. Some increase the risk of his developing complications during therapy. Certain medications—for example, steroids, aspirin, ascorbic acid, and vasodilators—promote oxygen toxicosis. If your patient's taking one of these medications, replace or discontinue it (or reduce its dosage) before therapy begins, as ordered.

Also, cautiously administer hypnotics, narcotics, sedatives, and digitalis to a patient receiving hyperbaric oxygen therapy. Concentrated oxygen potentiates these medications.

What other responsibilities do you have? Carefully study the following points.

Before therapy

- Tell the patient and his family why the doctor's ordered HBO therapy and how it'll help. Describe the chamber, so the patient knows what to expect. If your hospital supplies brochures or a patient-teaching aid explaining HBO therapy, give one to the patient and his family. Answer their questions.
- Explain how long each therapy session will last and how long the doctor expects treatment to continue. (This depends on the patient's condition.) For example, you might prepare him to spend 2 hours in the chamber once a day, for about 2 weeks.
- Warn him that when treatment begins, he may feel pressure in his ears, as though he were flying in an airplane. Instruct him to swallow, yawn, or move his lower jaw from side to side to relieve the discomfort. (These measures, called autoinflationary techniques, help equalize internal and atmospheric pressures.)
- Warn your patient he may experience visual changes, such as nearsightedness, double vision, and vision field contraction. Assure him that normal vision returns within a few weeks after therapy ends.

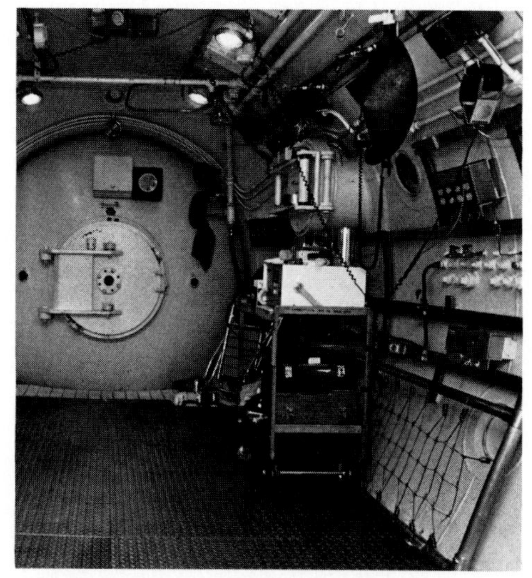

- If your patient's entering a multiplace chamber, tell him you'll place earmuffs on his ears to protect them against the high noise level.
- Warn him to avoid smoking until his course of treatment is complete. Explain that nicotine may alter the treatment's success.
- Inform him of the precautions you're taking to prevent fire (see box below).

During therapy

- Compress and decompress the chamber *slowly* to avoid barotrauma (problems associated with pressure changes). Rapid compression may cause inner ear congestion or tympanic membrane rupture; rapid decompression may cause pneumothorax. Encourage the patient to practice autoinflationary techniques. *Note:* If your patient has chronic sinus problems or difficulty clearing his ears, administer a decongestant before subsequent treatments, as ordered.
- Warn your patient *not* to hold his breath during compression. Doing so may cause air embolism.
- Don't give 100% oxygen at pressures higher than three times sea level pressure. Doing so may produce central nervous system (CNS) oxygen toxicosis, indicated by apprehensiveness, vision changes, and seizures. If your patient develops any of these signs and symptoms, notify the doctor.
- Provide attention and emotional support, according to your patient's needs. If appropriate, arrange for diversions, such as listening to music or watching television through transparent chamber walls.

Continuing care

Chances are, your patient's HBO therapy will last for several weeks. During this time, remember these points:

- Stay alert for possible complications associated with highly pressurized oxygen; for example, spontaneous pneumothorax, air embolism, CNS oxygen toxicosis, labored breathing, and barotrauma to the ears or sinuses (possibly causing pain, blockage, or temporary hearing loss).
- Assess the patient for such adverse psychological effects as claustrophobia or dependency neurosis (a fear that ending therapy will cause a relapse). If the patient develops claustrophobia, provide additional emotional support, teach relaxation exercises, and give a mild tranquilizer before each session, as ordered. *Remember:* Careful patient preparation *before* therapy begins can minimize this problem.

  If your patient develops dependency neurosis, provide additional patient teaching and emotional support. Inform him about his condition, so he understands why continued therapy isn't necessary. Your patient's less likely to develop dependency neurosis if he understands from the beginning of therapy that treatment will end within a specified time.
- Monitor hemoglobin and hematocrit levels, as ordered, to detect possible red blood cell damage and bone marrow suppression during prolonged treatment.

PRECAUTIONS

Minimizing fire hazards

Because the hyperbaric chamber contains high oxygen concentrations, be sure to take the following special precautions to prevent fire.

- Prevent static electricity by making sure all bed linens and towels inside the chamber are 100% cotton and the pillows are feather-filled.
- Make sure anyone entering the chamber is wearing all-cotton clothing.
- Don't allow combustible materials, including books, inside the chamber.

Note: If you're using a monoplace chamber that's partially transparent and your patient wants to read during therapy, place a book or magazine facedown on top of the chamber's outside.

- Don't permit pens, hearing aids, petrolatum-based products (for example, makeup and deodorants), matches, and smoking materials inside the chamber.
- Keep all electrical equipment, such as I.V. pumps, external pacemakers, and monitors, outside the chamber and connected to a common ground.

Kidney disease

Caring for a patient with kidney disease requires considerable knowledge and understanding. Can you meet the special challenges presented by such a patient? For example, can you determine if he's a candidate for continuous ambulatory peritoneal dialysis? Teach a patient who is blind to perform this procedure? Adjust drug dosage for a patient with kidney failure? You'll find the answers to these questions on the next few pages. Read them carefully.

Learning about continuous ambulatory peritoneal dialysis

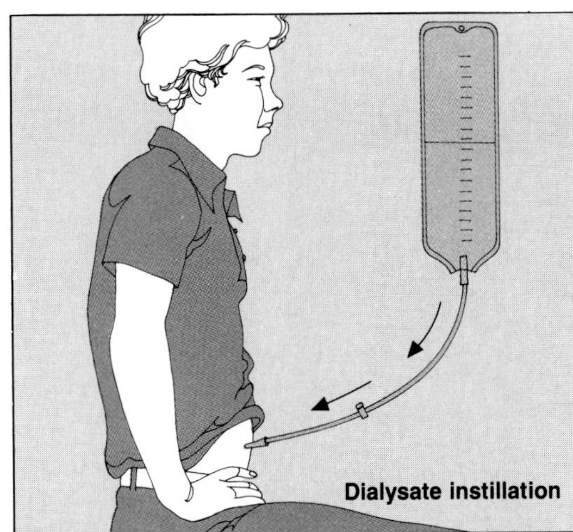

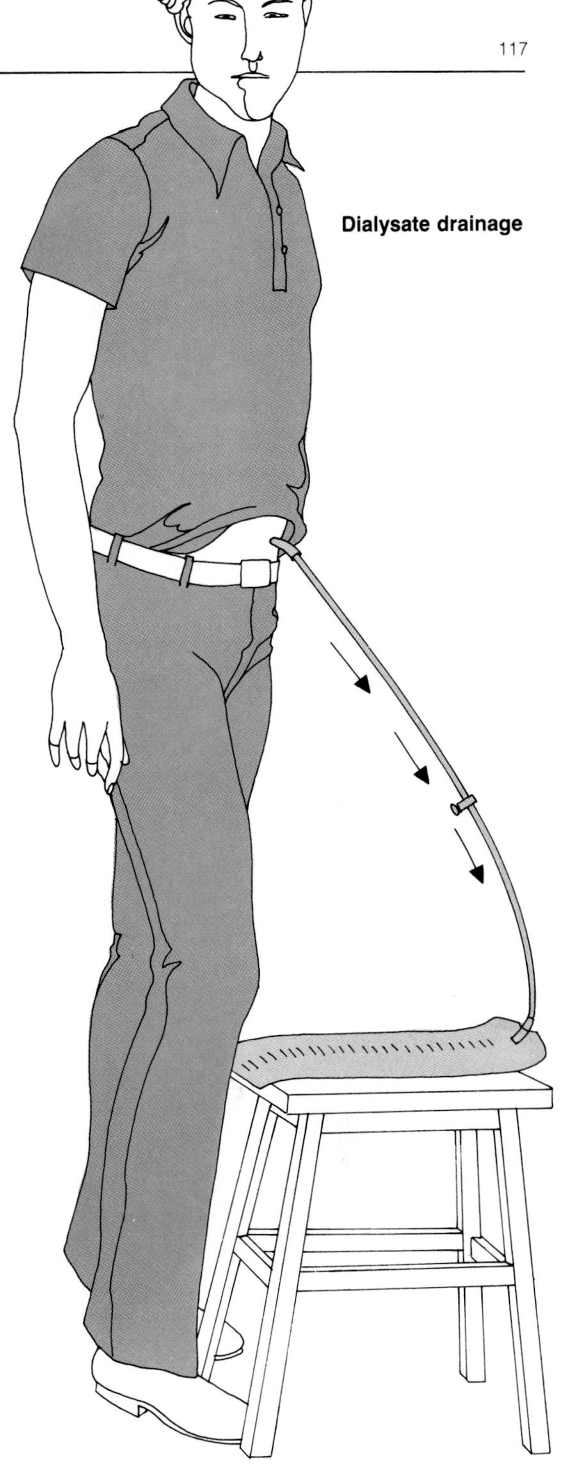

Remember our explanation of how the kidneys function as the body's filtering units, on page 10? Well, when the kidneys cease to perform this function, artificial filtering becomes necessary. One such method is continuous ambulatory peritoneal dialysis (CAPD).

First, the doctor inserts a Tenckhoff catheter into the peritoneal cavity. Similar to the Hickman catheter, the permanently implanted Tenckhoff catheter exits from the abdomen through a subcutaneous tunnel.

To perform CAPD, the patient hangs a container of dialysate (dialysis solution) on an I.V. pole or hook and instills the dialysate into the peritoneal cavity through tubing attached to the catheter as shown in the illustration above. When the bag's empty, he clamps the tubing and then folds the bag and puts it in a pocket. Now, through osmosis and diffusion, body wastes pass through the peritoneal membrane, which acts as a filter, and into the dialysate.

After 6 to 8 hours, the patient positions the empty dialysate bag below the catheter, unclamps the tubing, and drains the dialysate, as shown in the illustration at right. He performs this procedure (called an *exchange*) three to five times a day.

As the term CAPD suggests, this procedure enables a patient to be ambulatory throughout treatment, not confined to a bed or connected to a machine as he would be for hemodialysis or peritoneal dialysis. As you may know, freedom of movement's one of CAPD's primary advantages over other dialysis methods. Other advantages include:

- less stress on the patient's cardiovascular system, decreasing the risk of life-threatening complications
- fewer dietary restrictions
- less teaching time required than for hemodialysis.

CAPD's disadvantages include increased risk of peritonitis (primary disadvantage) and a slight change in the patient's physical appearance caused by fluid retention in the abdominal cavity. Also, the equipment requires meticulous care, to prevent infection.

Who benefits from CAPD?

Your patient with kidney failure may be a candidate for CAPD if he:

- is highly motivated and responsible.
- lives far from a dialysis treatment center.
- has coronary artery disease, arrhythmias, or diabetes mellitus.
- is a child. (Few children can tolerate hemodialysis.)

(For more detailed information on CAPD, see the NURSING PHOTOBOOK IMPLEMENTING UROLOGIC PROCEDURES.)

Kidney disease

Caring for a CAPD patient: Your role

Suppose you're caring for a patient undergoing continuous ambulatory peritoneal dialysis (CAPD). Do you know what special care he needs? If you're unsure, study these guidelines closely:

- Weigh your patient daily. If his weight's above or below the desired level, notify the doctor.
- Supply your patient with a high-protein diet.
- Make sure only specially trained health-care professionals perform dialysate exchanges. Remember, improper technique increases the risk of peritonitis.
- When changing a dialysate bag, make sure the work area's clean and free of dust and drafts. Also, provide adequate lighting and ensure privacy for the patient. Supply your patient and anyone else in the room with masks.
- If your patient routinely performs his own CAPD care, give him the equipment he'll need, including an I.V. pole for hanging the dialysate bag and an antimicrobial scrub for his hands. *Note:* Equipment and medication he brought from home may not be permitted at bedside. Check hospital policy, and explain the rules to him. Then, provide him with hospital supplies, as needed.
- Warn your patient that he may have to drain the dialysate from his abdomen before certain procedures; for example, biopsy, ultrasound, sigmoidoscopy, or X-ray dye tests. Instruct him not to replace the fluid until the test is completed.
- Before instilling the dialysate, make sure it's as close to body temperature as possible. Dialysate that's too warm may cause a burning sensation; dialysate that's too cold may cause chills. Additionally, your patient may experience abdominal cramping. If you detect any of these signs and symptoms, close the roller clamp immediately, drain the fluid that's been instilled, and perform the exchange with a new bag of fluid that's a comfortable temperature.
- Before injecting any medication into the patient's dialysate bag, follow the steps shown in the photos below. First, clean the medication vial's diaphragm with an alcohol swab. Then, clean the diaphragm with povidone-iodine swab for at least 5 minutes. When injecting the medication through the medication port, take care not to puncture the outlet port. Finally, mix the medication with the dialysate by inverting the bag several times.
- If you're adding more than one medication to the dialysate, use a separate needle and syringe to instill each medication.
- Because the risk of peritonitis is CAPD's biggest drawback, regularly assess your patient for this complication. Notify the doctor if you detect any of these signs and symptoms: dialysate outflow that's always cloudy; abdominal pain with tenderness; fever; nausea, vomiting, or diarrhea; and lethargy. *Important:* Teach your patient to watch for these signs and symptoms.
- If you detect bright red blood in your patient's outflow, notify the doctor immediately. If the blood's not bright red, perform two or three rapid dialysate exchanges; or, have the patient perform them. Check the outflow each time. If it remains bloody, call the doctor.

Troubleshooting

If your patient's dialysate bag isn't draining properly during an exchange, follow these steps: First, make sure the drainage clamp's open and check the catheter and tubing for kinks and leaks. Then, to improve drainage, have the patient walk around, cough, urinate, or move his bowels. You can also use these measures when the dialysate's instilling too slowly. Or, try raising the bag higher or squeezing it gently.

If you detect a leak in the tubing connecting the dialysate bag to the catheter, immediately close the roller clamp and tie two knots in the tubing between the patient and the leak. Then, call the doctor. He'll probably change the tubing.

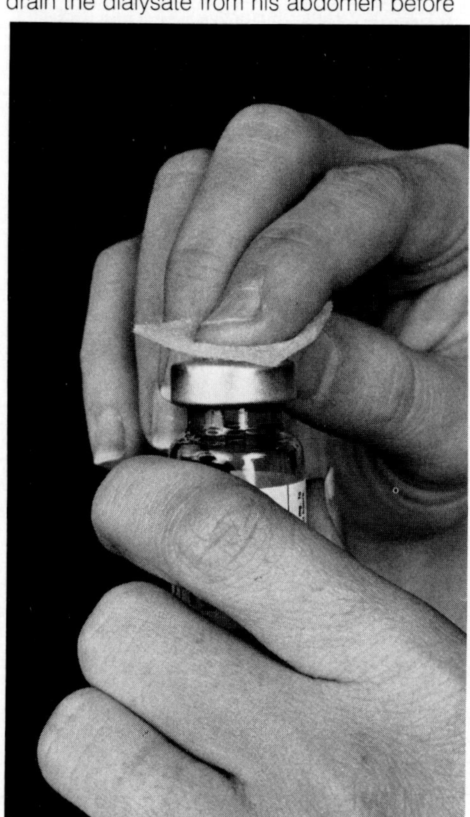

Cleaning with alcohol swab

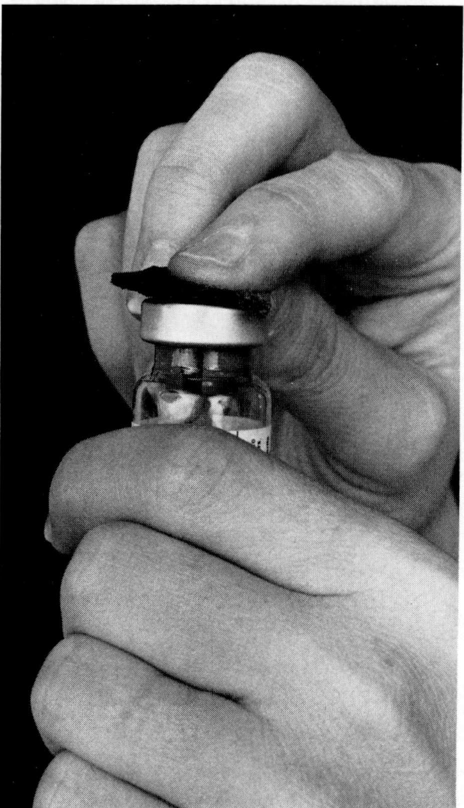

Cleaning with povidone-iodine swab

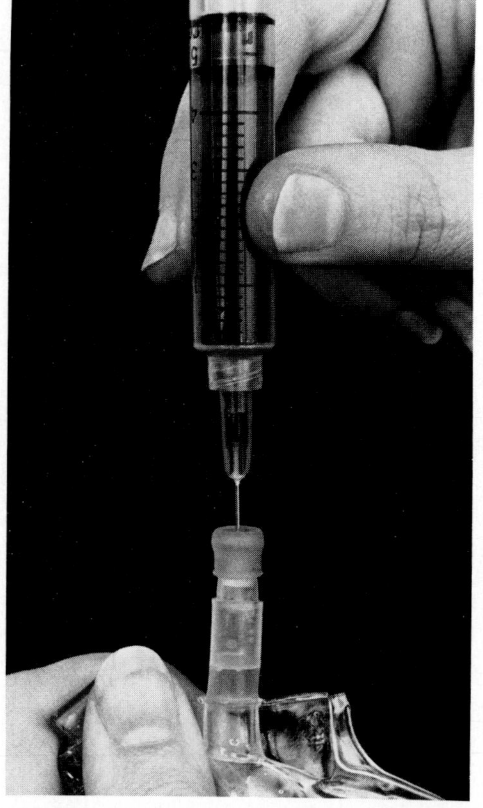

Injecting medication

PATIENT TEACHING

Teaching CAPD to a patient who's blind

Herb Shore, a 48-year-old high school English teacher, learned he had diabetes at age 19. Eventually, the disease blinded him. But he's never allowed this handicap to prevent him from leading an active, fulfilling life.

Recently, Mr. Shore's diabetes has caused kidney failure. As a result, he receives hemodialysis treatments three times a week. Mr. Shore says he detests the treatments because they limit his activity and make him feel helpless.

As you know, Mr. Shore's intelligence, independence, and motivation make him an excellent candidate for continuous ambulatory peritoneal dialysis (CAPD). Don't assume that his blindness is an insurmountable handicap. With the proper instruction and support, you can teach him to perform CAPD without increased risk of complications.

Begin teaching CAPD to a blind patient by familiarizing him with the equipment he'll use. Because he can't see the equipment, he'll have to use his sense of touch to memorize the form, content, and opening markings of various supplies. Allow him to practice as much as he wants. Plan to spend the first few weeks making mock exchanges.

Nursing tip: If your patient appears frustrated or depressed by his mistakes, ask another blind CAPD patient to talk with him. Someone who's mastered the CAPD procedure can empathize with your patient's frustration and encourage him to keep trying.

Mr. Shore will probably have trouble inserting the tubing spike in the dialysate bag's outlet port. Help him overcome this problem by following this procedure.

Have him place the spike and outlet port in a piece of plastic that has a groove down the middle, like the one shown in the top photo. To avoid contaminating the spike, make sure he keeps it raised slightly above the groove. Then, using the groove as a guide, tell him to bring the two together, until the spike's firmly secured in the outlet port.

Here's another method to try. First, have your patient wrap a povidone-iodine pad around the entry port of the bag containing fresh dialysate, as shown in the bottom photo. Tell him to hold the tubing spike between his two index fingers, and the entry port between his thumb and fingers. Then, have him pull the spike toward the port. Using this method, he can line up the spike with the entry port and correctly insert the spike without contaminating it.

Encourage your patient to wear sterile gloves while performing CAPD. Remember, he'll use his hands to feel the equipment; the gloves will ensure sterility. Teach him to don the gloves correctly, so he doesn't contaminate them.

How can a blind patient tell when outflow's complete? Tell him to assess for outflow completion during an exchange by feeling the catheter tubing for warmth and the bag for tautness.

Nursing tip: Consider placing braille markings on the dialysate bags to help him select the correct percentage of solution for exchanges.

Teaching a blind patient to perform CAPD takes a little extra time and effort, but for a patient like Mr. Shore, your efforts are well spent.

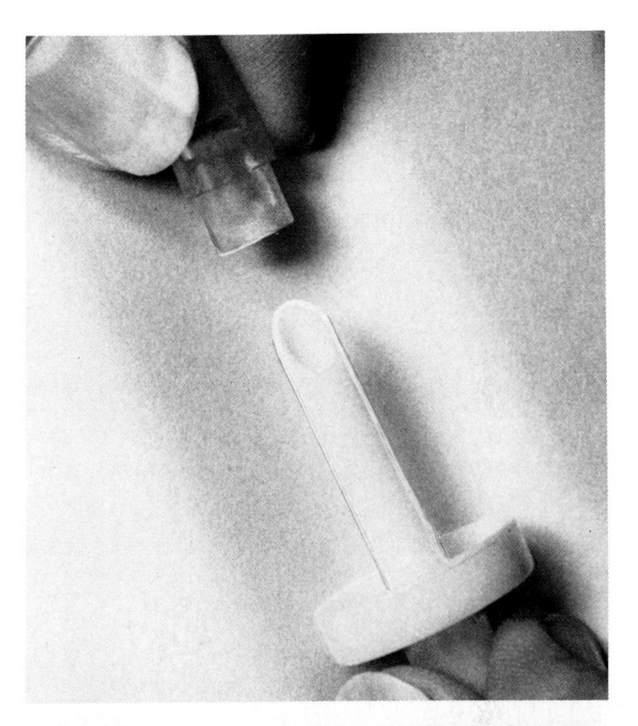

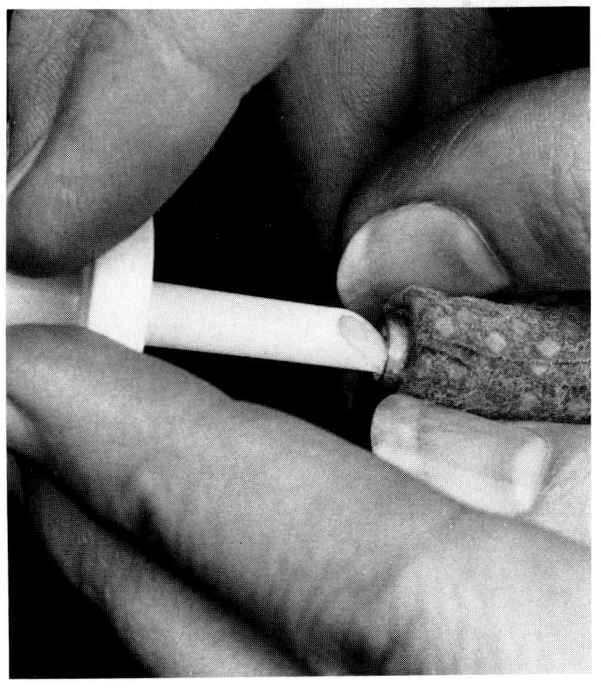

Kidney disease

Adjusting drug dosages with the interval extension method

As you know, the kidneys are a major excretory route for a number of commonly used drugs. So, when the kidneys fail to function properly, these drugs may be excreted slower than normal. Expect to adjust drug dosages for a patient with kidney failure, as ordered.

One way to adjust drug dosage is to lengthen the amount of time between doses. Known as the *interval extension method,* this adjustment allows normal-sized doses to be administered at longer intervals, which helps prevent toxicosis.

Although the doctor's responsible for ordering the correct drug dosage for your patient, you must make sure each dose is appropriate. The following chart lists some commonly used drugs that are normally excreted by the kidneys, the usual time interval between doses, and how this interval's altered for a patient with kidney failure. The chart also gives nursing considerations for administration to a patient with kidney failure.

Before studying the chart, review these general guidelines.

- Don't give any drug to a patient with kidney failure unless it's absolutely necessary.
- Ask yourself whether the drug's excreted by the kidneys, or whether it's likely to have an adverse effect on a patient with kidney disease. Also ask yourself whether the liver normally breaks down the drug. Remember, liver function may affect the kidneys' ability to excrete the drug.
- If you're not familiar with the drug, look it up. Follow the most specific and current dosage schedule for the drug. Keep in mind that drug companies continually update product information.
- Monitor your patient closely for signs of drug toxicosis. Make sure he's experiencing the drug's desired effects.

amphotericin B (Fungizone*)
Normal interval between doses
24 hours
Revised interval between doses
Moderate kidney failure: 24 hours
Severe kidney failure: 24 to 36 hours
Nursing considerations
- Drug is not removed by hemodialysis.
- Possible adverse effects include hypokalemia and further kidney damage.

amikacin sulfate (Amikacin*)
Normal interval between doses
8 to 12 hours
Revised interval between doses
Moderate kidney failure: 24 to 36 hours
Severe kidney failure: 36 to 48 hours
Nursing considerations
- Some of the drug's removed by hemodialysis or peritoneal dialysis.
- Administer the usual loading dose.
- Closely monitor drug levels in the blood.
- Adverse effects include ototoxicity and increased kidney damage.

gentamicin sulfate (Garamycin*)
Normal interval between doses
8 hours
Revised interval between doses
Moderate kidney failure: 12 to 24 hours
Severe kidney failure: 24 to 48 hours
Nursing considerations
- Same as for amikacin sulfate.

kanamycin sulfate (Kantrex*)
Normal interval between doses
8 hours
Revised interval between doses
Moderate kidney failure: 24 to 72 hours
Severe kidney failure: 72 to 96 hours
Nursing considerations
- Same as for amikacin sulfate.
- May cause respiratory paralysis; however, this complication is uncommon.

tobramycin sulfate (Nebcin*)
Normal interval between doses
8 hours
Revised interval between doses
Moderate kidney failure: 12 to 24 hours
Severe kidney failure: 24 to 48 hours
Nursing considerations
- Same as for amikacin sulfate.

phenobarbital (Gardenal*)
Normal interval between doses
8 hours
Revised interval between doses
Moderate kidney failure: 8 hours
Severe kidney failure: 8 to 16 hours
Nursing consideration
- Drug's removed by hemodialysis and peritoneal dialysis.

cefamandole naftate (Mandol)
Normal interval between doses
4 to 6 hours
Revised interval between doses
Moderate kidney failure: 6 to 9 hours
Severe kidney failure: 9 hours
Nursing considerations
- Some of the drug's removed by hemodialysis.
- Drug may cause further kidney damage when given with aminoglycosides, antibiotics, or diuretics or when your patient's dehydrated.

cefoxitin sodium (Mefoxin)
Normal interval between doses
6 to 8 hours
Revised interval between doses
Moderate kidney failure: 8 to 12 hours
Severe kidney failure: 24 hours
Nursing considerations
- Same as for cefamandole naftate.

cephalothin sodium (Keflin Neutral*)
Normal interval between doses
6 hours
Revised interval between doses
Moderate kidney failure: 6 hours
Severe kidney failure: 8 to 12 hours
Nursing considerations
- Same as for cefamandole naftate; however, further kidney damage isn't likely when the drug's given alone.

ampicillin (Amcill*)
Normal interval between doses
6 hours
Revised interval between doses
Moderate kidney failure: 6 to 12 hours
Severe kidney failure: 12 to 16 hours
Nursing considerations
- Drug may cause allergic interstitial nephritis.
- Seizures and coagulopathy are possible when high levels are present in the blood.
- Normal dosage is required to treat urinary tract infections.

carbenicillin disodium (Geopen)
Normal interval between doses
4 hours
Revised interval between doses
Moderate kidney failure: 12 to 24 hours
Severe kidney failure: 24 to 48 hours
Nursing considerations
- Same as for ampicillin.
- Drug's removed by hemodialysis or peritoneal dialysis.
- Drug can be added to peritoneal dialysate.

*Available in both the United States and Canada

penicillin G potassium (Novopen-G*)
Normal interval between doses
8 hours
Revised interval between doses
Moderate kidney failure: 8 to 12 hours
Severe kidney failure: 12 to 18 hours
Nursing considerations
- Same as for ampicillin.
- Drug's removed by hemodialysis but not by peritoneal dialysis.
- If patient has severe kidney failure, maximum dose of 4 to 6 million units is suggested.

---

ticarcillin disodium (Ticar)
Normal interval between doses
4 to 6 hours
Revised interval between doses
Moderate kidney failure: 12 to 24 hours
Severe kidney failure: 24 to 48 hours
Nursing considerations
- Drug's removed by hemodialysis and peritoneal dialysis.
- Same as for carbenicillin disodium.

---

minocyaline hydrochloride (Minocin*)
Normal interval between doses
12 hours
Revised interval between doses
Moderate kidney failure: 18 to 24 hours
Severe kidney failure: 24 to 36 hours
Nursing considerations
- Drug is not removed by dialysis.
- Drug may increase catabolism or raise serum phosphate and BUN levels.

---

acetaminophen (Tylenol*)
Normal interval between doses
4 hours
Revised interval between doses
Moderate kidney failure: 4 hours
Severe kidney failure: avoid using if possible
Nursing considerations
- Drug is not removed by peritoneal dialysis or hemodialysis.
- Drug may cause additional kidney damage.

---

aspirin (A.S.A.)
Normal interval between doses
4 hours
Revised interval between doses
Moderate kidney failure: 4 to 6 hours
Severe kidney failure: 8 to 12 hours
Nursing considerations
- Drug's removed by hemodialysis and peritoneal dialysis.
- Drug may cause gastrointestinal irritation.

quinidine sulfate (CinQuin)
Normal interval between doses
6 hours
Revised interval between doses
Moderate kidney failure: 8 to 12 hours
Severe kidney failure: 12 to 18 hours
Nursing considerations
- Drug's removed by hemodialysis and peritoneal dialysis.
- May exacerbate uremic gastrointestinal symptoms; for example, nausea and vomiting.

---

digoxin (Lanoxin)
Normal interval between doses
12 hours
Revised interval between doses
Moderate kidney failure: 24 to 36 hours
Severe kidney failure: 36 to 48 hours
Nursing consideration
- Drug's not removed by hemodialysis or peritoneal dialysis.

---

ethacrynic acid (Edecrin)
Normal interval between doses
6 hours
Revised interval between doses
Moderate kidney failure: 6 hours
Severe kidney failure: avoid giving
Nursing consideration
- Drug may be partially removed by hemodialysis or peritoneal dialysis, but effectiveness of dialysis is uncertain.

---

mercurial diuretics; for example, mercaptomerin sodium (Thiomerin)
Normal interval between doses
24 hours
Revised interval between doses
Moderate kidney failure: avoid giving
Severe kidney failure: avoid giving
Nursing consideration
- Watch patient for signs and symptoms of mercury accumulation; for example, metallic taste, thirst, severe abdominal pain, vomiting, and bloody diarrhea.

---

meprobamate (Meprocan)
Normal interval between doses
6 hours
Revised interval between doses
Moderate kidney failure: 9 to 12 hours
Severe kidney failure: 12 to 18 hours
Nursing considerations
- Drug's removed by hemodialysis and peritoneal dialysis.
- Patient may become oversedated.

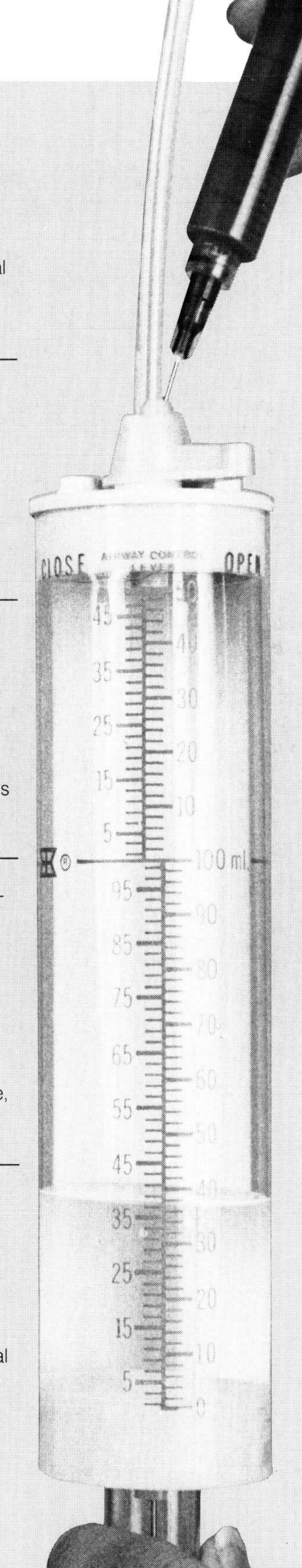

Radiation therapy

One out of two patients with cancer will receive radiation treatment. Yet, many of these patients know little about the treatment and have difficulty understanding how it can help them. As a nurse, you can fill in the information gaps and give your patient the special care he needs.

To refresh your knowledge of radiation therapy, read the following pages. On them, you'll learn:
- how radiation therapy works.
- how to prepare your patient for radiation therapy.
- how to recognize radiation's adverse effects.

Understanding radiation therapy

Of course, you know that radiation is an effective cancer treatment—especially if it can be used with surgery or chemotherapy. But do you know *why* radiation works? Consider the following points.

How radiation kills tissue

Radiation capable of destroying tissue is called *ionizing radiation.* Examples include X-rays, gamma rays, and beta rays. Ionizing radiation kills or damages tissue cells by removing an orbital electron from each cell atom it interacts with, causing physical and chemical changes within the cell. Unavoidably, both normal and cancer cells are damaged or destroyed by radiation. Cancer cells, however, have less ability to withstand radiation, probably because they have less ability to repair damage. As a result, they are especially vulnerable.

Cancer cells tend to divide more rapidly than normal cells, which increases their vulnerability to radiation (radiosensitivity). Some cancer cell types divide more quickly than others. These types are especially radiosensitive.

Among the most highly radiosensitive cancers are lymphoma, Hodgkin's disease, seminoma, and dysgerminoma. Moderately radiosensitive cancers include squamous and basal cell skin carcinomas and adenocarcinomas of the breast and endometrium. Osteosarcoma, neurogenic sarcoma, and malignant melanoma tend to resist radiation therapy.

Certain normal tissues and organs are also highly radiosensitive; for example, the kidneys and liver.

To minimize damage to healthy tissue, the doctor or radiation therapist calculates a precise radiation dose for each patient, taking into account the tumor's size and location, the cancer's radiosensitivity, and the radiosensitivity of surrounding normal tissue.

Types of radiation therapy

A patient may receive radiation therapy from an external or an internal source. External therapy's delivered with one of many types of machine; for example, a linear accelerator, a betatron, or a cyclotron. Why so many types? Because tumors of different types and depths necessitate different treatments. A highly specialized machine can deliver precise radiation doses to a tumor, while sparing as much normal tissue surrounding the tumor as possible. For example, a patient with skin cancer needs treatment with a low-energy machine that delivers high radiation doses to the skin and minimal doses to deep structures; a patient with bladder cancer needs a higher-energy machine that can deliver high doses to the bladder, while sparing the skin and other overlying tissues from high radiation doses.

Before therapy, the doctor uses an X-ray simulator to determine how to direct the radiation beam. Then, if possible, shields are custom-made to protect surrounding normal tissue. The doctor also marks the patient's skin at the site of beam entry. This mark remains on the skin throughout treatment, to ensure accurate and consistent radiation doses.

Internal radiation therapy is delivered by radioactive material that's surgically or percutaneously implanted in or near the tumor. Examples of radioactive materials are radium needles, radon, iodine, gold seeds or pellets, and iridium wires. Most of these materials are removed from the patient at the end of therapy. An exception is gold seeds or pellets, because they remain radioactive for only a short time.

The advantage of internal radiation therapy is that it delivers a high radiation dose relatively quickly. Unlike external therapy, it doesn't adversely affect large areas of surrounding tissue. A possible disadvantage is that the patient may have to be isolated during therapy.

Understanding therapy goals

The goal of radiation therapy may be curative or palliative. *Curative* therapy, when successful, destroys all cancer cells in the primary tumor and surrounding lymph nodes, with minimal damage to normal tissue. Most patients undergoing curative therapy receive radiation treatments 4 days a week for 5 to 7 weeks.

Palliative therapy is prescribed to improve the quality of the patient's life when a cure isn't possible. It relieves or prevents symptoms by shrinking tumor size, reducing pressure exerted by the tumor on surrounding tissues; by stopping or decreasing bleeding; and by promoting the healing of ulcerations. Most patients undergoing palliative therapy receive high radiation doses in 3 to 10 treatments.

Your role

When caring for a patient undergoing radiation therapy, you'll have to meet both his physical and emotional needs. Remember, radiation therapy—and the disease itself—can greatly stress your patient.

First, provide your patient with accurate

information about the treatment. Fear of the unknown needlessly heightens his anxiety. Your teaching should include what's going to be done, how it'll be done, and why it's necessary. Suggest that he visit the radiation therapy department before therapy begins. By becoming familiar with the area, he may be more relaxed. Also, explain the possible side effects, so he'll be prepared for them and won't be alarmed. Encourage him to ask questions, and answer them fully.

Important: Don't forget to explain these points to the patient's family as well. Because most patients receive external radiation therapy on an outpatient basis, they'll need their families' care and support.

When caring for a patient receiving *external* radiation therapy, follow these general guidelines:

- Assure your patient that he isn't radioactive and doesn't endanger those around him.
- Tell him that he won't see, hear, or feel the radiation. But warn him that the machine administering the radiation may make a loud noise.
- Inform your patient that the doctor or radiation therapist will ask him to sit or lie in a special position during treatment. Tell him to remain motionless in this position during treatment and breathe normally.
- Although he'll be alone during the procedure, you or a co-worker will observe him either through a specially designed window or a video device.
- Take care not to wash off the skin marking indicating the beam's entry site. If the marks are removed for any reason, don't attempt to redraw them.

Follow these guidelines when caring for a patient receiving *internal* radiation therapy:

- Inform him that his activity will be limited while the radioactive material's in place.
- Tell him, as well as his family, that visits will be limited to 30 minutes within a 24-hour period.
- Also inform your patient that no children or pregnant women will be allowed to visit.
- Assure your patient that he won't be radioactive after the implanted material's removed or, in the case of seeds or pellets, after the material has lost its radioactive property.

Important: No matter which type of therapy your patient's receiving, carefully monitor his nutritional status, as you learned on pages 35 through 45.

SPECIAL CONSIDERATIONS

Minimizing radiation risks

Radiation exposure increases your health risks; for example, the risk of cancer or reproductive system damage. So, if you're working around radioactive equipment or materials, take precautions to protect yourself. (Of course, you'll also take measures to protect others who may be exposed to radiation, including co-workers and the patient's visitors.)

Three factors affect the amount of radiation you receive: the length of time you're exposed, your distance from the radiation source, and how well you're shielded. Keep these factors in mind as you review the following guidelines.

Caution: Avoid all radiation exposure if you are (or may be) pregnant. Radiation can cause birth defects.

Taking precautions

If you're caring for a patient receiving external radiation, you're at risk only if you help him hold still during X-ray simulator use to determine radiation beam direction. In this situation, wear protective equipment, such as lead gloves or a lead apron. Also, alternate such duties with a co-worker, so you're not continually exposed.

Note: Follow similar precautions when caring for a patient receiving diagnostic X-rays or fluoroscopy.

You're at greater risk when caring for a patient undergoing *internal* radiation therapy, because his radioactive implant constantly emits radiation. Keep these important points in mind:

- Obtain a film badge to measure the amount of radiation you receive, and attach it to your clothing where it's exposed to the same amount of maximum radiation as you. (For example, if your head is constantly exposed, wear it on your collar.)
- Place warning signs showing the universal radiation symbol (see illustration at right) on the door to the patient's room and at the foot of his bed.
- Instruct your patient to wear a yellow wristband with a radiation symbol, according to your hospital's policy. This warns other hospital personnel that he's receiving internal radiation treatment.

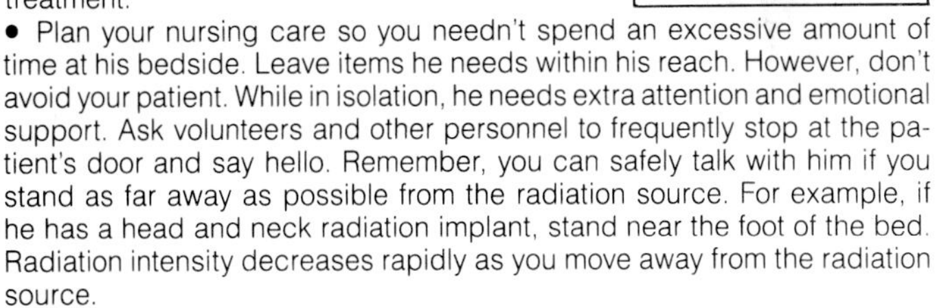

- Plan your nursing care so you needn't spend an excessive amount of time at his bedside. Leave items he needs within his reach. However, don't avoid your patient. While in isolation, he needs extra attention and emotional support. Ask volunteers and other personnel to frequently stop at the patient's door and say hello. Remember, you can safely talk with him if you stand as far away as possible from the radiation source. For example, if he has a head and neck radiation implant, stand near the foot of the bed. Radiation intensity decreases rapidly as you move away from the radiation source.
- Thoroughly wash your hands after performing patient care. If you're wearing gloves, wash them with soap and water before removing them.
- If possible, make sure the nursing staff's rotated regularly, so the same nurses aren't continually exposed to a patient undergoing internal radiation therapy.
- Carefully monitor your patient's visitors. Don't allow children and pregnant women to visit or a visitor to stay with the patient for longer than 30 minutes in a 24-hour period. Suggest to his family and friends that they send cards or letters, or call on the telephone. Inform visitors that these precautions are for their protection.
- Place thick lead shields, if available, at the patient's bedside to protect visitors and health-care professionals.
- Depending on the implant's location, regularly check emesis basins, bed linens, and dressings for implant parts that may have been dislodged and expelled. If you find any radioactive material, immediately notify the radiologist. *Caution:* Never allow such material to touch your skin; handle it with long-handled forceps.
- To lessen the risk of implant dislodgment, encourage your patient to stay in bed as much as possible.

Radiation therapy

Nurses' guide to adverse radiation effects

Most patients undergoing radiation therapy don't suffer *serious* adverse effects. But the incidence and severity of effects vary greatly, depending on the patient's age and condition, his tolerance of the treatment, the extent of the cancer, and the extent of radiation damage to normal tissue. As a rule, the better your patient's general health, the better he'll tolerate therapy. Also, younger patients tolerate therapy better than older patients.

Adverse local effects are limited to the body area receiving treatment. For example, if your patient's receiving radiation therapy on his leg, he won't suffer adverse effects in his mouth or lungs.

As indicated in the following chart, adverse effects are classified as either early or late. Early effects are usually temporary and occur during or immediately after radiation therapy; these include lethargy, anorexia, nausea, and vomiting. Late effects may occur months or years after treatment.

Study the following chart to learn more about adverse effects of radiation therapy, according to the area being treated.

Note: Adverse effects are the same for both external and internal radiation therapy.

Skin

Early effects
- Localized dryness
- Mild to severe erythema
- Increased skin pigmentation
- Localized itching and peeling
- Localized hair loss

Late effects
- Localized dryness, from permanently damaged sweat or sebaceous glands
- Increased pigmentation
- Leathery skin, caused by decreased elasticity from fibrosis
- Epithelial thinning
- Telangiectasia (tissue reddening caused by capillary dilation)
- Narrowing of small blood vessels
- Change in local hair pattern

Nursing interventions

For early effects:
- Assess the patient's skin before each treatment.
- Tell the patient to prevent skin breakdown by keeping his skin dry. Also tell him to avoid skin trauma.
- Advise the patient not to use soaps, powders, perfumes, oils, or creams on affected skin, unless the doctor says it's O.K.
- Remind your patient to expose the affected area to air as much as possible. Doing so keeps the skin dry and lessens the risk of infection. Suggest that he wear loose cotton clothing over the site and that he avoid clothing that irritates his skin.
- If your patient irritates his skin by scratching it while sleeping, advise him to wear gloves or socks over his hands. Also tell him to clip his nails and keep them short.
- Emphasize that hair loss will occur only in the area directly in the path of radiation. Reassure the patient that hair loss usually isn't permanent and that his hair will probably grow back in 2 to 3 months. Explain that some permanent changes in hair thickness and hair pattern may result. For example, hair shafts may become thinner and hair may grow slower. Also, the color may change slightly.

For late effects:
- Tell your patient to gently cleanse the affected area daily, using a half-strength hydrogen peroxide solution and sterile cotton-tipped swabs, and to gently dry the area after cleansing it.
- Tell the patient to apply a moisturizing agent, such as baby oil, to his skin about three times a day. Doing so helps keep skin in the affected area soft and pliable. Remind him to remove excess ointment before applying a new layer.
- Warn your patient to avoid prolonged exposure to direct sunlight. If he plans to leave the affected area exposed to the sun for longer than 10 minutes, advise him to protect his skin by applying a sunscreen ointment with a sun protection factor rating of 15.
- Warn your patient to avoid trauma to the affected area to lessen the risk of infection. Also instruct him to protect the affected skin from heat and cold. Because of vascular changes in the skin, he's particularly susceptible to frostbite and burns.

Head and neck

Early effects
- Dry mouth; thick, scant saliva
- Mucous membrane inflammation
- Decreased sense of taste
- Tooth hypersensitivity
- Trismus (inability to fully open the mouth, resulting from muscle fibrosis)
- Mild hearing loss
- Pain or sensation of fullness in ears

Late effects
- Dry mouth, with increase in saliva acidity
- Mucous membrane fibrosis
- Tooth decay, usually at the gum line
- Possibly trismus
- Greatly increased risk of infection of bones exposed to radiation during treatment

Nursing interventions

For early effects:
- Assess affected area before each treatment.
- Urge patient to maintain high fluid intake—at least 2 qt (1.9 liters) per day.
- Check your patient's mouth for irritations and signs and symptoms of infection.
- Emphasize the importance of maintaining meticulous oral hygiene. Suggest that the patient rinse his mouth frequently with a solution of ½ tsp of salt and ½ tsp baking soda dissolved in 1 qt (0.95 liter) of warm water. Tell him to avoid commercial mouthwashes, which may irritate his throat.
- Remind him to continue meticulous oral hygiene and dental care. Tell him to notify his dentist of the radiation treatments. Because of the treatments, his risk of infection during a tooth extraction or surgical procedure increases.
- To help your patient minimize tooth hypersensitivity and radiation dental caries, have him treat his teeth and gums daily with a fluoride solution. He can use custom-made, plastic carriers that fit over his teeth. First, he'll fill the carriers with a 1% sodium fluoride gel and place them over his teeth. He'll leave the carriers in place for 5 minutes. Then, he'll remove them and rinse his mouth. Or, he can use a cotton-tipped swab to brush a 0.4% stannous fluoride solution on his teeth. He'll leave the solution on for 5 minutes, and then rinse his mouth to remove the excess fluoride. Warn him not to swallow the excess fluoride. Also, tell him to brush his teeth thoroughly, using a soft-bristle toothbrush, before applying the fluoride.
- Advise him to avoid trauma to the affected area.
- Assess his nutritional status. Help him find foods that taste good to him. Tell him to try a variety of flavorings and seasonings on his food. Suggest that he moisten his foods with gravies or sauces. Advise him to eat small, frequent meals and to perform oral hygiene before meals to make food taste better.
- Once a week during treatment, assess his ability to open his mouth wide. To help prevent trismus, encourage your patient to frequently exercise by opening his mouth as wide as possible 20 times.
- Periodically, assess his hearing. If you detect any problems, notify the doctor.

For late effects:
- Perform a detailed assessment of the patient on follow-up visits. Weigh him and assess his nutritional status. Observe his mucosa for signs and symptoms of ulceration and infection. Advise your patient to avoid smoking, alcoholic beverages, extremely hot or cold food and drinks, spicy foods, and foods with rough edges, such as potato chips.
- Instruct him to continue mouth exercises.

Chest

Early effects
- Difficulty swallowing and burning or pain on swallowing caused by esophageal irritation (esophagitis)
- Pain or burning sensation when breathing caused by lung irritation (pleuritis)

Late effects
- Difficulty swallowing and substernal pain caused by esophageal fibrosis
- Fistula formation
- Bleeding
- Perforation of esophagus or trachea
- Chest pain, cough, and dyspnea from pulmonary fibrosis, usually visible on X-ray
- Pericarditis, myocardial fibrosis, or coronary artery damage

Nursing interventions

For early effects:
- Tell the patient he can avoid irritating his esophagus by eating a soft, bland diet; by avoiding alcohol, tea, coffee, and extremely hot or cold foods; by chewing his food thoroughly; and by eating slowly.
- To relieve pain, administer a chewable analgesic as well as other local analgesics, such as lidocaine hydrochloride (Xylocaine viscous*), as ordered.
- Watch for any change in your patient's respiratory status. If lung inflammation develops, urge the patient to rest and administer antibiotics, as ordered.

For late effects:
- On follow-up examination, assess the patient's nutritional status. Check his weight and ability to swallow. Also ask about his eating habits.
- Assess the patient's respiratory status.
- Tell him to inform the doctor or X-ray technologist of his radiation therapy before any chest X-rays are performed.
- Assess for chest pain, peripheral edema, blood pressure decrease, and other signs and symptoms of heart failure.
- Check his stool and vomitus for occult blood.

Abdomen

Early effects
- Pain and heartburn caused by stomach inflammation (gastritis)
- Diarrhea and abdominal cramping from intestinal inflammation
- Bone marrow depression, as indicated by blood studies
- Elevated blood pressure, malaise, dull back pain, vomiting, anemia, proteinuria, or hematuria (from radiation nephritis)
- Weight gain, enlarged liver, ascites, abdominal pain, and abnormal liver function studies (from radiation hepatitis)

Late effects
- Reduction in gastric secretions, possibly accompanied by pain, bleeding, and decreased peristalsis
- Edema or fibrosis of the wall of the small intestine, possibly resulting in thickening and narrowing of the intestine; may eventually cause stricture or obstruction
- Nephritis (uncommon); usually not evident until 6 to 13 months after treatment
- Hepatitis (uncommon); usually not evident until 2 to 6 weeks after treatment

Nursing interventions

For early effects:
- Weigh your patient frequently to assess his nutritional status.
- Urge him to eat small, frequent meals consisting of bland foods, to relieve nausea. Low-residue foods also allow the intestine to rest. Suggest that he maintain a high-protein, high-calorie diet.
- Ensure adequate fluid intake.
- Administer an antiemetic, such as prochlorperazine maleate (Compazine), as ordered.
- Administer an antidiarrheal, such as diphenoxylate hydrochloride (Lomotil*), as ordered.
- Watch for signs and symptoms of bowel damage; for example, cramping, diarrhea, fat globules in stool from fat malabsorption, nausea, and vomiting.
- Test stool specimens and vomitus for occult blood.
- Watch for signs of infection or bruising, which may indicate bone marrow depression.
- If your patient develops hemorrhoids, tell him to use suppositories to relieve discomfort.

For late effects:
- On follow-up examination, weigh patient and determine whether his eating habits have changed. Ask him whether he's experienced abdominal pain, cramping, nausea, or vomiting. Also ask whether he's noticed blood in his stools or vomitus.
- Check for signs and symptoms of radiation nephritis and radiation hepatitis.

Pelvis

Early effects
- Diarrhea and cramping caused by intestinal irritation
- Cystitis
- In a woman, pain or discomfort during vaginal examination or intercourse; atrophy of the ovaries, accompanied by sterility, genetic changes in ova, and decrease or loss of hormone production
- In a man, destruction of sperm in the testes, resulting in temporary or permanent sterility and genetic changes in sperm

Late effects
- Diarrhea, telangiectasia, ulceration, perforation, and obstruction or fistula formation of intestine from thickening of intestinal wall
- Chronic cystitis
- Possibly ureteral obstruction and fibrosis, ulceration, fistula formation, and atrophy of the uterus, cervix, and vagina
- Pale, dry vulval tissues
- Depending on dose received, possibly permanent sterility and genetic changes in ova or sperm

Nursing interventions

For early effects:
- Assess patient's nutritional status, hydration, and bowel habits.
- Recommend a low-residue diet to allow bowel to rest.
- Advise him to drink plenty of fluids—2 qt (1.9 liters) per day—to help prevent urinary tract infection. Also remind him to avoid substances that may irritate his bladder, such as coffee, tea, and alcoholic beverages.
- Watch for signs and symptoms of cystitis: urinary frequency and urgency, pain on urination, and decreased bladder capacity.
- Determine whether patient has experienced any change in urinary habits since therapy began.
- If you suspect an infection, obtain a urine specimen for culture.
- Check the perineal area for signs and symptoms of inflammation.
- Tell the patient to keep the perineal area dry and to expose it to the air as much as possible.
- Make sure the patient's aware of the possibility of sterility, and suggest appropriate counseling, if necessary.
- Tell a female patient that douching helps reduce irritation. Instruct her to douche twice daily with a solution of 1 tb (15 ml) of white vinegar and 1 qt (0.95 liter) of warm water.

For late effects:
- On follow-up examination, assess the patient's nutritional status and bowel habits. Ask him whether he has experienced abdominal pain or tenderness.
- Determine the patient's voiding habits and whether he experiences pain or discomfort when he urinates or during intercourse.
- Recommend to a female patient that she use a vaginal dilator on days when she doesn't have intercourse, to help prevent fibrotic narrowing of the vagina.
- Examine vaginal area for ulceration.

Brain and spinal cord

Early effects
- Possibly cerebral edema, resulting in increased intracranial pressure
- Loss of sensation or movement caused by irreversible spinal cord damage

Late effects
- Possibly atrophy of brain
- Change in vascular supply of spinal cord

Nursing interventions

For early effects:
- Watch for signs and symptoms of increased intracranial pressure and spinal cord damage.
- Emphasize the importance of taking prescribed corticosteroids to decrease cerebral and spinal edema.

For late effects:
- Assess the patient's mental function.
- Assess for signs and symptoms of spinal cord damage (usually temporary).

*Available in both the United States and Canada

DIC

Disseminated intravascular coagulation (DIC) is a complex and potentially fatal condition that may result in widespread hemorrhaging.

How familiar are you with all aspects of DIC? For example, do you know:
- how DIC affects the blood's normal clotting cascade?
- which disorders may result in DIC?
- how to recognize DIC's early indications?

If you're unsure of the answers to these questions, read the next few pages carefully. The information you find may help save your patient's life.

Understanding DIC

Imagine you're caring for Howard Peterson, a 62-year-old truck driver who has recently undergone a lobectomy for lung cancer. As you're checking on Mr. Peterson, you notice a greater-than-normal amount of drainage coming from his incision. You also observe blood oozing from his I.V. site and petechiae across his arms and chest. Of course, you quickly notify the doctor, who orders a series of tests. Test results reveal that Mr. Peterson has decreased hemoglobin and hematocrit levels, along with prolonged clotting times.

After studying the results, the doctor orders heparin administered by I.V. drip—an order that puzzles you. After all, isn't the order contradictory—giving an anticoagulant to a patient already unable to clot?

If you question the doctor's order, you're probably unfamiliar with Mr. Peterson's problem: disseminated intravascular coagulation (DIC). In DIC, the blood's normal clotting capability goes awry; the administration of heparin may help restore it.

What happens in DIC

To fully understand DIC, you must first know how blood clots. Review the information about the clotting cascade on pages 30 and 31. As we said earlier, when bleeding occurs, changes in the vascular system and extravascular tissue activate the clotting cascade. The body balances the clotting process with physical and chemical anticoagulant forces. Together the clotting factors and anticoagulant forces prevent total vessel clotting or uncontrolled hemorrhaging. DIC upsets this balance and allows both conditions to occur.

In DIC, normal clotting is accelerated. As a result, clotting factors (fibrinogen, prothrombin, Factor V, Factor VIII, and platelets) are used up, form microthrombi, and lodge in capillaries and small vessels. Before the body can replace these factors, normal anticoagulant factors are released in response to the now-missing clotting factors. The result is an overabundance of anticoagulant factors, which trigger uncontrolled bleeding.

As you can see, DIC is a dangerous paradox: Most of the visible symptoms are caused by the patient's inability to clot, yet the real problem's uncontrolled clotting.

What causes DIC?

Although DIC's cause isn't known, it's not a primary disorder. DIC results from or is a complication of an underlying disorder that releases a triggering substance into the bloodstream. The following types of disorders may lead to DIC. They include:
- *Infection:* gram-negative or gram-positive septicemia; viral, fungal, or rickettsial infection; protozoal infection
- *Obstetric complications:* abruptio placentae, amniotic fluid embolism, toxemia, retention of dead fetus, septic abortion
- *Neoplastic disease:* acute leukemia, metastatic cancer
- *Disorders that produce necrosis:* extensive burns and trauma, brain tissue destruction, transplant rejection
- *Others:* heatstroke; hypovolemic shock; poisonous snakebite; cirrhosis; fat embolism; incompatible blood transfusion; cardiac arrest; crushing injuries; some types of surgery, especially neurosurgery, cardiopulmonary bypass surgery, prostatic surgery, and thoracic surgery; hemangioma; severe venous thrombosis; purpura fulminans.

Your role in DIC

Because bleeding caused by DIC can be fatal, your ability to quickly recognize its signs and symptoms is crucial.

As DIC exhausts the blood's clotting factors, the first signs you'll see are hematuria, decreased arterial blood pressure, and increased levels of fibrin split products (fibrin fragments that result from clot breakdown).

After DIC depletes the clotting factors, the anticoagulant factors that are normally present take over. During this stage, a patient may exhibit petechiae, ecchymosis, epistaxis, hemoptysis, and signs of hemorrhaging from the brain, the adrenal gland, the heart, or other organs. (To learn how DIC may affect many body systems, study the illustration on pages 128 and 129.)

Besides watching your patient for signs and symptoms of DIC, you may have to assist the doctor with heparin administration. If administered early enough, heparin may limit clotting by blocking thrombin's clotting action. But if heparin's administered after clots have formed, much of its effectiveness will be reduced.

Other treatment of DIC involves correcting the underlying disorder and controlling bleeding. In general, follow these guidelines when caring for a patient with DIC:
- Monitor blood study results, especially hemoglobin and hematocrit values, and coagulation time.
- Administer replacement blood or blood

products, as ordered. Blood products include fresh-frozen plasma, clotting factors, and platelets. Watch for transfusion reactions and fluid overload.
- Administer oxygen, as ordered.
- To determine blood loss, weigh any dressings and linen, and record the amount of drainage.
- Weigh the patient daily for fluid assessment, especially if he has a kidney disorder. In acute DIC, monitor intake and output hourly.
- Watch for bleeding from the gastrointestinal and genitourinary tracts. If you suspect intra-abdominal bleeding, measure the patient's abdominal girth every 4 hours. Test specimens of gastric secretions, stool, and urine for occult blood.
- Monitor the patient closely for signs and symptoms of hypovolemic shock, if appropriate.
- Check I.V. and venipuncture sites frequently for bleeding.
- Limit the number of intramuscular injections your patient receives. Apply pressure to injection sites for at least 10 minutes to control bleeding.
- To prevent clots from dislodging and causing fresh bleeding, don't scrub bleeding areas. Use pressure, cold compresses, and topical hemostatic agents—for example, absorbable gelatin sponge (Gelfoam)—to control bleeding.
- Monitor heparin administration, if appropriate.
- Protect the patient from injury. Turn and position him carefully. Enforce bed rest during bleeding episodes. If the patient's agitated, pad the bed's side rails. Also, provide emotional support for the patient and his family.
- Advise co-workers of the patient's tendency to hemorrhage.
- Provide gentle mouth care for your patient. Remember, his gums may bleed easily, causing him to swallow blood and become nauseated.
- Avoid using adhesive tape; the pulling action of tape removal may cause bleeding.
- Because DIC may cause bleeding into your patient's major organs, watch for signs and symptoms of further complications from the bleeding. For example, if blood accumulates in your patient's brain, watch for signs and symptoms of cerebrovascular accident, such as aphasia, weakness, sensory changes, and altered level of consciousness.

By learning to recognize such signs and symptoms, you can learn where bleeding is occurring.

Laboratory tests results for DIC

Certain laboratory test results can help you detect DIC in a patient. Study these carefully. Keep in mind that no single diagnostic test confirms DIC.

Also, a patient with liver disease may have similar values for the tests below. Confirm DIC by comparing test results with other assessment findings.

Screening tests	Normal values	Values indicating DIC	Nursing considerations
Prothrombin time (PT)	12 to 15 seconds	Times exceeding 15 seconds	• PT is also prolonged in patients with vitamin K deficiency or liver disease and in those receiving coumarin therapy. • Fill a 7-ml blue-top collection tube. Send the specimen to the lab immediately.
Plasma fibrinogen level	195 to 365 mg/dl	Levels less than 150 mg/dl	• Collect a specimen in a 7-ml blue-top collection tube, and send it to the lab immediately. • Handle the specimen gently. Hemolysis affects test results.
Platelet count	130,000 to 370,000/mm^3	Count of less than 150,000/mm^3. Progressively falling platelet count also indicates DIC, even if absolute value doesn't.	• Collect a specimen in a 7-ml lavender-top tube. Handle the specimen carefully and send to the lab immediately. • Check patient medications. Many commonly used drugs decrease platelet count.
Fibrin split products (FSP)	Less than 10 mcg/ml	Level greater than 40 mcg/ml	• Collect a specimen in a special tube provided by the lab. Handle the specimen carefully and send to the lab immediately. • Some drugs raise FSP levels; for example, urokinase. • Heparin causes false-positive results.
Plasma thrombin time	10 to 15 seconds	Prolonged thrombin times ranging from 20 to 40 seconds	• Fill a 7-ml blue-top tube. Handle the specimen carefully and send to the lab immediately.
Whole blood clotting time	5 to 15 minutes	Whole blood clotting time longer than 15 minutes	• Patient with vitamin K deficiency will have a similar result.
Activated partial thromboplastin time (APTT)	25 to 36 seconds	Times exceeding 36 seconds	• Collect the specimen in a 7-ml blue-top collection tube. Gently invert the tube several times to mix the sample and anticoagulant. • Patient receiving heparin therapy may have similar results.

DIC

Recognizing signs and symptoms of DIC

As we stated on the previous page, your most important role in caring for a patient with disseminated intravascular coagulation (DIC) is early detection of the condition's signs and symptoms. DIC can affect almost every body system, which means you may detect dozens of signs and symptoms caused by massive clotting or massive hemorrhaging. To become familiar with them, study the following chart carefully.

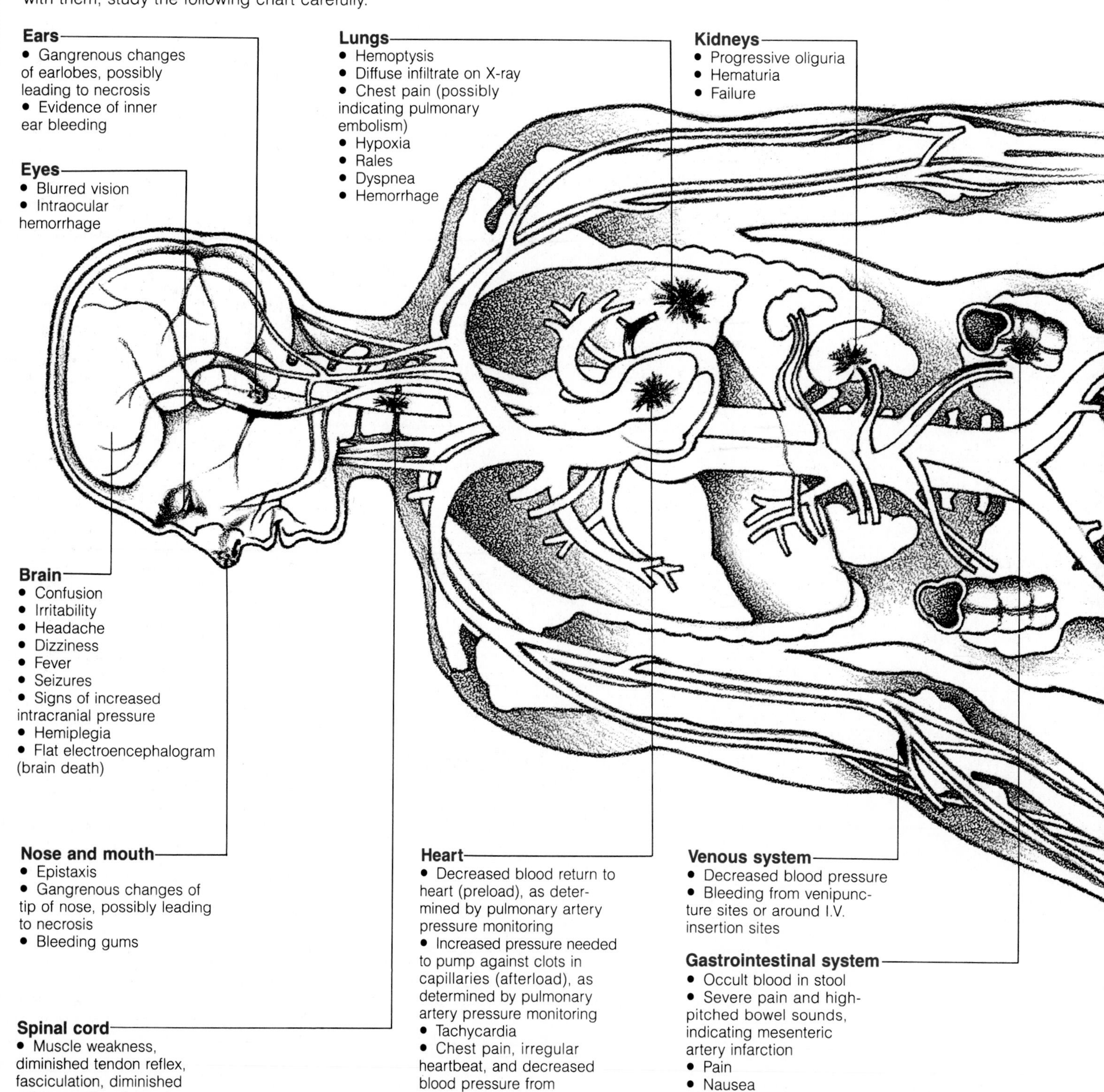

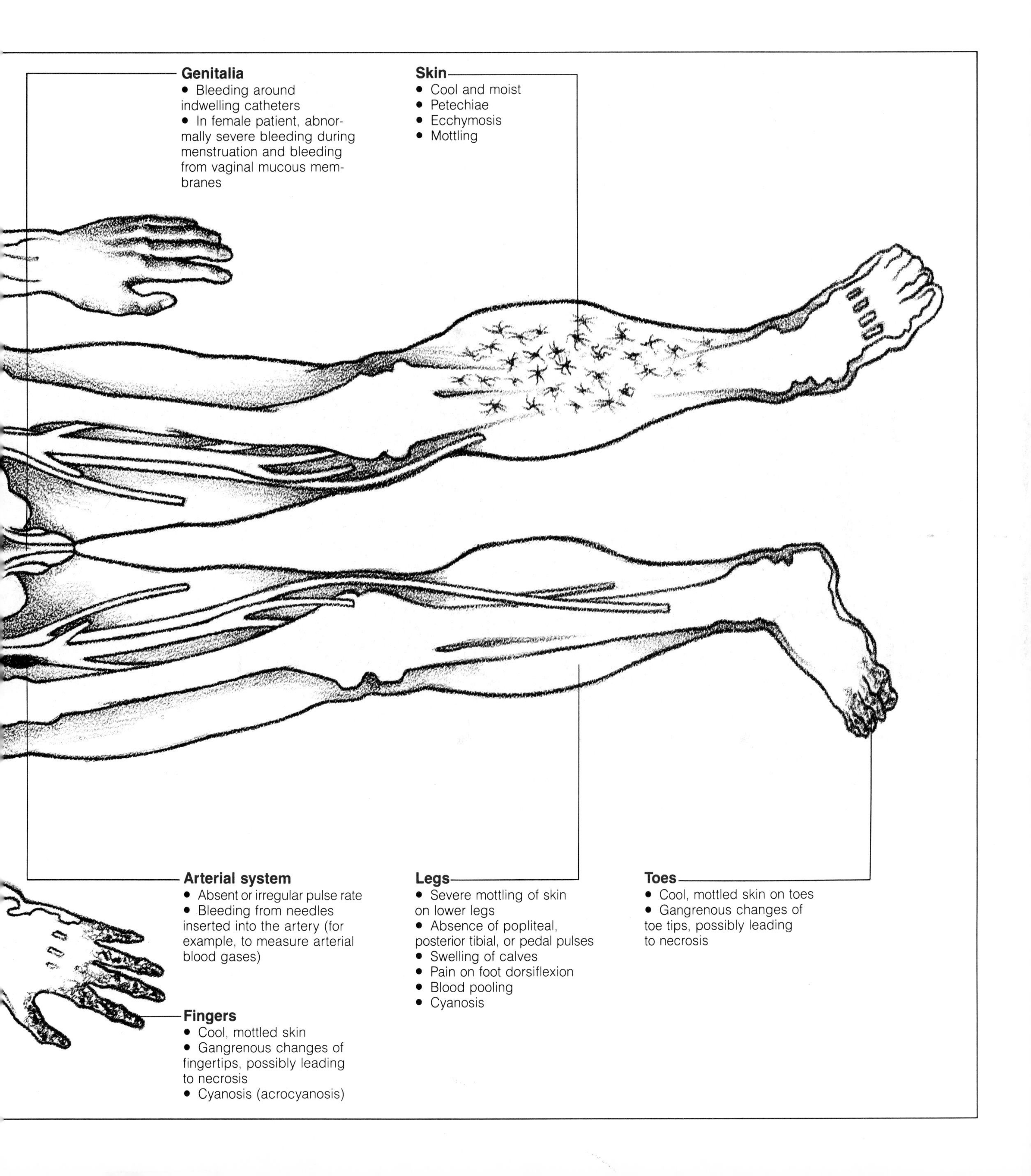
Genitalia
• Bleeding around indwelling catheters
• In female patient, abnormally severe bleeding during menstruation and bleeding from vaginal mucous membranes
Skin
• Cool and moist
• Petechiae
• Ecchymosis
• Mottling
Arterial system
• Absent or irregular pulse rate
• Bleeding from needles inserted into the artery (for example, to measure arterial blood gases)
Fingers
• Cool, mottled skin
• Gangrenous changes of fingertips, possibly leading to necrosis
• Cyanosis (acrocyanosis)
Legs
• Severe mottling of skin on lower legs
• Absence of popliteal, posterior tibial, or pedal pulses
• Swelling of calves
• Pain on foot dorsiflexion
• Blood pooling
• Cyanosis
Toes
• Cool, mottled skin on toes
• Gangrenous changes of toe tips, possibly leading to necrosis

Coma

If you've ever taken care of a comatose patient, you know that he presents a special challenge to your nursing skills. Such a patient can't express his needs or wants. As a result, he's dependent on you. Your skilled nursing care may have a substantial impact on your patient's chances for recovery.

Be prepared to meet this challenge by reading the next few pages. You'll learn how to:

- develop your patient care plan.
- perform nose and mouth care.
- prevent corneal irritation.
- meet your patient's psychosocial needs.

Formulating a patient care plan

Nineteen-year-old Donna Holmes has been in a coma since she was admitted to the ICU after an automobile accident 3 weeks ago. She has a fractured right leg, fractured ribs, and a closed head injury. Because her condition's stabilized, she's being transferred to your unit within the hour.

When you read her records, you see that she has a nasogastric tube in place for tube feeding, an I.V. line in her left arm, and a long leg cast on her right leg. Do you have time to provide the care a patient like Donna needs? A comprehensive care plan will help you organize her care.

To develop a care plan that meets Donna's needs and your unit's staffing, review and revise Donna's ICU care plan. Then, schedule a conference with the health-care team that will be caring for your patient—physical therapist, dietitian, doctors, and nurses—to review her care and set new goals, if necessary. Be sure appropriate long- and short-term goals are set.

Keep in mind that a well-planned, clearly written care plan offers these advantages for you and your patient:

- details when to perform a procedure
- ensures continuity of care
- lays the groundwork for problem-oriented assessment.

Plan format

An effective patient care plan includes this information:

- personal data, such as the patient's name and age and the name of her doctor
- the doctor's diagnosis, as well as special problems that may have arisen during hospitalization. Include the date the problem was identified. Doing so helps differentiate chronic from acute problems and helps determine how long problem solving will take.
- specific goals of nursing care so you can determine if your interventions have succeeded.

Important: Don't restate a problem as a goal. For example, don't write that your patient's 50 lb (22.7 kg) overweight. Develop a plan to reduce her weight by a certain amount each week, and then weigh her frequently to determine whether the goal's being attained.

Note: Be sure to explain the transfer to her family and reassure them. When you speak with her family, be alert for comments or clues that may help you personalize Donna's care; for example, food preferences and personal habits.

Review the sample care plan on the next page. Use it as a guide for developing your own plan. Remember that each plan varies according to the patient's condition and needs, the doctor, and your hospital's policy.

DOCUMENTING

Tips for a good care plan

What's wrong with the care plan below?

If you answered that it's too general, then you already have an idea of what a good care plan looks like. The plan won't succeed in directing patient care.

To ensure quality care for your patient, keep these care-plan tips in mind:

- Check your hospital policy to determine whether your patient's care plan is part of her permanent record. If so, write the plan in ink. Don't forget to sign your name.
- Avoid wordiness when writing, but don't be so brief that the plan's intentions aren't clear.
- Make notes on a piece of scrap paper as you care for your patient. Then, at the end of your shift, transfer those ideas to the plan. By doing so, you avoid forgetting to add important information.
- Make sure all abbreviations and numbers are written clearly, so they don't confuse co-workers.
- Review and update your patient's care plan daily. Try doing so during a shift change, because it gives you an opportunity to share ideas with co-workers.

DATE	PATIENT PROBLEMS	NURSING ACTIONS	EXPECTED OUTCOME	TARGET DATE
	Skin care	Turn every 2 hours		
		Back rub		
	Nutrition	Tube feedings	Weight gain	

DATE	PATIENT PROBLEMS	NURSING ACTIONS	EXPECTED OUTCOME	TARGET DATE
2/3/83	Alteration in consciousness	Provide stimulation	Prevent postcoma depression	Duration of
		Explain all procedures		hospitalization
		Encourage visits by friends		or altered
		and family		state of
		Orient to time, place,		consciousness
		and person		
		Prevent self-injury	Prevent self-removal of NG tube	Duration of intubation
		Restrain arms, as needed	Reduce number of scratches on arms	2/7/83
		Keep fingernails short	Prevent bruises of head and arms	2/7/83
		Pad bed rails, as needed	Prevent skin breakdown from	Duration of
		Pad left ankle	rubbing left ankle on cast	right leg cast
2/3/83	12-lb weight loss from	Weigh patient daily	Early recognition of any further	Duration of
	admission weight	Maintain tube feeding schedule	weight loss	hospitalization
		50 ml blenderized tube	Reverse weight loss trend	2/6/83
		feeding every hour		
		30 ml fruit juice on even hours		
		30 ml water on odd hours		
			(continued)	

LONG-TERM GOALS ① Prevent further weight loss ② Maintain present skin integrity

SHORT-TERM GOALS ① Prevent contractures ② Family performs daily care

DIAGNOSIS	ALLERGY	PAGE
1/13/83 Auto accident – Fx Ⓡ leg, Fx ribs, closed head injury 1/14/83 open reduction Ⓡ leg	None known	PAGE ____ OF ____

ROOM	NAME	AGE	DOCTOR
736 A	Holmes, Donna	19	Mendelson

Coma

How to wash your patient's hair

As you know, your nursing responsibilities include providing for Donna Holmes' personal hygiene as well as meeting her other physical and emotional needs. Of course, performing relatively simple personal hygiene tasks becomes increasingly difficult when the patient's in a coma. For example, do you know how to wash a comatose patient's hair? If you're unsure how to proceed, review the following photostory.

Begin by gathering the following equipment: three towels, shampoo (preferably one with cream rinse), two large pitchers filled with warm water, large basin, and overbed table. Make sure all the equipment's within easy reach.

Explain to your patient what you're going to do and reassure her. Ask a co-worker to help position her flat on the bed. Raise the bed to a height that enables you to work comfortably. Then, remove the bed's headboard.

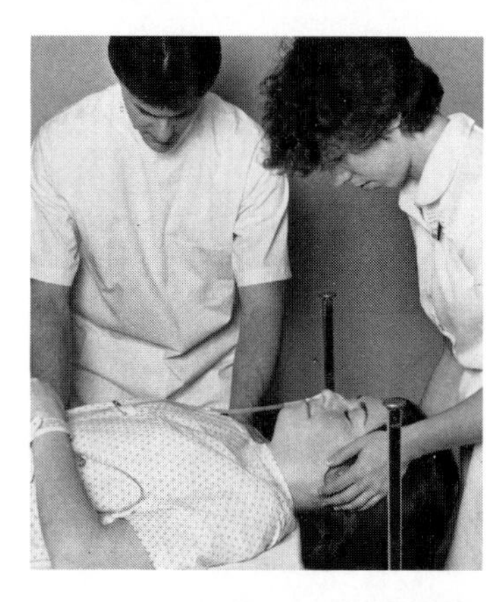

1 With a co-worker's help, position Donna so her head extends slightly beyond the mattress, as shown here. Make sure you or your co-worker supports her head at all times.

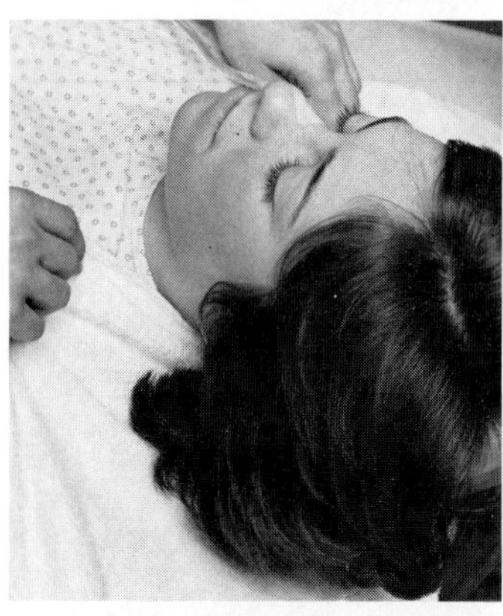

2 Place a towel under Donna's shoulders and neck to keep the bed linens dry.

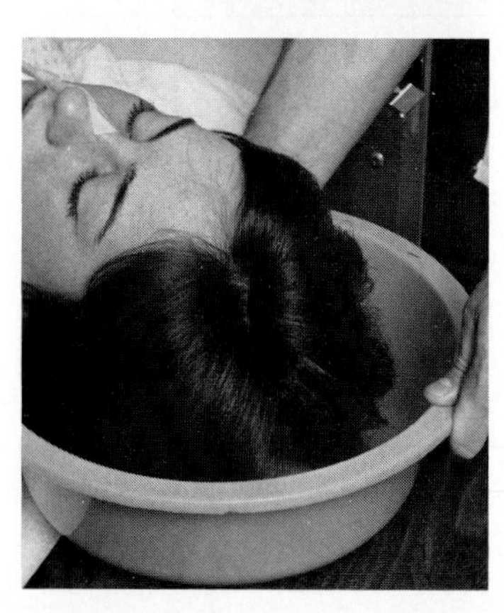

3 Position the basin on the table, directly under your patient's head.

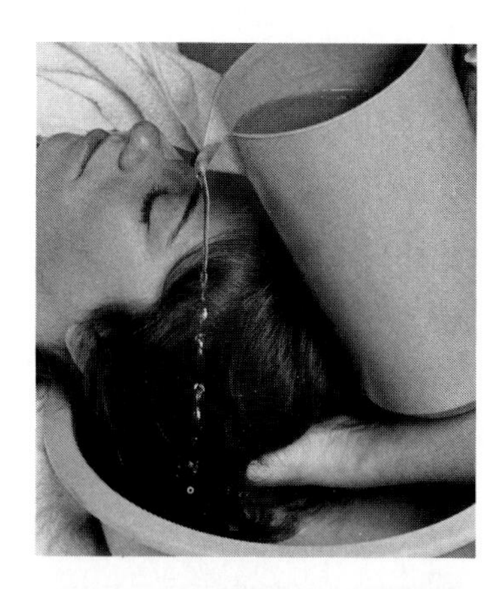

4 Pour warm water from one of the pitchers over Donna's hair. Make sure you wet her hair thoroughly.

Note: Always check to be sure the water is a comfortable temperature.

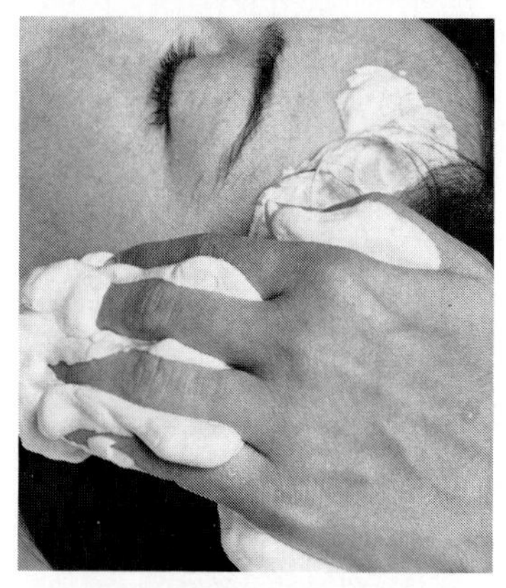

5 Now, apply the shampoo to her hair. Thoroughly work the shampoo into her scalp. Take care not to get shampoo or water in her eyes or ears.

Note: Blot any water on her forehead, face, or neck with a towel.

If necessary, empty the basin before proceeding.

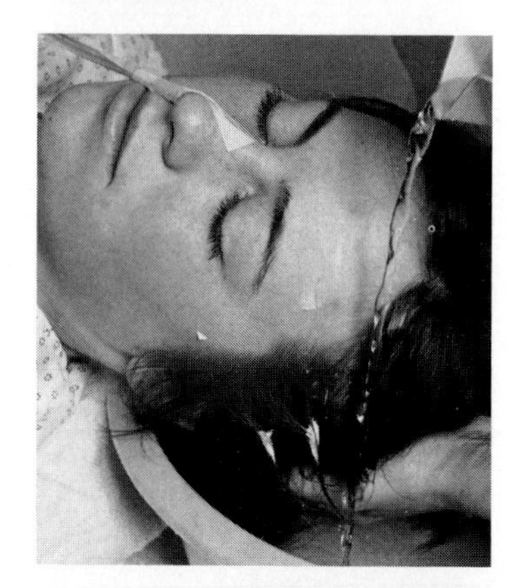

6 Pour the second pitcher of water over your patient's hair. Make sure you rinse all the shampoo from her hair; shampoo residue may irritate her scalp.

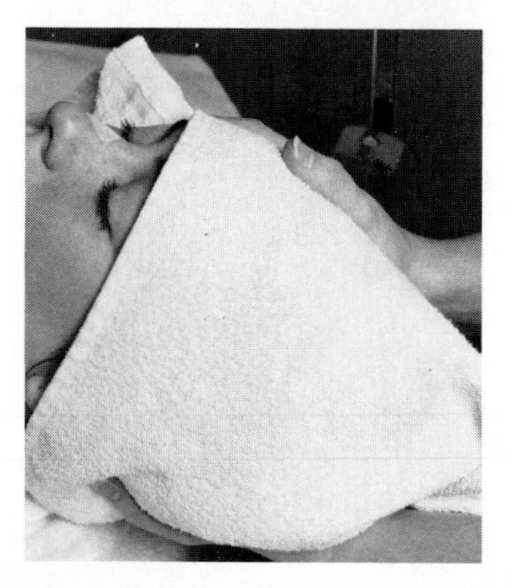

7 Wrap a towel around her hair. Then reposition Donna on the bed. Replace the headboard.

Remove the towel from her head. Then, dry her hair thoroughly and comb it. If your hospital policy allows, use a hair dryer. After you're finished, dispose of the equipment, according to hospital policy. Document the procedure, including how well Donna tolerated it.

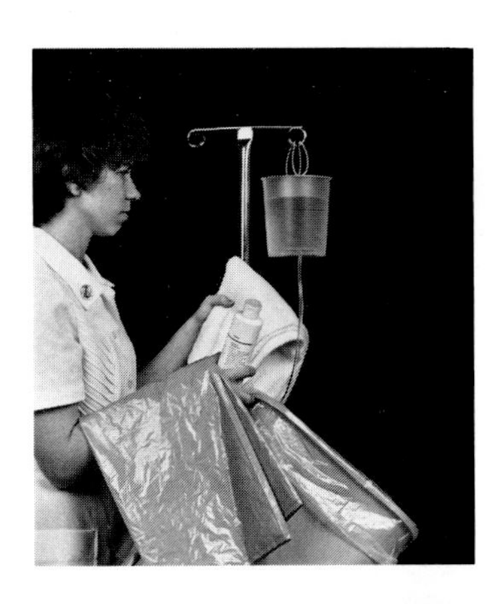

8 Here's another way to wash your patient's hair. Begin by gathering this equipment: three towels, shampoo, clean enema bucket filled with warm water, I.V. pole, large plastic trash bag, and trash can. Enlist the aid of a co-worker to help you remove the bed's headboard and position your patient at the head of the bed. Make sure you or your co-worker supports the patient's head at all times.

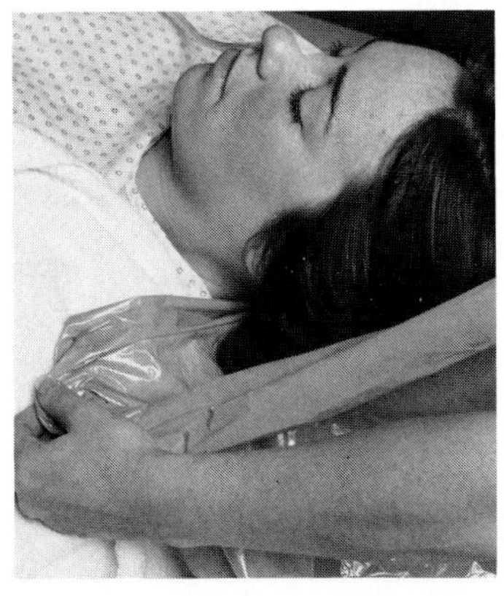

9 Place a towel under your patient's shoulders and head. Position the open end of the plastic trash bag under her head, as shown here.

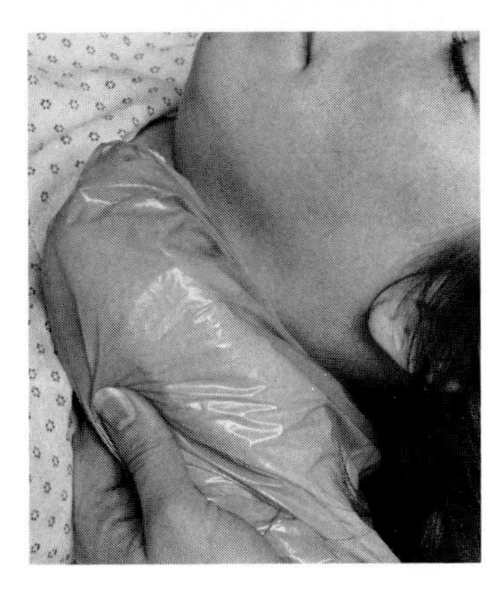

10 Use the towel to raise the trash bag around your patient's ears.

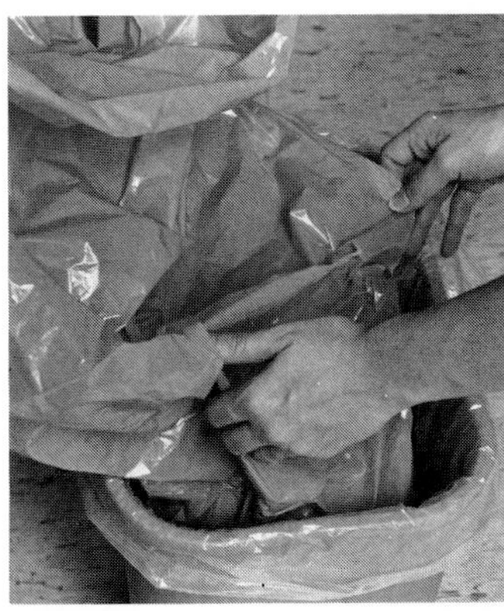

11 Place the closed end of the trash bag into the trash can to hold the water.

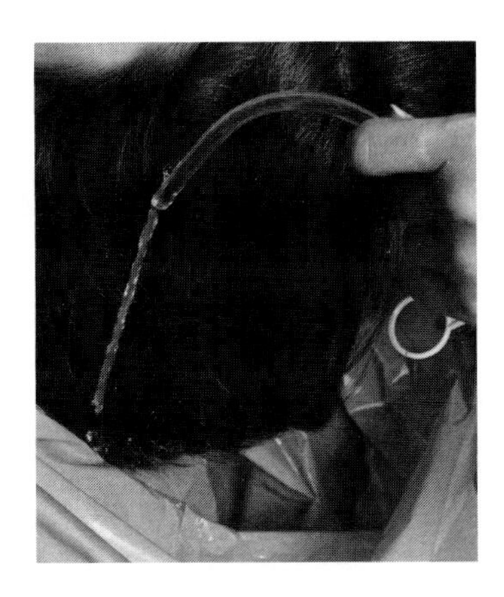

12 Hang the filled enema bucket on the I.V. pole. Hold the bag's tubing over your patient's hair, and open the clamp to release the water. Wet her hair thoroughly; then, close the clamp.

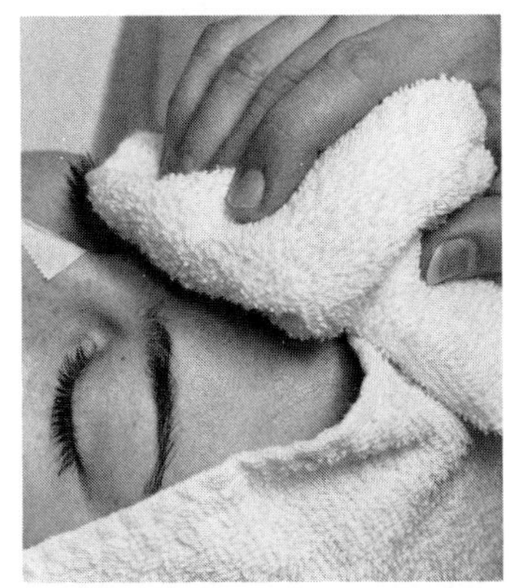

13 Next, apply the shampoo and work it through her hair. Release the tubing clamp and rinse her hair. But, avoid getting water in her eyes or ears.

After you're finished rinsing her hair, close the clamp. Wrap a towel around her hair. Use another towel to blot any water that may have splashed on her face or neck.

Have a co-worker help you reposition your patient on the bed and replace the headboard.

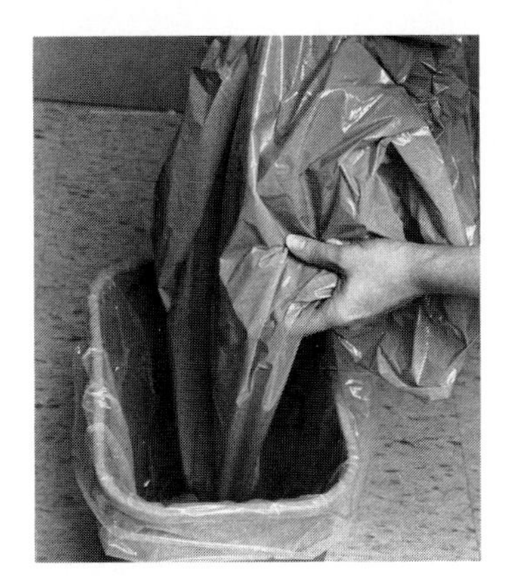

14 Carefully remove the trash bag from the trash can. Empty the bag into the sink, and then dispose of the bag properly.

Remove the towel from your patient's head, and dry her hair thoroughly. Then, comb it.

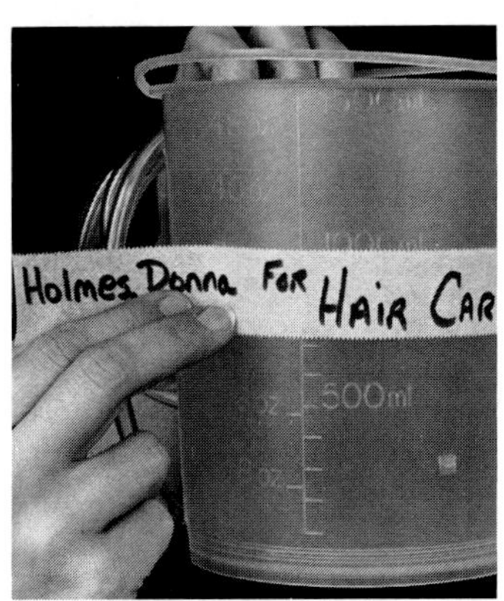

15 Finally, empty the enema bucket. Label this bucket "For Hair Care Only," and store it in the patient's bedside stand. Document the procedure.

Coma

Nurses' guide to eye lubrication products

Because a comatose patient may not blink enough to sufficiently lubricate her eyes, she's susceptible to corneal irritation and scratching. By administering an eye lubricant, you can help prevent corneal damage. Besides temporarily lubricating your patient's eyes, such lubricants help protect against irritation and infection. To become more familiar with eye lubricants, review the examples listed below.

Note: For detailed information on administering eye medications, see the NURSING PHOTOBOOK GIVING MEDICATIONS.

Artificial tears
(Hypotears, Lacril*, Tears Naturale*)

Indication
To provide temporary lubrication of dry eyes when tear production's insufficient

Interaction
If artificial tears containing polyvinyl alcohol are used with eye irrigation solutions containing borate, gel or gummy deposits may form on eyelids.

Nursing considerations
- Check patient's history and product label to make sure your patient's not allergic to the drug's active ingredients or preservatives.
- Don't touch your patient's eye with the drug container's tip or use the same container for more than one patient.
- Warn your patient that the drug may temporarily cause blurred vision.

Eye irrigation solutions
(Dacriose, Murine Eye Drops)

Indication
To cleanse eyes and eyelids, remove eye film, and provide temporary lubrication

Interaction
Eye irrigation solutions containing borate used with artificial tears products containing polyvinyl alcohol may cause gel or gummy deposits to form on eyelids.

Nursing considerations
- Check patient's history and product label to make sure your patient's not allergic to the drug's active ingredients or preservatives.
- Don't touch your patient's eye with the drug container's tip or use the same container for more than one patient.
- As ordered, flush the eye with irrigation solution every 2 hours. Most products provide only short-term lubrication.
- Check the drug's expiration date to be sure it's fresh.
- Store in tightly closed, light-resistant containers.
- When using an eye irrigation solution, turn your patient's head slightly to the side and irrigate from the inner to the outer canthus. Use tissues to wipe excess solution.

Ocular lubricant ointments
(Duolube, Lacri-Lube S.O.P)

Indication
Long-term eye lubrication

Interaction
None

Nursing considerations
- Check patient's history and product label to make sure your patient's not allergic to the drug's active ingredients or preservatives.
- Don't touch your patient's eye with the drug container's tip or use the same container for more than one patient.
- To prevent buildup of ocular lubricant ointment in your patient's eyes, remove previously applied ointment with an eye irrigating solution before each administration.
- Warn your patient that the drug may cause blurred vision for several minutes.

*Available in both the United States and Canada

Taping your patient's eyes

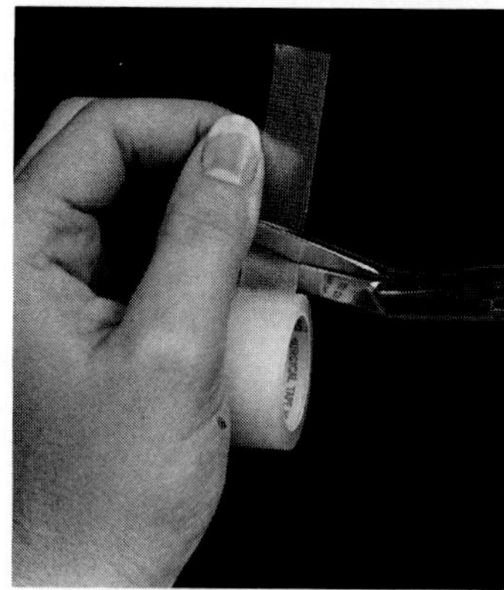

1 While performing morning care, you notice that Donna Holmes isn't blinking. A second look tells you that her eyes are slightly open and losing lubrication, which increases the risk of corneal damage. Instillation of an eye lubricant provides a temporary solution. But to protect Donna's eyes and prevent serious damage, tape them shut. First, cut two 1½" (3.8-cm) strips of ½" wide, transparent, nonallergenic tape. Explain the procedure.

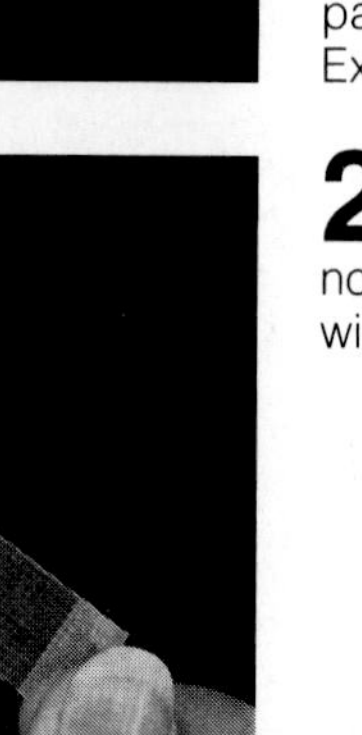

2 Fold one tape end back on itself, forming a ¼" long nonsticky tab. Repeat this step with the other tape strip.

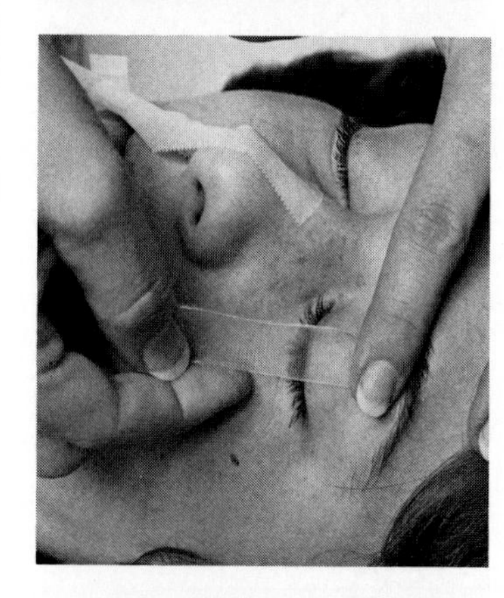

3 Place the sticky end of one strip on your patient's left upper eyelid, just below the eyebrow. (Make sure the tape doesn't touch her eyebrow.) Gently press the tape down over your patient's eyelid until the end with the tab rests on her cheek. Make sure the tape's tight enough to keep her eye closed.

Repeat the procedure on her right eye.

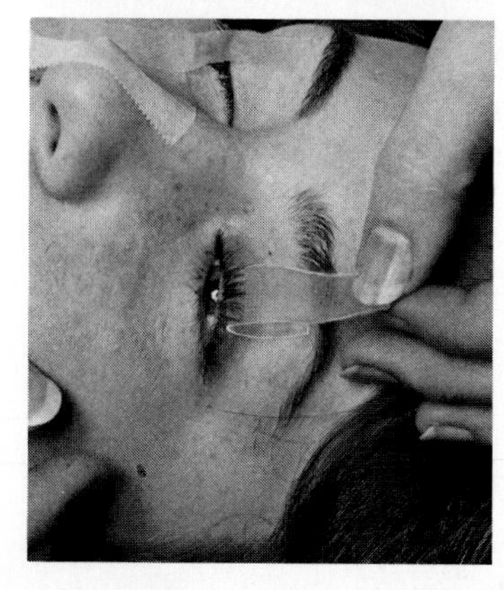

4 To assess your patient's eyes and her pupillary response, gently lift the tab ends from her cheeks until you can see her eyes. After completing your assessment, reapply the tape. Replace the tape every 6 to 12 hours, or as needed.

Remember: If your patient blinks on her own, don't tape her eyes closed. Doing so will make her extremely anxious.

Performing nose care

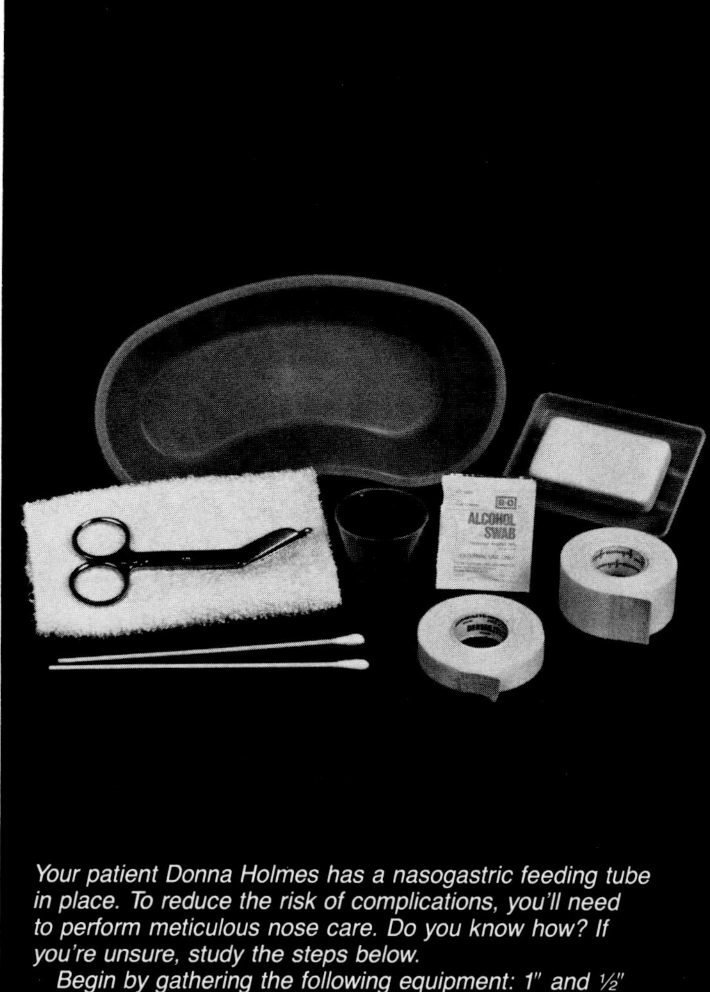

Your patient Donna Holmes has a nasogastric feeding tube in place. To reduce the risk of complications, you'll need to perform meticulous nose care. Do you know how? If you're unsure, study the steps below.

Begin by gathering the following equipment: 1" and ½" wide nonallergenic tape (or other adhesive tape), scissors, washcloth, soap, emesis basin filled with warm water, alcohol swab, cotton-tipped applicators, and medicine cup containing mineral oil. Place the equipment on a nearby bedside stand. Then, explain the procedure to Donna, even though she's in a coma.

Note: *For more information on nasogastric tube care, see the* NURSING PHOTOBOOK PERFORMING GI PROCEDURES.

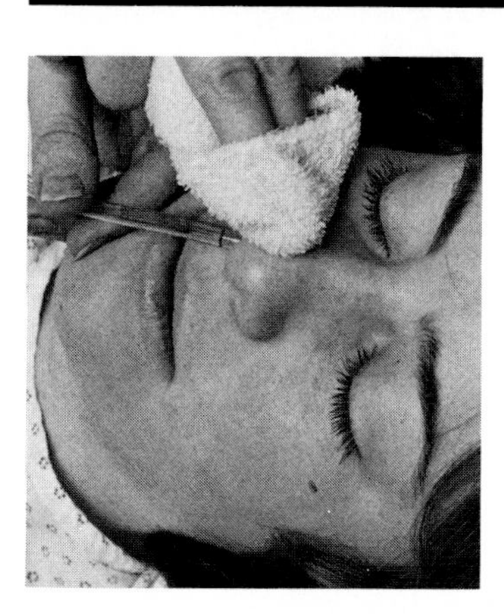

1 First, remove any tape from your patient's nose and tube. Immerse the washcloth in the basin until it's thoroughly wet. Rub some soap on the washcloth and cleanse Donna's nose, nostrils, and upper lip. *Important:* Make sure you don't dislodge the tube while you're cleansing the area.

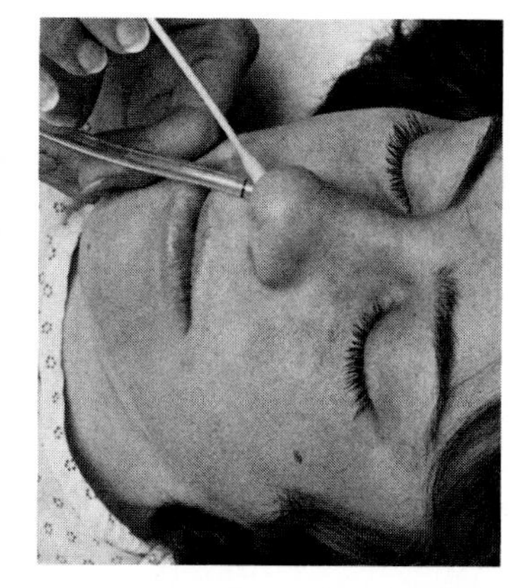

2 Next, check for a buildup of crusted secretions inside Donna's nostrils. If you notice any crusts, soften them by applying mineral oil liberally with a cotton-tipped applicator. Then, remove the crusted material using another cotton-tipped applicator.

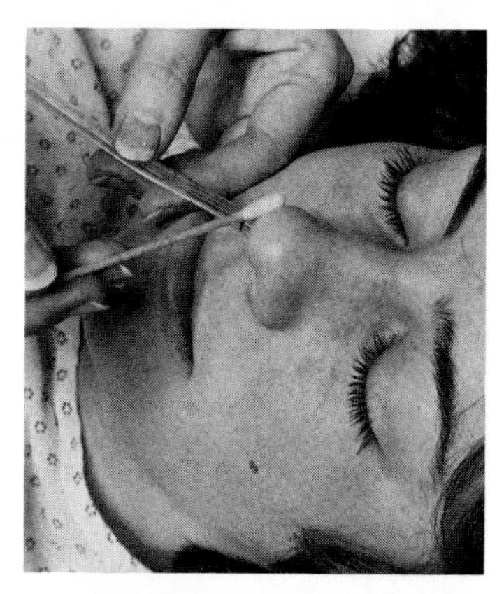

3 After removing the crusted secretions, use another cotton-tipped applicator to apply mineral oil to the inside edge of Donna's nostrils. Doing so keeps the skin soft and prevents irritation.

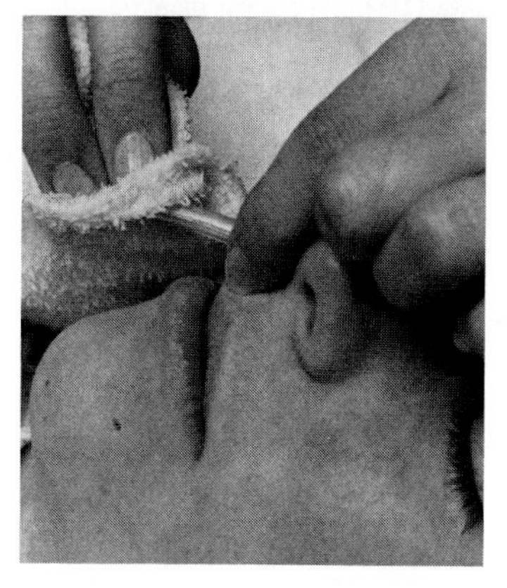

4 Next, clean the nasogastric tube with soap and water. If any mineral oil or old adhesive tape is still on the tube, remove it with an alcohol swab. Then, make sure you thoroughly dry the tube, so the tape will adhere better.

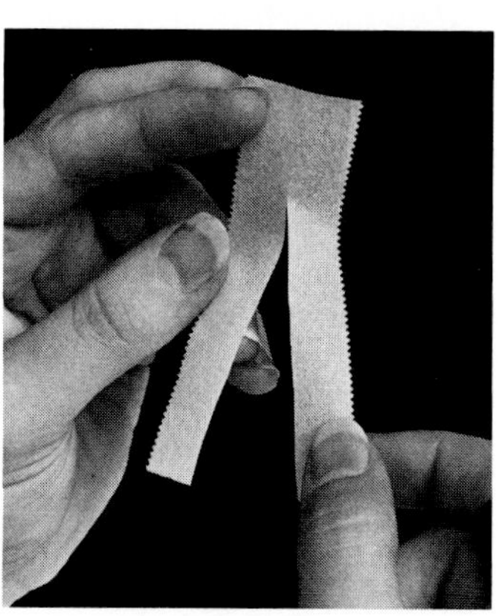

5 Cut a 3½" (9-cm) strip of 1" wide nonallergenic tape. Split the tape lengthwise, leaving a small piece of tape intact at one end.

Coma

Performing nose care continued

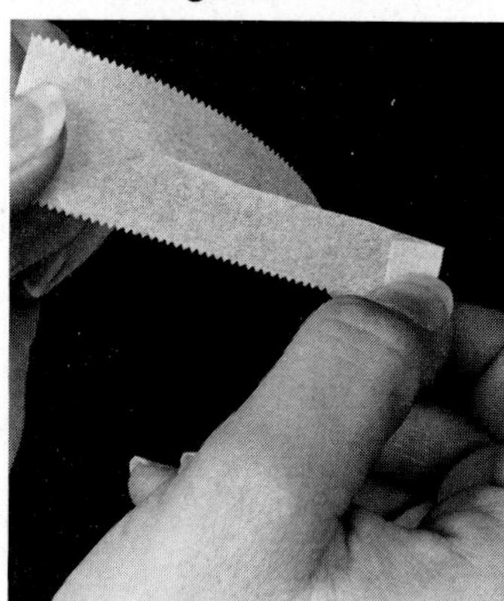

6 Fold the split tape ends as shown here, making two small, nonsticky tape tabs.

Note: If your patient's restless, split the new tape before removing the old tape. This way you can quickly interchange the tape pieces and prevent your patient from removing the tube.

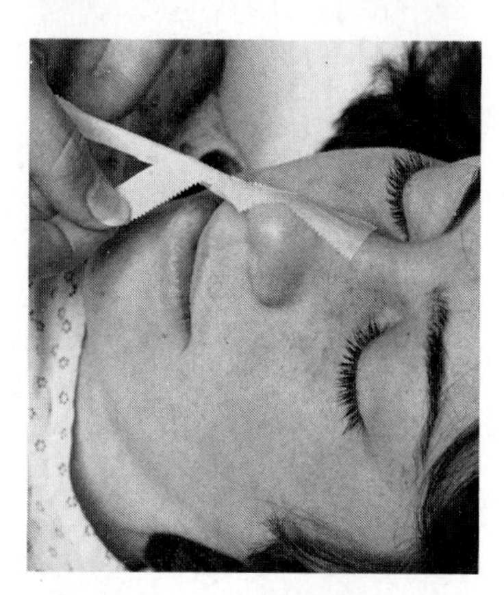

7 Apply the tape's uncut end to your patient's nose. Place half the cut end along the tube and wrap the other half around the tube.

After 8 hours, you or a coworker will remove the old tape, cleanse the patient's nose, and prepare new tape. Tape the tube in the same manner as above, but switch the position of the tape's cut ends.

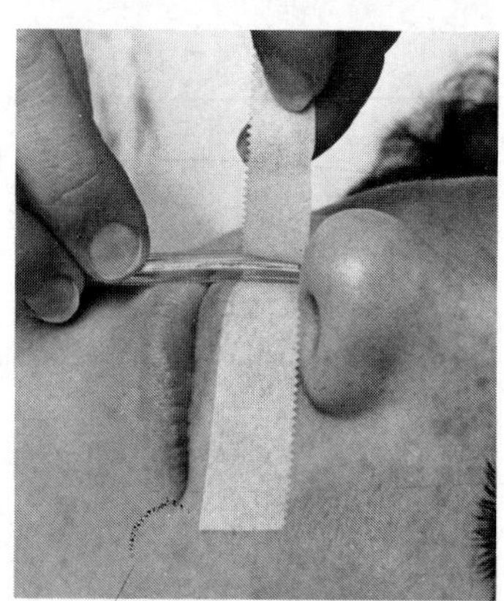

8 After another 8 hours, remove the old tape and cleanse your patient's nose and upper lip again. Then, cut two 2" (5-cm) strips of ½" tape. Apply one strip over her upper lip and then tape the tube over the first tape strip, as shown.

Be sure to alternate the taping sites every 8 hours.

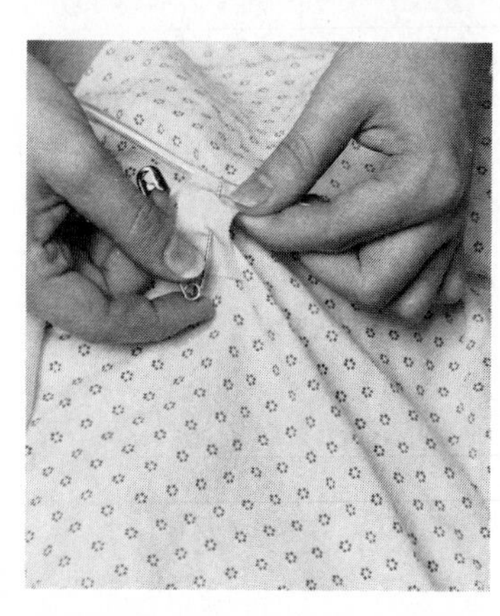

9 Finally, provide further protection by cutting a 2" (5-cm) strip of 1" tape and wrapping it around the tube's distal end. Place two sticky sides of the tape together to make a nonsticky tab. Pin the tab to Donna's gown with a safety pin. Be sure to allow slack for the tube to accommodate any head movements.

Document the procedure.

Performing mouth care

Meticulous mouth care's important for any patient—particularly one who's in a coma. Secretions accumulate quickly in a comatose patient's mouth, increasing the risk of infection or aspiration. If you're not sure what's involved in providing mouth care for a comatose patient, read the following photostory.

First, gather this equipment: nonsterile examination gloves; small, padded tongue blade; soft-bristle, child-sized toothbrush; toothpaste; petrolatum; cotton-tipped applicator; and towel. You'll also need a large syringe (without the needle) filled with water, roll of 1" wide adhesive tape, suction catheter, and suction source.

To protect your patient's gown, place a towel across her chest. Then, turn on the suction machine and attach the catheter.

Nursing tip: *Convert an intermittent-suction catheter to a constant-suction catheter, necessary for mouth care, by applying a tape strip over the whistle tip.*

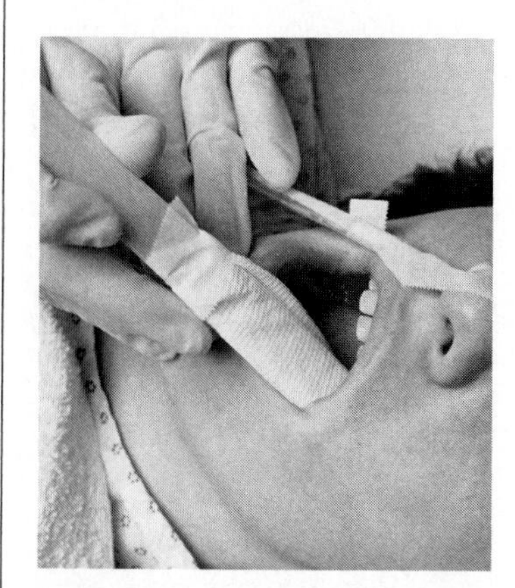

1 Explain the procedure to your patient. Then, wash your hands and put on gloves. To keep your patient's teeth apart during cleaning, insert a padded tongue blade between her upper and lower teeth, as the nurse is doing here.

Important: Take care when placing your fingers near a comatose patient's teeth; she may unknowingly bite down.

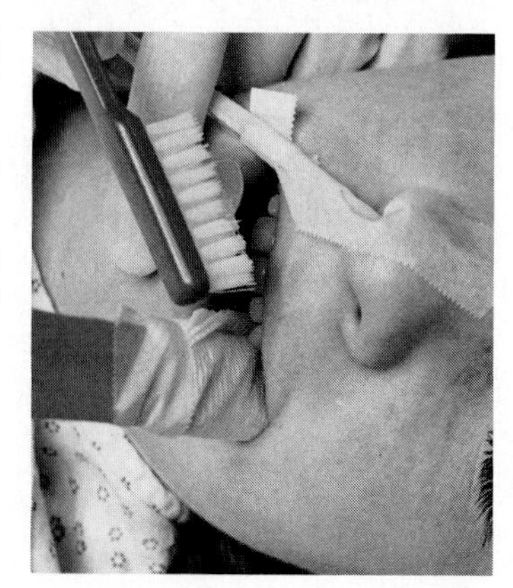

2 Reduce the risk of secretion aspiration by turning your patient's head to one side. Doing so helps pool secretions in her cheek. Apply a *small* amount of toothpaste to the toothbrush and gently brush her teeth and gums. Intermittently, suction secretions and toothpaste from her mouth. Or, position the catheter at the back of her mouth while you brush. But don't position the catheter so far back that you cause her to gag.

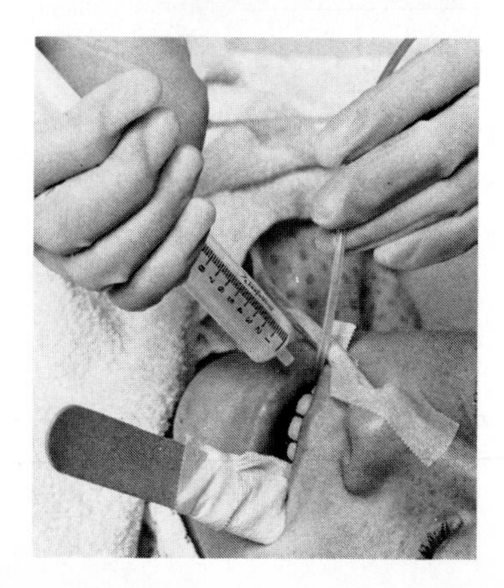

3 Then, use the syringe to rinse her teeth and gums. Don't direct the water toward the back of her throat, or she may gag. Remember to suction secretions frequently. Also be sure to suction between her gums and cheeks and under her tongue.

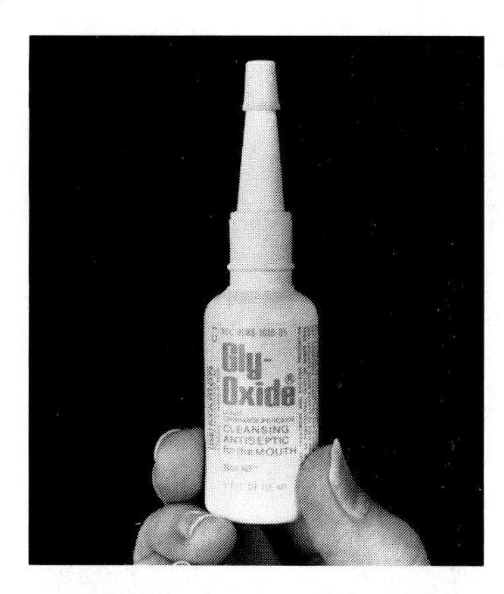

4 If you can't brush your patient's teeth (for example, because they're clenched), treat them with carbamide peroxide (Gly-Oxide*). This liquid coats the teeth and gums and helps destroy bacteria that may cause an infection. *Note:* You may have to obtain a doctor's order to use Gly-Oxide. Check your hospital policy.

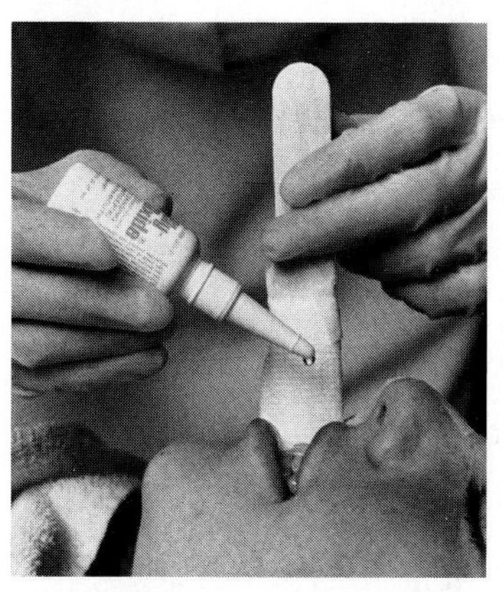

5 To administer Gly-Oxide, remove the protective cap and place 10 drops on your patient's tongue and around her mouth, as the nurse is doing here. Gly-Oxide will begin to foam in a few seconds. Allow the solution to act for about 1 minute, and then suction it from her mouth.

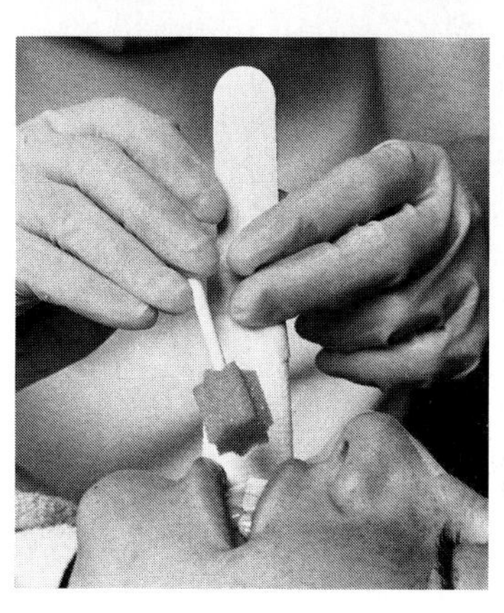

6 Consisting of a small sponge attached to a short paper applicator stick, a Toothette is another way to protect your patient's teeth from infection. A Toothette may come premoistened or you can moisten it yourself in normal saline solution with peppermint flavoring added. To use, dip the Toothette into the solution, and gently brush your patient's teeth and gums. Then, use the water-filled syringe to rinse her mouth.

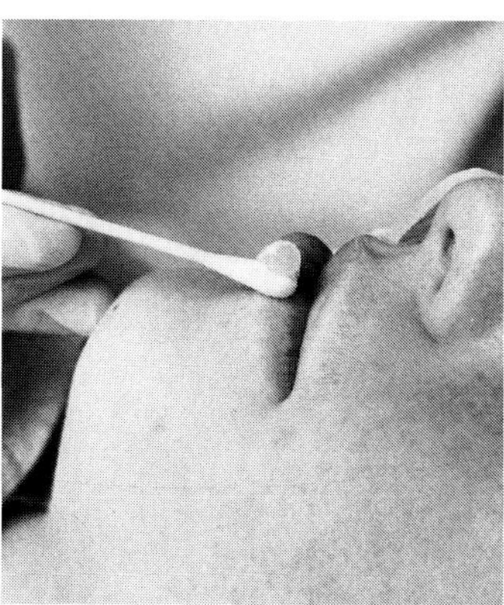

7 Finally, use a cotton-tipped applicator to apply a lubricant, such as petrolatum, to your patient's lips and around her mouth. Doing so prevents drying and cracking.

Repeat mouth care at least every 4 hours, or as needed. When you're finished, dispose of all equipment according to hospital policy and document the procedure.

*Available in both the United States and Canada

SPECIAL CONSIDERATIONS

Meeting your patient's psychosocial needs

A week has passed since Donna Holmes was transferred to your unit. During this time, you've achieved one of your care plan's major goals: preventing physical complications. But now you'd like to do more with another aspect of Donna's care: meeting her psychosocial needs. How can you achieve this goal? Read on for some answers.

First, keep in mind that although Donna can't communicate, she still thinks, feels, and hears. Don't be tempted to ignore her identity and classify her by her condition. Every time you enter her room, be sure to talk to her; tell her which day it is, what the weather's like. Explain all procedures before you perform them. And don't say anything near her you wouldn't want her to hear. Advise other staff members of your plan and ask their cooperation. After recovery, some patients who were comatose recall details of their care.

Include your patient's family in her care. Find out which activities Donna enjoys, which are her favorite foods, and if she has any clothing she enjoys wearing. Then, try working this knowledge into your care plan. Talk to Donna about her favorite activities. If possible, obtain one of her favorite foods and place it near her. Determine whether she responds to the aroma. If her family brings a robe that she enjoys wearing, put it on her. Although she may not respond to these gestures, she may enjoy them.

In addition, encourage Donna's family to participate in her physical care; for example, washing her face and hair. Before you do, check your hospital's policy and evaluate the family's ability and desire to participate. But remember, the family will probably be distraught because of the uncertainty of Donna's condition. By explaining the details of her care and encouraging the family to help as much as possible, you can help ease the tension.

Here are other ways you can give your patient the benefit of outside stimuli:

- If possible, seat your patient in a chair by the window.
- Turn on a radio or television, when appropriate, for your patient to listen to.
- Keep a calendar in her room, and each day tell her the day and date. Ask her family to mark special dates, such as birthdays and anniversaries, on the calendar, and tell her about them.
- Ask your patient's friends to visit and talk or read to her.
- Consider posting a sign over the patient's bed reminding all personnel that your patient, even though comatose, can hear what's said. Include a reminder to explain all procedures.

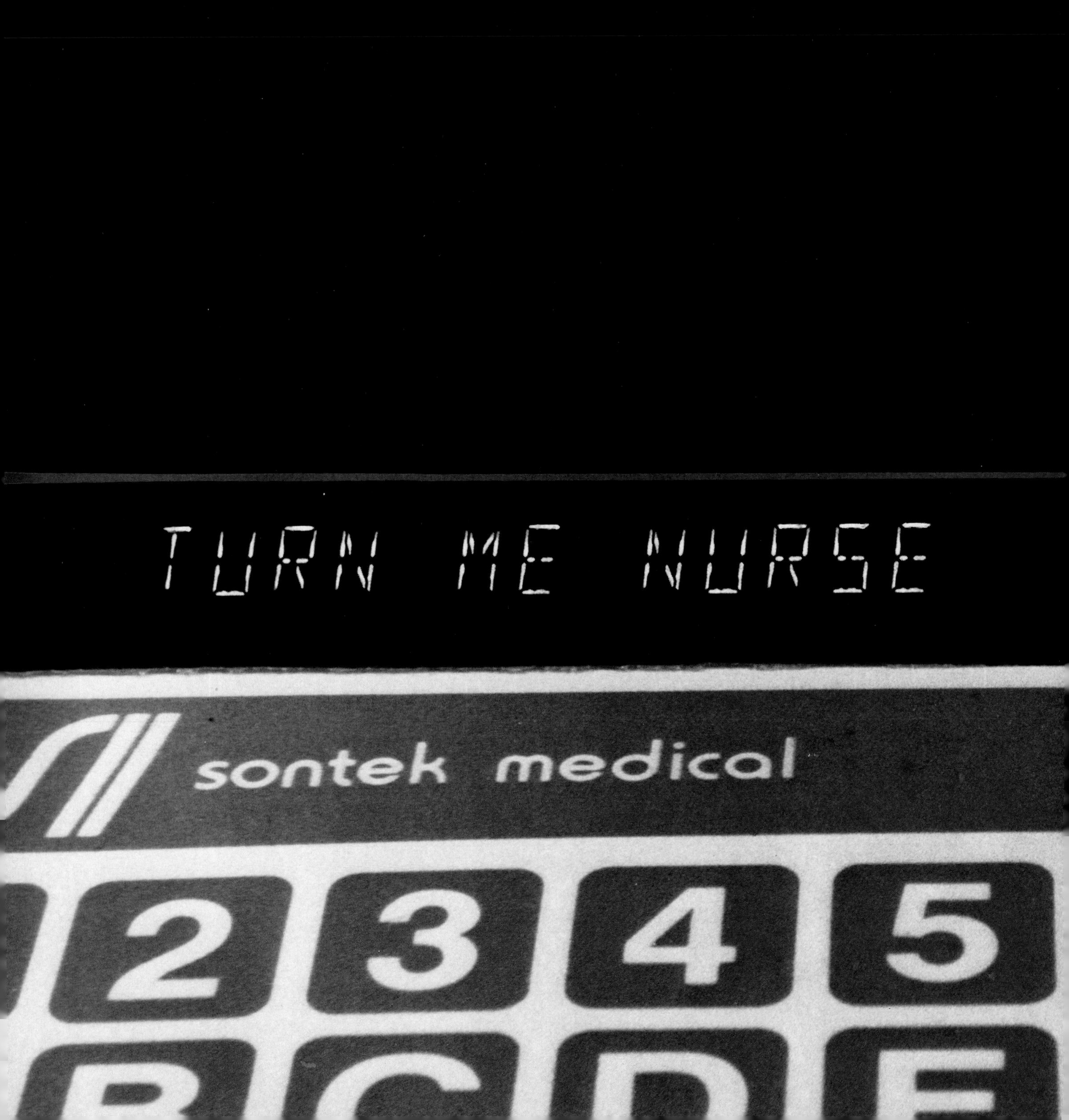

TURN ME NURSE

sontek medical

2 3 4 5

Meeting Special Challenges

Communication problems

Braces and prostheses

Alternate pain control

Postmortem care

Organ donation

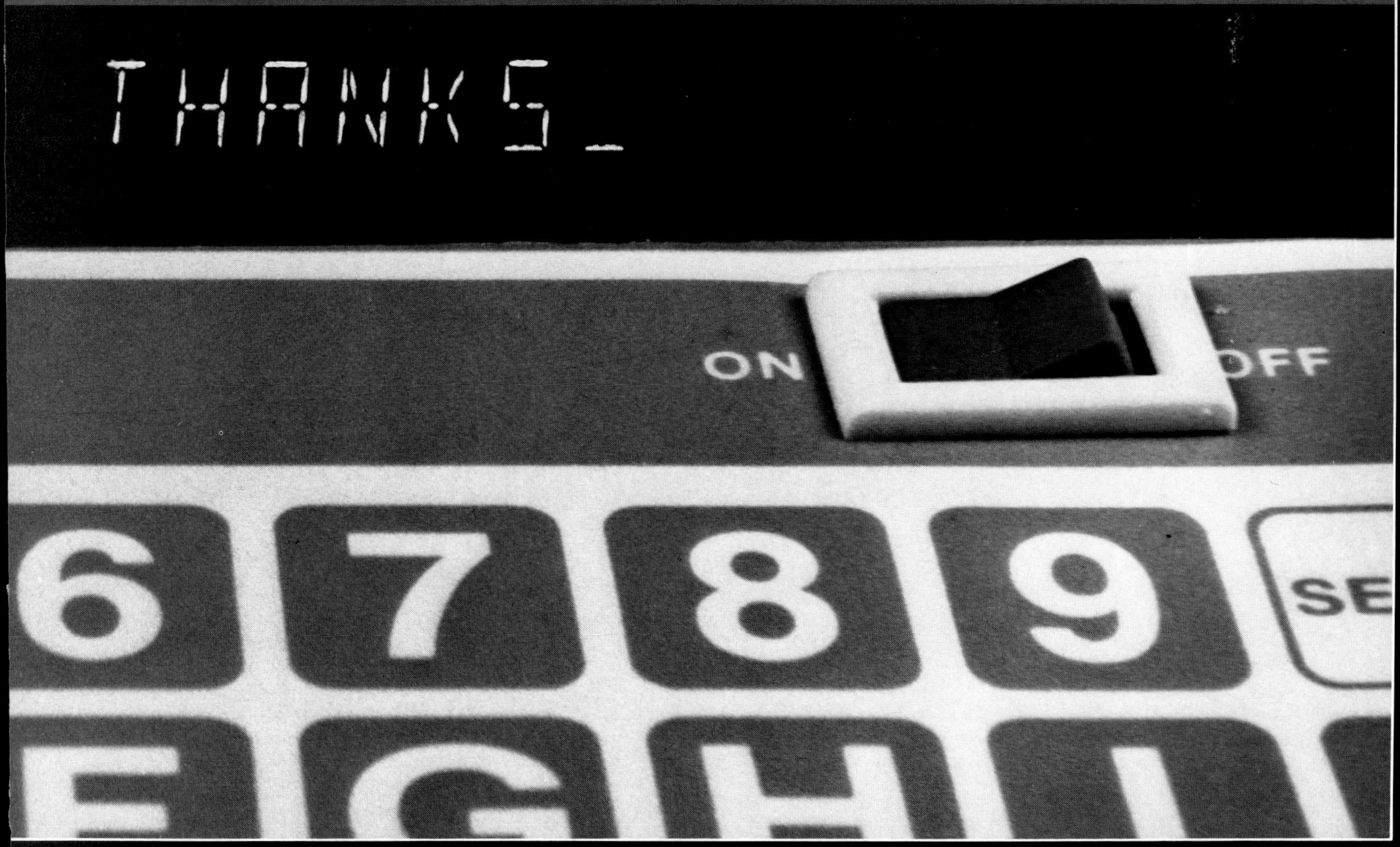

THANKS_

ON OFF

6 7 8 9 SE

F G H I

Communication problems

As you know, understanding what your patient wants to communicate isn't always easy. For instance, he may not speak English. Or perhaps he can't speak because of trauma; for example, from a paralyzing accident or such a disease as amyotrophic lateral sclerosis.

Regardless of the cause, coping with a communication problem is your responsibility. On these pages we give you valuable insights into techniques for meeting this special challenge. Read the material carefully.

Coping with communication problems

Sooner or later you'll probably care for a patient who has a problem communicating. And if you do, will you be prepared to make the necessary provisions to cope with the problem? To learn how to manage these communication challenges, study the case histories below.

The patient who can't speak

Harry Robins, a 58-year-old maintenance foreman, has cancer of the trachea. During the past 2 years, Mr. Robins' condition has been deteriorating. Now, Mr. Robins is in the terminal stage. Because he has a tracheostomy and is breathing with the assistance of a ventilator, he can only mouth a few words. Although you understand most of Mr. Robins' communication by reading his lips, you aren't always accurate.

What can you do? Gently remind your patient to speak slowly and to use phrases instead of complete sentences. If you rush him, he may become frustrated and silent. Always give Mr. Robins a chance to complete his message, instead of trying to finish his thoughts for him.

Wondering how to ensure communication accuracy? Have your patient write his message on paper. Not only does this method improve communication, but it also saves time. Provide Mr. Robins with the supplies he'll need, such as pen, paper, clipboard (or other firm writing surface), and a trash can (for note disposal).

An alternative to the pen-and-paper method is a Magic Slate (shown at right). This handy communication tool provides a hard writing surface, erases with a lift of the acetate coversheet, and responds to the lightest touch of the small writing stick.

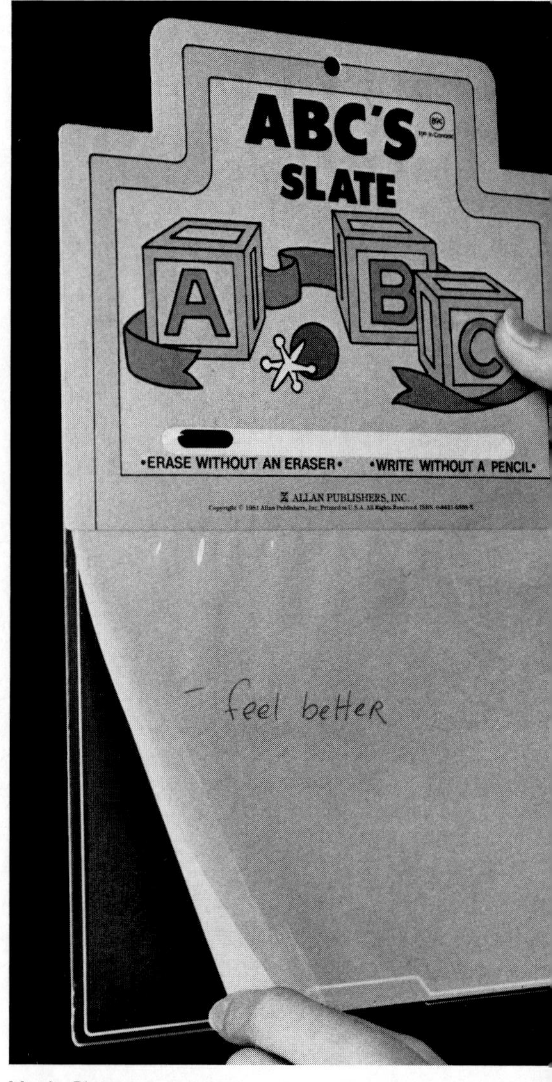

Magic Slate

The patient who speaks only a foreign language

Hester Ramirez has been admitted to your unit after a total abdominal hysterectomy 2 days ago. She appears withdrawn, frightened, and in pain. When you approach her, you realize she speaks only Spanish. How can you communicate with her?

Perhaps Ms. Ramirez has a friend or family member who is bilingual. Or maybe a co-worker can act as an interpreter. If you work in a large hospital, the social service department can probably provide a list of volunteers and employees who can act as interpreters.

While you're trying to locate an interpreter, attempt to communicate with Ms. Ramirez through simple gestures. But remember, Ms. Ramirez is frightened and in pain. In a strange environment, she may be self-conscious about using gestures.

Suppose you're caring for several patients who—like Ms. Ramirez—don't speak English. Consider starting a flash card collection to improve communication. To do this, print the word or concept you're trying to convey (in the patient's language) on one side of a sturdy piece of paper, such as cardboard. On the card's other side, print the English translation and the phonetic pronunciation of the word. Keep the concept brief and concise; this way your patient can answer *yes* or *no*. As soon as the patient understands the flash card system, try putting several phrases together to form more complete thoughts.

Nursing tip: If the patient can't read, select a magazine or newspaper picture that indicates the thought you wish to convey, attach it to the card, and print the phonetic pronunciation next to it.

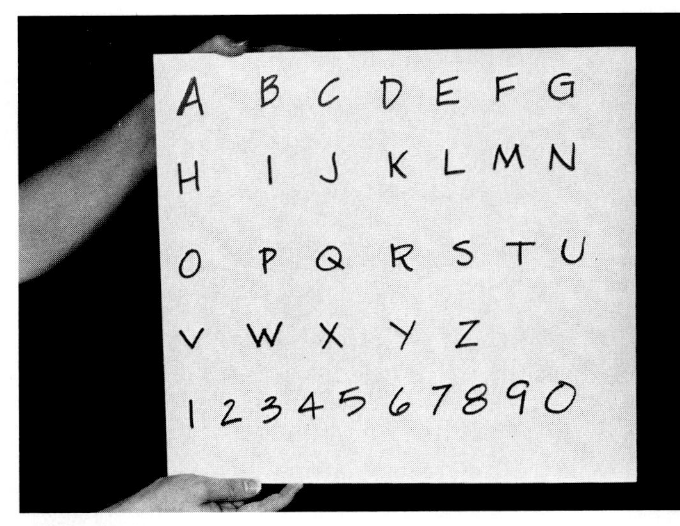

Letter-number board

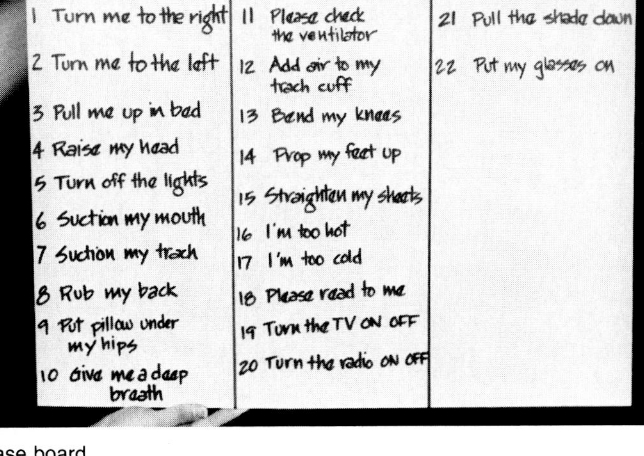

Phrase board

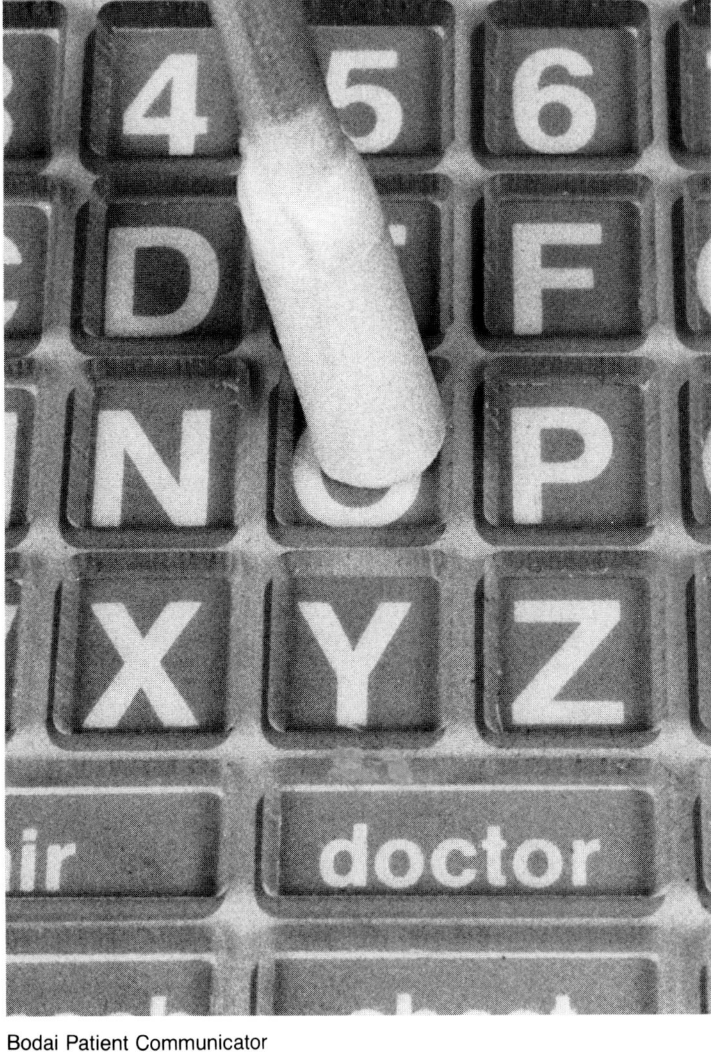

Bodai Patient Communicator

The patient who can't speak or move
Sixty-two-year-old Mark Chun has had amyotrophic lateral sclerosis for the last 3 years. Day by day, the disease has impaired more and more of Mr. Chun's body functions. Because of increasing facial weakness, he can only blink. Mr. Chun blinks once to say *hello* and once to answer *yes* to a yes-or-no question. Of course, you have to be an alert observer not to confuse a yes blink with a normal eye-lubricating blink. Although this system usually works O.K., it still is inadequate because of the many thoughts Mr. Chun can't express with a simple yes or no.

To help you and your patient improve communications, consider designing a letter-number board. Be sure to list on the board the letters in the alphabet, arranged in four rows, and numbers one through nine and zero (see top photo at left). Also design a phrase board, including the patient's most common communications, such as *suction my mouth* and *rub my back*. Number each phrase, and combine them in lists of 10 phrases per column (see bottom photo at left). Mr. Chun can indicate which board he wants to use by staring at the appropriate board. If he indicates the letter-number board, start by asking him if he wants the first, second, third, or fourth row. Then, say each letter in the row until he blinks yes. Suppose he indicates the phrase board. Point to each column, until he indicates which one he wishes. Then, count down from the top of the column until he blinks yes for a number. Compare the number with the phrase.

Consider for a moment the case of 45-year-old Bill Johnson. As the result of an automobile accident, Mr. Johnson is paralyzed from level C2. He's in a Stryker frame and needs a mechanical ventilator to breathe. Although you can read his lips when he's lying on his back, you can't even see his face when you turn him over. How do you communicate with Mr. Johnson?

The Bodai Patient Communicator, by Sontek Medical Inc., can make the task easier for both you and your patient. By using a straw or stick, your patient can press the appropriate letter or number on the Communicator's keyboard (see photo directly above) to form words on a two-sided display panel. Preprogrammed buttons at the screen's base enable the patient to convey frequently communicated phrases without spelling them out letter by letter. For more details on operating the Communicator, read the following photostory.

Communication problems

How to use a Bodai Patient Communicator

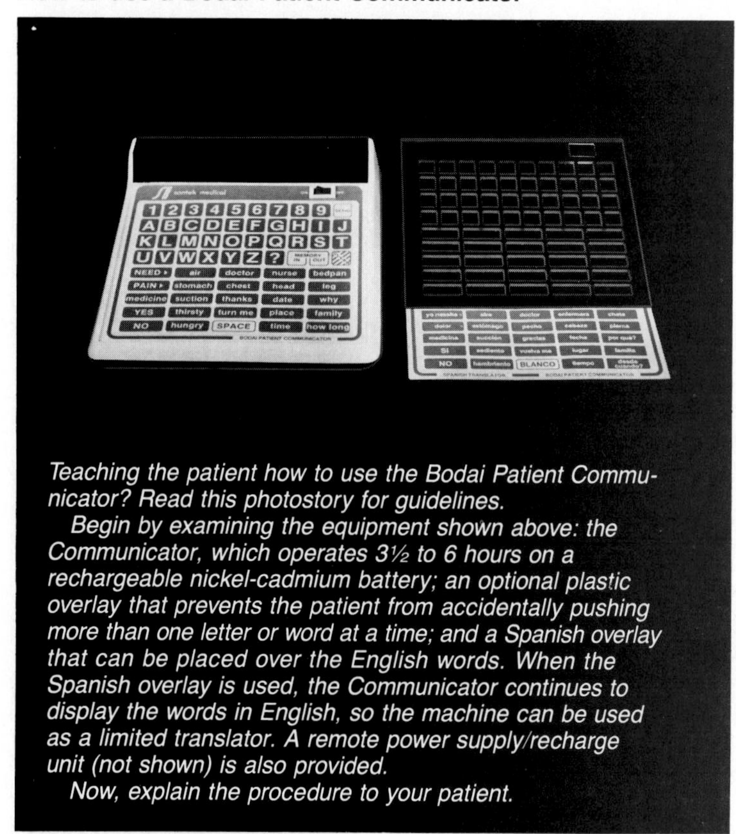

Teaching the patient how to use the Bodai Patient Communicator? Read this photostory for guidelines.

Begin by examining the equipment shown above: the Communicator, which operates 3½ to 6 hours on a rechargeable nickel-cadmium battery; an optional plastic overlay that prevents the patient from accidentally pushing more than one letter or word at a time; and a Spanish overlay that can be placed over the English words. When the Spanish overlay is used, the Communicator continues to display the words in English, so the machine can be used as a limited translator. A remote power supply/recharge unit (not shown) is also provided.

Now, explain the procedure to your patient.

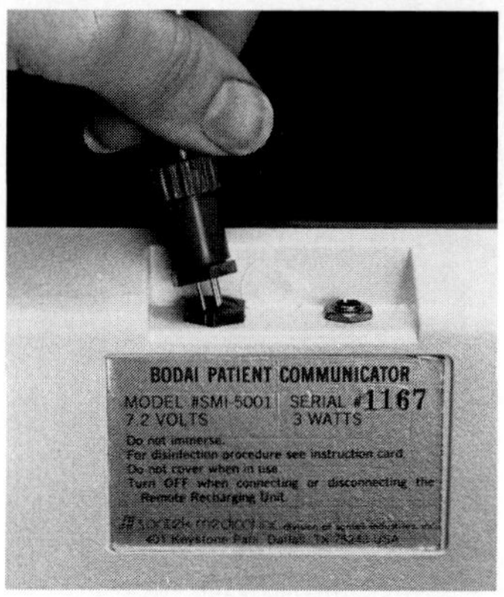

1 Next, check to be sure the remote power supply and Communicator switches are OFF. Plug one end of the remote power supply cord into a wall outlet. Plug the cord's other end into the unit, as shown. Press the remote power supply switch to ON and press the Communicator's power switch to ON. You'll see a horizontal cursor bar at the display panel's far left. The cursor indicates where the next letter or word will appear.

2 Instruct your patient to lightly press the key corresponding to the word, letter, or number he wishes to communicate. When he does, the Communicator will beep softly to confirm key depression.

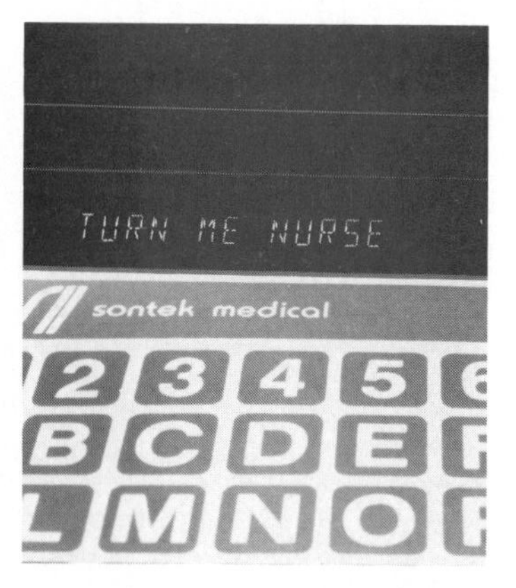

3 As you can see in this photo, the patient has written, *TURN* (space) *ME* (space) *NURSE*. The dual display panel enables you to read the patient's message as he composes it, without looking over his shoulder.

Note: Tell your patient that he doesn't have to press the space key for preprogrammed phrases.

4 Explain to your patient that the three keys at the base of the whole-word column are reprogrammable. To reprogram a word, have your patient slide the program switch, located under the unit, to the right.

Then, have him press the key he wishes to reprogram. Tell him to input the new word or thought in 10 characters or less. If he makes a mistake, instruct him to slide the program switch to the left and start again.

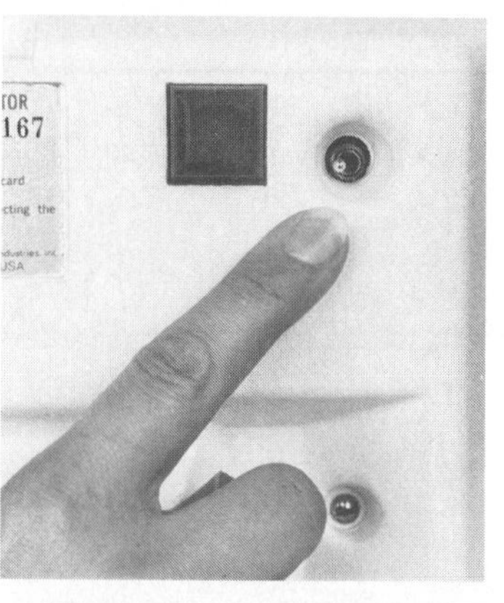

5 Does your patient want to change the newly programmed words back to the original ones? Have him switch the long-term storage button to OFF, wait 30 seconds, and then turn the button to ON. If he does everything correctly, the original words should appear.

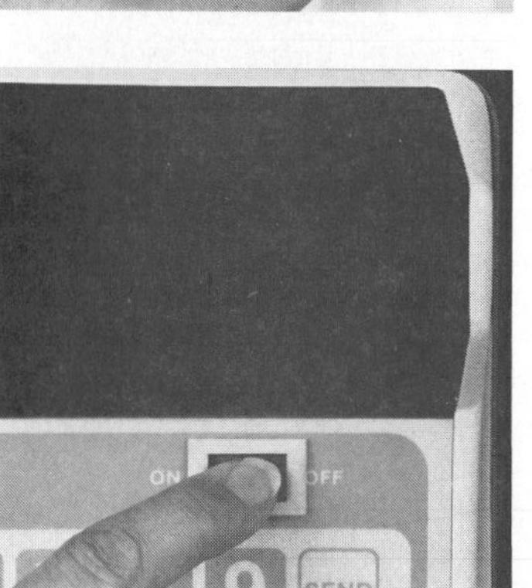

6 After each day's use, turn the Communicator's power switch to OFF, as shown here.

Important: For more detailed operating information, read the manufacturer's instructions.

Braces and prostheses

Caring for a patient with a brace or limb prosthesis? If you are, you need to know how to apply, remove, and care for his mobility aid.

Read this section for guidance. In it, you'll learn:
- why the doctor may order a leg brace for your patient.
- how to identify the four parts of an arm prosthesis.
- how baby powder can help you assess the fit of an above-the-knee prosthesis.

In addition, you'll find information on caring for a patient's stump. Review these pages carefully.

Learning about braces

You can see that 78-year-old Anton Jacoby is upset. And you can understand why. About 2 years ago he suffered a cerebrovascular accident that caused left-sided hemiplegia and aphasia. Now he's been admitted to your unit with a urinary tract infection.

Because you've already read the initial report on Mr. Jacoby, you know the doctor wants him to walk three times a day. You also know Mr. Jacoby wears a brace on his left leg. But do you know which type of brace he wears? Or how to help him apply and remove it properly?

The following information will refresh your memory of braces so you know how to help a patient like Mr. Jacoby.

Brace basics

As you know, a brace supports, aligns, or holds a body part in correct position. Specifically, a patient may wear a brace to:
- protect weak muscles
- prevent or correct a deformity
- control involuntary movement
- protect a diseased or injured joint
- support body weight.

Brace models are available in two general classifications.
- *Below-the-knee brace.* Designed to support the ankle joint, this type of brace consists of two upright bars positioned bilaterally on either side of the leg. Each bar is secured at the upper end by a calf strap. The bars' lower ends are attached to a stirrup, which, in turn, connects to a metal or plastic shoe insert or to a metal plate that attaches to the shoe's sole. A mechanical ankle joint is positioned between the upright bars and the stirrup, at the normal ankle joint. The joint moves harmoniously with the patient's normal ankle joint.
- *Above-the-knee (or long leg) brace.* As you can see in the illustration at right, this brace consists of two bilateral upright bars; one end of each bar is attached to a sturdy shoe and the other ends are secured to the patient's calf with a calf strap. A mechanical ankle joint is positioned between the bars and the shoe, at the normal ankle joint. The mechanical knee joint fits next to the normal knee joint and connects to two bilateral thigh bars, which, in turn, are secured to the patient's leg with a thigh strap.

Although the mechanical knee joint assists in knee flexion, it doesn't precisely imitate normal knee movement. Why? A normal knee joint has a changing axis of rotation; a mechanical knee joint is fixed. As a result, the brace shifts—to some degree—during the flexion and extension of the knee joint.

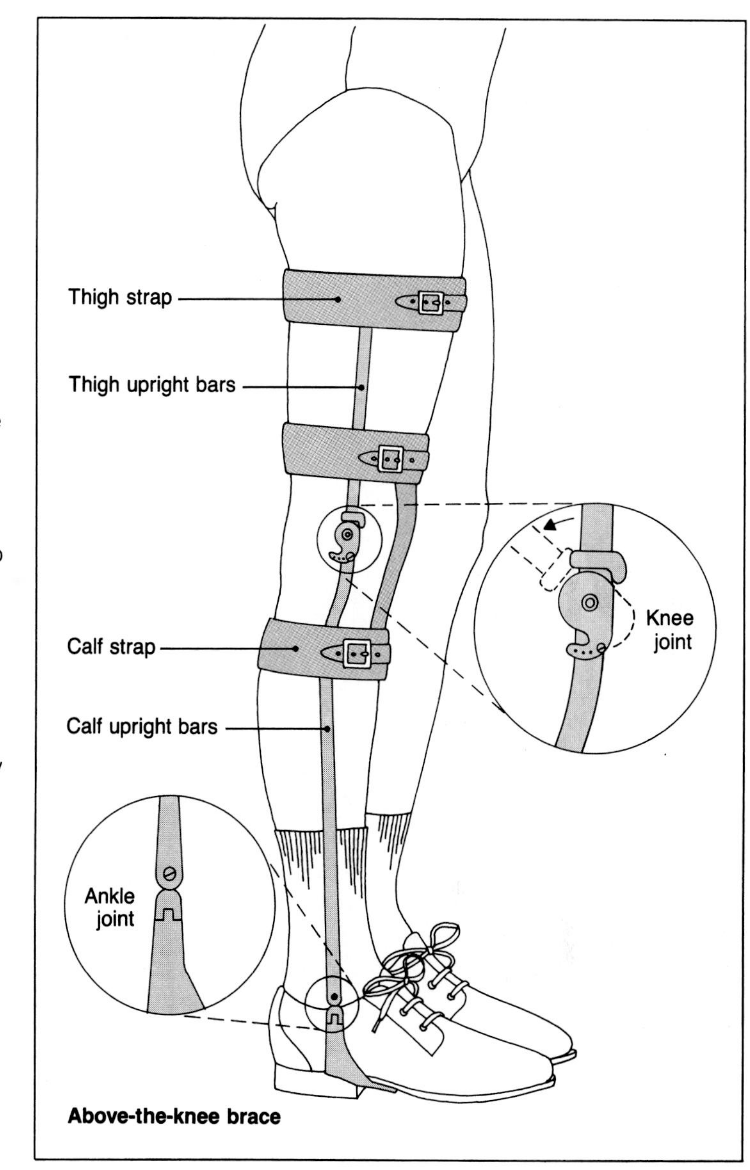

Above-the-knee brace

Understanding knee locks

A knee lock controls knee flexion. Four types are available.
- *Drop ring:* drops into place manually or by gravity when the knee is fully extended
- *Spring-loaded pull rings:* attach to a drop ring for manual positioning without necessitating the patient's bending over
- *Plunger lock or spring-loaded pull rod:* locks manually when the leg is extended
- *Cam lock:* uses a lever to simultaneously lock or unlock both sides of the knee.

To learn how to help a patient apply a below-the-knee brace, read the following photostory.

Braces and prostheses

How to apply a below-the-knee brace

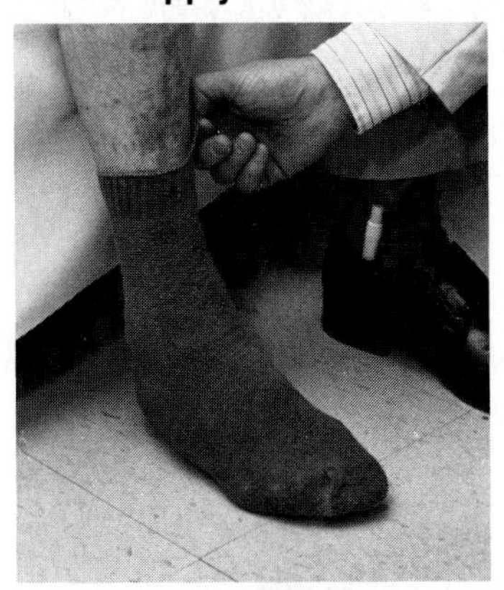

1 Caring for a patient with a below-the-knee brace? He'll need to apply the brace every time he walks. Make sure you can help him, if necessary, by reviewing these steps.

First, help him to a sitting position at the edge of the bed. Next, check the affected leg and foot to be sure they are clean and dry. Then, inspect his brace and shoe for signs of unusual wear.

Put clean socks on his feet, as the nurse is doing here.

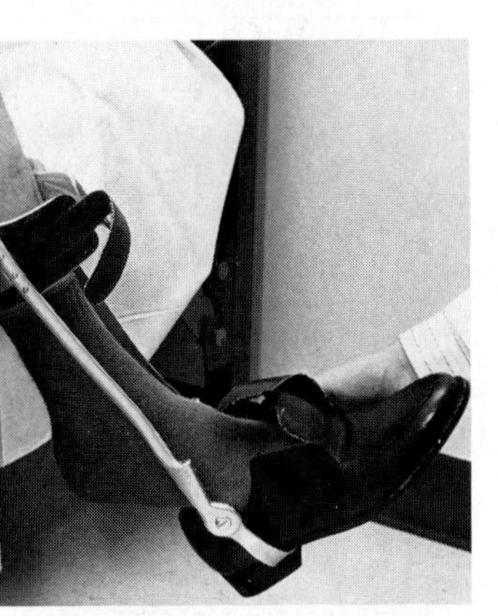

2 Unbuckle the brace's leather cuff and open the calf band. Have the patient cross his affected leg over his other leg. Doing so makes applying the brace easier. Position the brace under the patient's affected leg so the bilateral bars are at either side of his leg. Then, insert his foot into the brace's shoe.

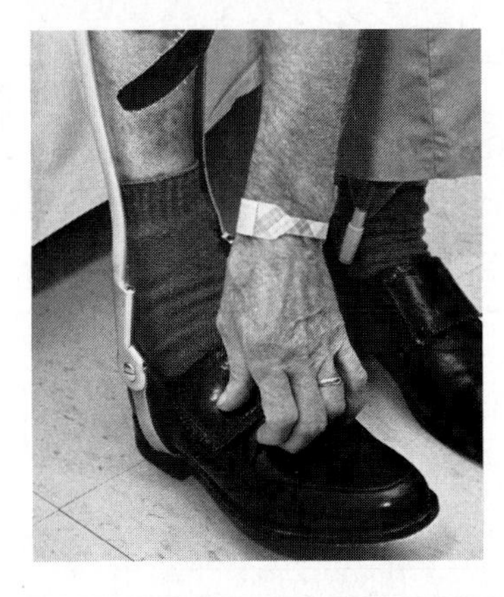

3 Now, have your patient uncross his leg and place the shoe flat on the floor. Adjust the strap on the shoe so the shoe fits snugly, as the patient is doing here.

Remember: Encourage your patient to do as much as possible for himself.

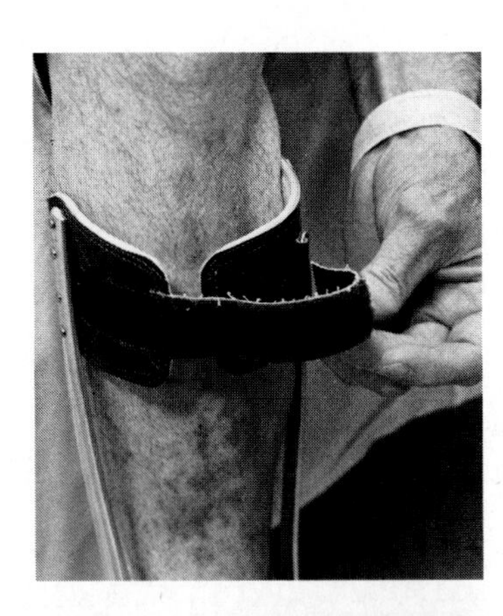

4 Next, ask the patient to adjust the leather cuff to his calf size.

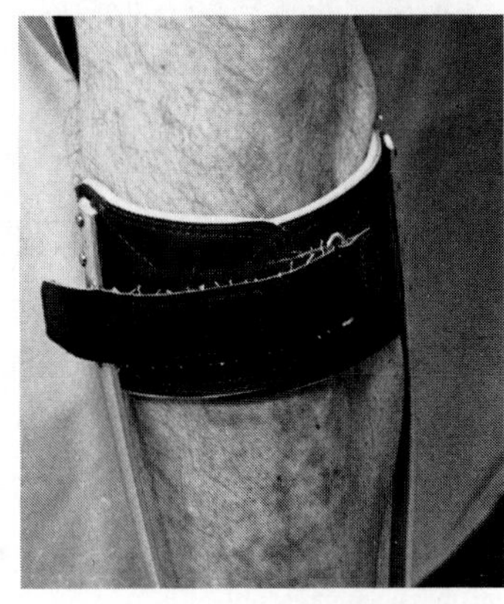

5 Be sure the band's snug but not too tight and that the metal bars aren't touching the patient's calf.

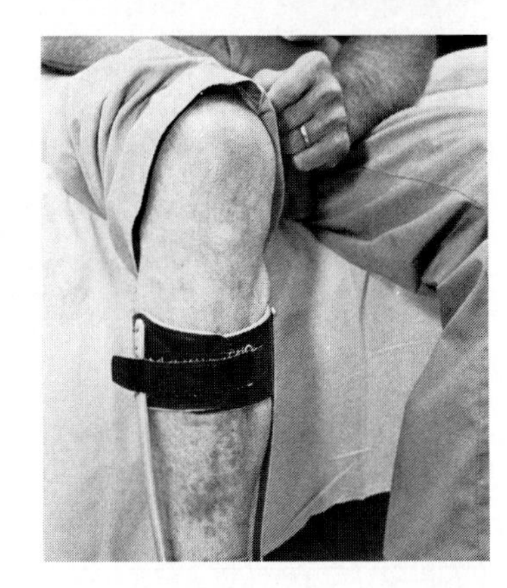

6 Now, help him adjust his pant leg over the brace and assist him to standing position for walking.

Applying an above-the-knee brace

Forty-nine-year-old Stella Fink wears an above-the-knee brace on her left leg as a result of an injury. Now, she's recovering from a partial colectomy. Her overall condition is such that she can walk on her own. You want to assist her.

To do this, help with the brace application, as follows:

- Place your patient in a supine position.
- Inspect the affected leg and foot to be sure they are clean and dry. Also, inspect the brace and shoe for signs of wear or damage. Expect the brace's metal calf and thigh bands to be free of rough edges, the leather cuffs to be clean and smooth, and the mechanical ankle and knee joints to align with her anatomic joints.
- Help your patient put clean socks on her feet.
- Unbuckle the straps on the calf and thigh bands, and open the bands and knee pad.
- Place the brace under the affected leg, so the bilateral upright bars extend up either side of the leg.
- Insert her foot in the shoe.
- Close and adjust the leather straps securely around her leg. Now, close the knee pad, and manually lock the knee joint so her leg's straight. Doing so keeps the mechanical knee rigid, so your patient can easily swing her leg and the brace over the bed's edge. Unlock the knee joint when she's ready to walk.

Reviewing prosthesis types

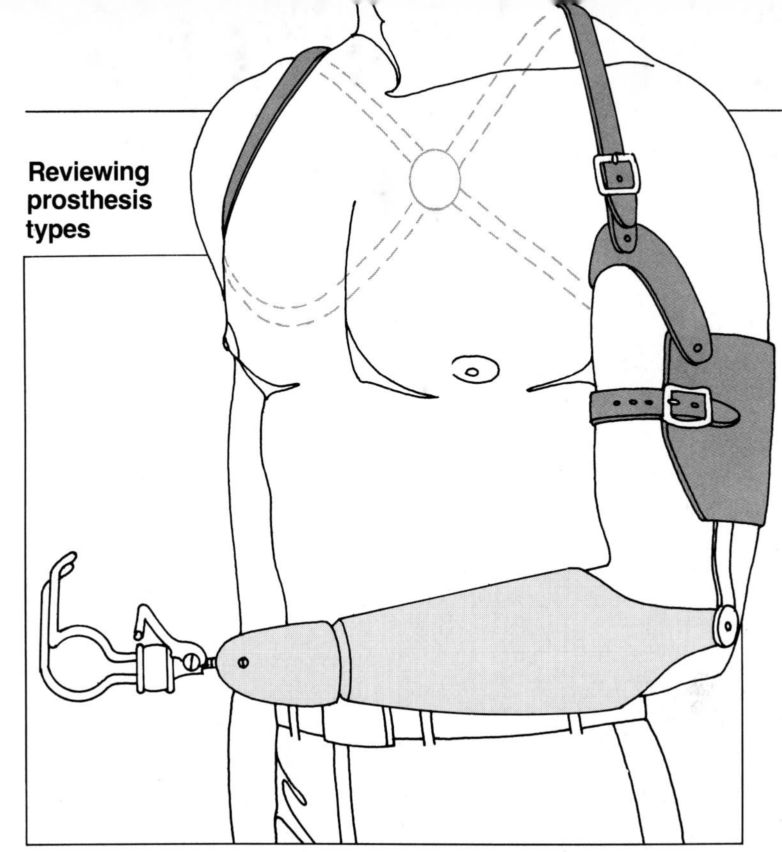

Whenever you care for a patient with a prosthesis, be prepared to help him apply, remove, and care for his mobility aid, if necessary. To ensure your patient's comfort and safety while you perform these tasks, familiarize yourself with the prosthesis types and models detailed below.

Arm prosthesis

As you can see in this illustration, an arm prosthesis consists of four basic parts:

- terminal appliance, such as a hook (more versatile than an artificial hand), a hand, a cosmetically covered hook, or a double hook
- arm component (size depends on the level of amputation)
- socket (depression in the prosthesis into which the stump fits)
- harness (secures the prosthesis to patient's upper body).

A patient with a below-the-elbow amputation or a wrist disarticulation powers the prosthesis by way of a Bowden cable, which is stimulated by bicep muscle movement or pronation of the forearm. But suppose your patient has had an above-the-elbow amputation or a shoulder disarticulation. In either case, his prosthesis has a shoulder lock that can be engaged or disengaged manually or with shoulder movement against the prosthesis. Control of the terminal device on this prosthesis is achieved by shoulder or forearm movement.

Leg prosthesis

Whenever we refer to a leg prosthesis, we're speaking about one of two types: above the knee or below the knee. Specific models depend on the level of amputation.

- *Ankle disarticulation.* Prosthesis slides on the base of patient's leg like a boot and can be secured to the leg with laces, straps, or a suction socket.
- *Below-the-knee amputation.* Prosthesis has a foot and lower-leg component, as well as a socket and thigh corset.
- *Knee disarticulation.* Prosthesis has a suction socket that joins the lower-leg component and stump.
- *Above-the-knee amputation.* Prosthesis has a foot and lower-leg component, a manual locking or variable friction knee, an upper-leg component with a socket, and a suspension belt that fits around the lower trunk.
- *Hip disarticulation and hemipelvectomy.* Prosthesis has a foot and leg component with a knee lock, upper-leg component, hip lock (not on all models), and a molded bucket to fit pelvic girdle and suspend ischial tuberosity.

Stump care: Some guidelines

You know one of your nursing responsibilities is to help your patient put on his prosthesis. But your responsibilities don't end there. You also need to help your patient care for his prosthesis and stump. Doing so promotes patient comfort and prevents complications.

Here are some guidelines to keep in mind:

- Unless contraindicated, try to get your patient out of bed and walking within 48 hours, regardless of why he was admitted to your unit.
- Once each day, check your patient's stump for signs of skin breakdown, such as swelling or redness, especially around the incision site. (Don't neglect this step, even if the incision is healed.)
- Cleanse the stump daily, using warm water and a mild soap. Rinse the area and dry thoroughly.
- Encourage your patient to do as much as possible for himself and praise him for his efforts.
- To ensure proper prosthesis fit, don't apply alcohol, oil, or body lotion to your patient's stump.
- When you remove your patient's prosthesis, use a damp cloth to wipe out its inside. Thoroughly dry the dampened area with a towel. *Important:* Never immerse the prosthesis in water, because water will cause the prosthesis' leather and joints to deteriorate.
- When your patient's not wearing his prosthesis, wrap his stump in an elastic bandage to prevent swelling. If your patient's stump begins to swell, elevate it above heart level for several hours.
- Don't shave your patient's stump. Doing so may cause skin irritation, a rash, or infection.
- Wash stump socks daily in warm water and a nondetergent soap. Squeeze out excess water and lay socks flat on a towel to dry.

Nursing tip: For faster drying, punch holes in a plastic bottle, and place the sock over it.

- Regularly assess your patient for weight gain or loss. Remember, weight changes affect how the prosthesis fits. If necessary, temporarily improve the fit by changing the number of socks he wears between the prosthesis and his stump. But remember that, in time, a prosthesis that fits poorly causes irritation and pressure sores. Encourage the patient and his family to contact a prosthetist for adjustments.

Applying an arm prosthesis: Learning the basics

Although applying an arm prosthesis may be difficult at first, with a little practice, you can become skilled at it. To begin, check that your patient's stump and the prosthesis socket are clean and dry. Inspect his stump for signs of skin irritation, such as swelling and redness. Then, make sure he's wearing an undershirt, to prevent irritation from the harness rubbing against his skin.

Now you're ready to slide the sock onto your patient's stump. If he has a shoulder disarticulation, have him wear a clean, dry undershirt with sleeves to cover the area, instead of a stump sock. Then, carefully slip the stump into the prosthesis socket, and buckle the biceps cuff. Now, extend the unbuckled figure-eight strap diagonally across your patient's back, under his arm, and to the center of his chest. Secure the buckle.

To remove the prosthesis, reverse these steps.

Braces and prostheses

How to apply an above-the-knee prosthesis

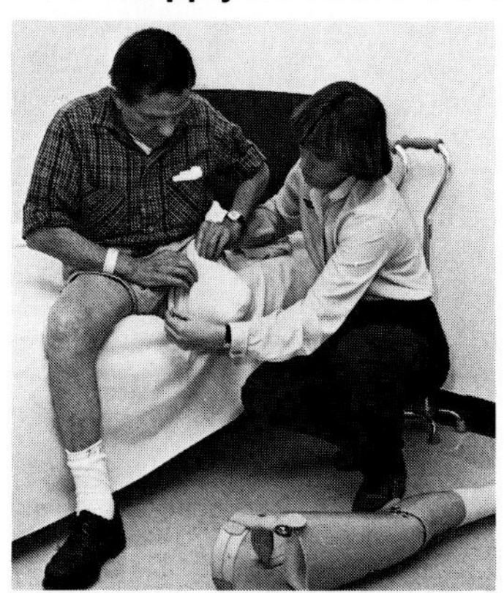

1 Several years ago, Sam Posen had his left leg amputated because of diabetic complications. Today he's recovering from surgery to remove a skin lesion. The doctor asks you to help Mr. Posen walk three times a day.

Begin by making sure the prosthesis socket and stump socks are clean and dry and that his stump's not irritated. Have Mr. Posen sit at the bed's edge and apply his two stump socks.

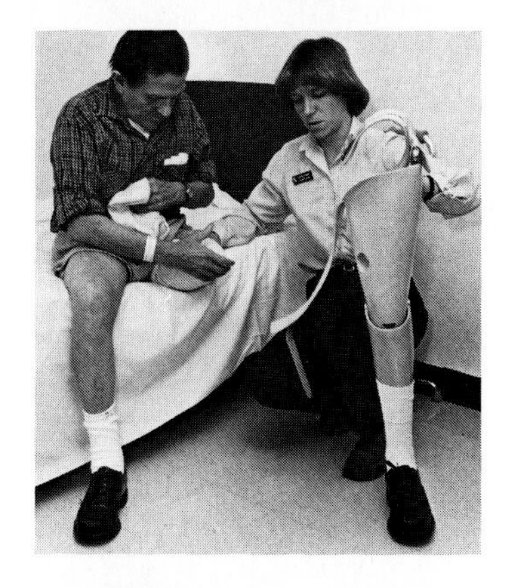

2 Make sure the socks fit properly; smooth out any wrinkles.

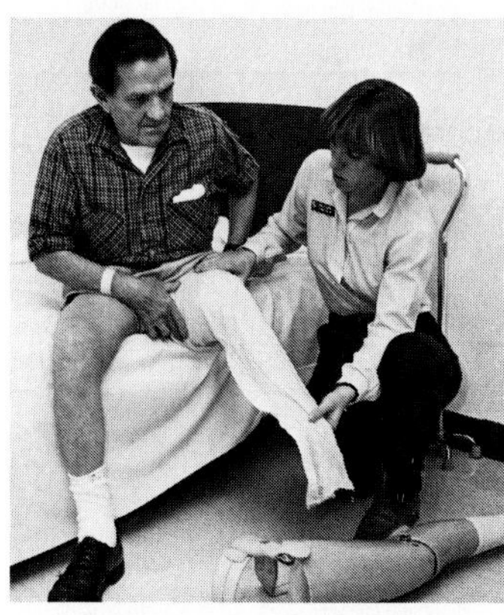

3 Now, apply stockinette over the stump socks. This additional sock will help position the stump deep into the prosthesis' socket.

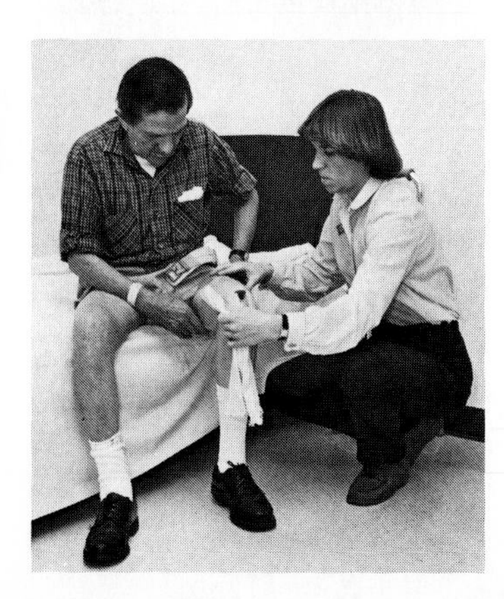

4 Help Mr. Posen push the prosthesis onto the stump. Pull the stockinette's free end through the valve hole on the prosthesis' medial aspect, as the nurse has done here.

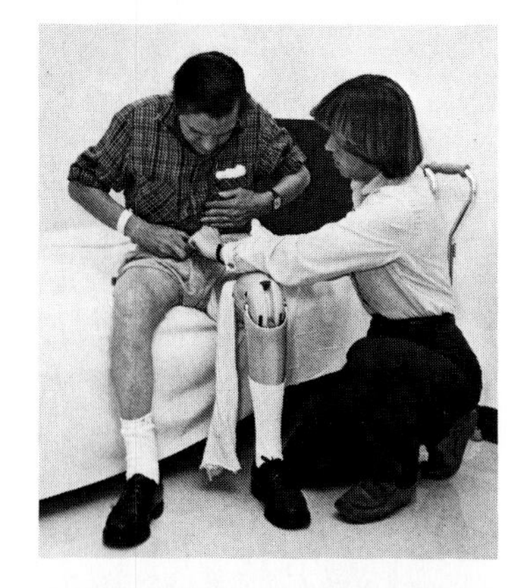

5 Put the suspension belt around Mr. Posen's waist, and help him tighten the belt, as shown.

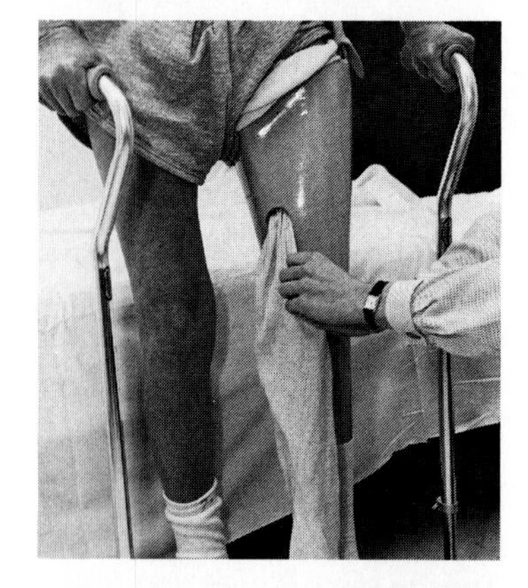

6 Help Mr. Posen stand. Now, pull down the stockinette. As you do, you'll pull the stump deeper into the socket. Continue pulling until the stockinette comes off the stump.

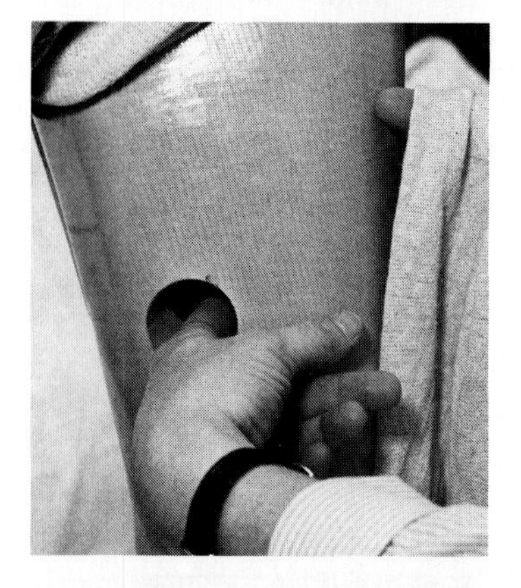

7 To confirm proper fit, insert your finger into the valve hole and note the stump's position. If your patient has a prosthesis without a valve hole, confirm proper fit in this manner: First, dust the socket with baby powder. Next, help your patient put on the prosthesis and take a short walk. Then, remove the prosthesis without disturbing the sock. If the sock's nearly covered with powder, the stump's in total contact with the socket.

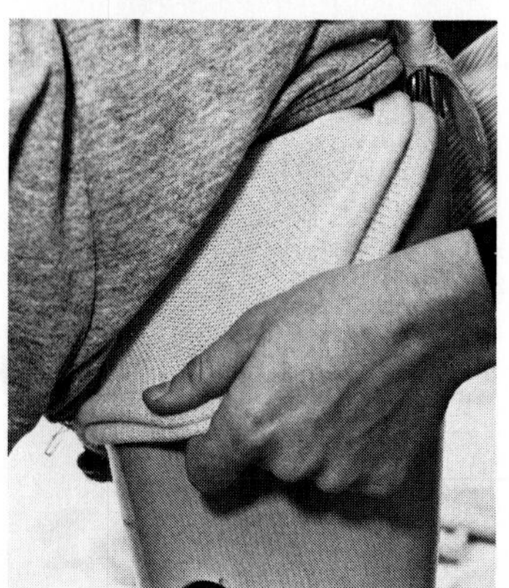

8 Finally, pull the tops of the stump socks down over the prosthesis. Doing so eliminates wrinkles from stockinette removal.

Alternate pain control

Several days have passed since Elsie Granger, a 35-year-old legal secretary, was admitted to your unit for diagnostic testing. Today, the doctor has confirmed that she has a tumor on her stomach wall.

Ms. Granger says she is relieved that the testing is over, but you're less so, because you know she'll have to cope with the pain and anxiety of complex treatment. You can help her deal with the possibility of surgery, as well as a prolonged recovery period, by using alternate pain-control techniques.

To refresh your memory of the growing field of alternate pain control, on the next few pages we review:

- how to use conscious suggestion effectively.
- when a patient may benefit from hypnosis.
- which pain-control methods necessitate special training.
- advantages and disadvantages of alternate pain-control methods.

Read this information carefully.

Learning about alternate pain control

Yesterday Elsie Granger appeared to take the doctor's news about her condition matter-of-factly, but today is a different story. When you enter Ms. Granger's room to help with morning care, you find her extremely anxious, and when you question her, she admits she has abdominal pain.

Of course, you want to help her relax and to relieve the pain she's experiencing. But don't reach for a sedative or narcotic; consider some form of nonnarcotic pain relief. Which form is appropriate for your patient?

Begin by assessing Ms. Granger's pain and anxiety level. The following guidelines will aid your assessment.

- Consider your patient's condition. Different types of conditions cause different types of pain.

After a hysterectomy, for example, your patient may experience incisional or abdominal pain, as well as a feeling of loss. Take care not to let your preconception of her condition affect your assessment. Listen to her comments. Remember, she's the one experiencing pain and anxiety.

- Observe your patient for physical and psychological signs that may indicate pain, such as restlessness, irritability, wincing, grimacing, and body stiffening. Be alert for telltale changes in vital signs, such as an increase in heart rate, blood pressure, and respiratory rate. Also watch for pupillary dilation, skin color and temperature changes, and diaphoresis.
- If your patient's alert, ask her to describe the quality of her pain; for example, is it keeping her awake?
- Ask her if she has any feelings associated with the pain or anxiety; for example, does she become depressed?

As you talk with Ms. Granger about her feelings, keep in mind that, in most cases, a person in pain or distress wants to feel more relaxed. Create a relaxing atmosphere by encouraging her to turn frequently, attending to her personal needs, giving her back rubs, and spending time with her. Then, explain to Ms. Granger the relationship between relaxation and pain relief. Emphasize that when the body relaxes, it releases a natural, narcoticlike painkiller (endorphin), which'll help make her more comfortable. (For more information on relaxation and pain relief, see the chart on the next two pages.)

SPECIAL CONSIDERATIONS

Hypnosis: Fact and fiction

Although almost everyone's seen hypnotic trances depicted on television and in the movies, few persons have had firsthand experience with this effective pain-control method. If you're like most people, you could use some help sorting out fact from fiction. Read the following to learn some basic points.

Fiction
Only a few, highly susceptible people are good subjects for hypnosis.
Fact
A skilled hypnotist can lead almost any consenting individual of normal intelligence into a hypnotic state. A patient who is psychotic or has limited intelligence may be difficult or impossible to hypnotize.

Fiction
Hypnosis is a party trick that has little or no therapeutic value.
Fact
Hypnosis has been used successfully to control or eliminate pain in the emergency department, at accident scenes, and during major surgery. In dental surgery, hypnosis can be used to control bleeding as well as pain. In high-risk patients and during childbirth, it's also employed as an anesthetic.

Fiction
Hypnosis puts a person to sleep.
Fact
Hypnosis is a state of extreme concentration that minimizes most distractions.

Fiction
A person in a hypnotic state behaves unpredictably.
Fact
Except under extraordinary circumstances, a person who's hypnotized won't do anything against his conscious morals. If hypnosis is administered inappropriately, a person who's prepsychotic may gain insight into a problem he can't cope with and enter a psychotic state.

Fiction
A person must be coached into a hypnotic state.
Fact
With practice, a person can put himself into a hypnotic state (autohypnosis).

Fiction
Hypnosis can cure a disease or help a person solve a problem.
Fact
Hypnosis can't cure a disease. It may alter a patient's perception of a problem or pain but not the problem or pain itself.

Alternate pain control

Nurses' guide to alternate pain-control methods

Relaxation

How to perform
Use the power of suggestion to distract the patient's attention from his pain, reduce his anxiety level, and give him a sense of control over pain. Controlled breathing's the most common technique.

Indication
- Chronic pain or short-term pain, such as during childbirth

Advantages
- Reduces anxiety, muscle tension, pain, and fatigue
- May enhance analgesic effects

Disadvantage
- Doesn't completely relax skeletal and smooth muscles

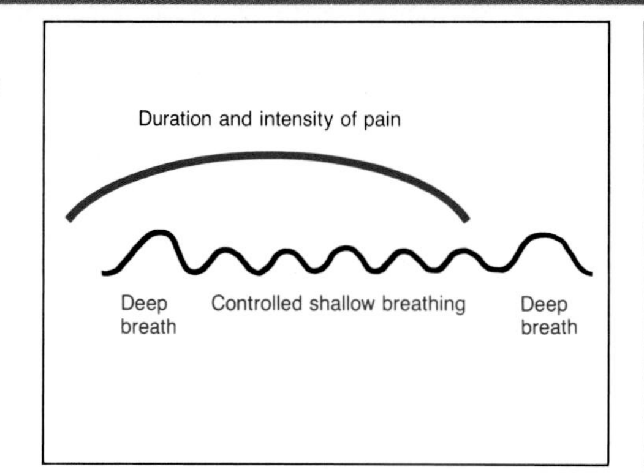

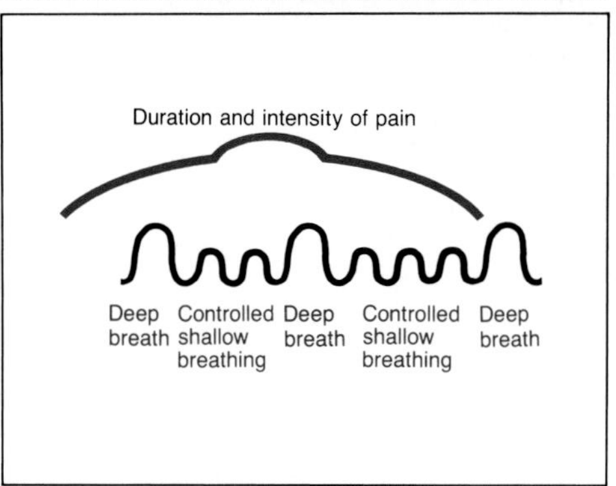

Cutaneous stimulation

How to perform
Directly stimulate the patient's skin by applying fingertip pressure (effleurage), cold or warm packs, or menthol ointments over the affected area or at the same site on the opposite side of the body (contralateral stimulation).

Indications
- Intense, chronic pain
- Short-term pain, such as during childbirth

Advantages
- Doesn't necessitate patient training
- Can be performed by patient without assistance

Disadvantages
- May require a doctor's order
- Applying menthol ointment to a patient's incision may cause itching and lead to burning and excoriation.

Distraction

How to perform
Divert the patient's attention from his pain by asking him to relate an interesting or pleasant experience or by having him listen to a favorite musical tape, sing, or practice rhythmic breathing.

Indication
- Acute, episodic pain

Advantages
- Doesn't necessitate patient conditioning
- Can be learned quickly

Disadvantage
- Doesn't relieve chronic pain

Guided imagery

How to perform
Have patient relax as much as possible. Then, ask him to describe his pain. For example, he may say, "I feel like my back is on fire." Encourage him to find a way to put out the fire, such as wading into a cool lake. Then, guide him step by step into the lake.

Indication
- Chronic pain

Advantage
- Can be performed by patient without assistance

Disadvantages
- Requires trust between therapist and patient
- Effectiveness depends on patient's suggestibility.

Conscious suggestion

How to perform
Use vocal tone, volume, and word choice to disarm patient with statements that seem to come from his own mind. For example, "You want to relax, don't you? You're going to let yourself relax, aren't you? You're going to relax, aren't you?"

Indication
- Chronic pain
- Short-term pain, such as during childbirth
- Short-term pain, such as during suturing of a laceration

Advantage
- Can be used by any health-care professional at any time

Disadvantages
- Effectiveness depends on patient's suggestibility.
- Doesn't completely relax skeletal and smooth muscles

Hypnosis

How to perform
Use suggestion to induce the patient's conscious and unconscious mind into a psychological state that alters normal body function. This procedure has three parts: induction, therapeutic suggestion segments, and awakening.

Indication
- Chronic pain
- Short-term pain, such as during childbirth

Advantages
- Provides deep, significant, long-lasting relief
- After appropriate teaching, technique can be performed by patient without assistance (autohypnosis)
- Provides anesthetic for procedures where deep muscle relaxation is unnecessary, such as dental surgery, dilation and curettage, or childbirth.
- Modifies behavior for smoking, weight control, and enuresis

Disadvantages
- Requires special training for participants, usually with a therapist
- Effectiveness may depend on patient's suggestibility.
- In chronic conditions, patient may become dependent on therapist.
- In rare cases, may push patient who's prepsychotic into psychosis

Acupuncture

How to perform
A trained acupuncturist applies a stimuli to identified points on the patient's body. The stimuli transmits and alters messages to the somatic and autonomic nervous system's efferent fiber.

Indication
- Acute or chronic pain

Advantage
- Relieves pain in one or two treatments

Disadvantage
- Must be performed by a trained acupuncturist

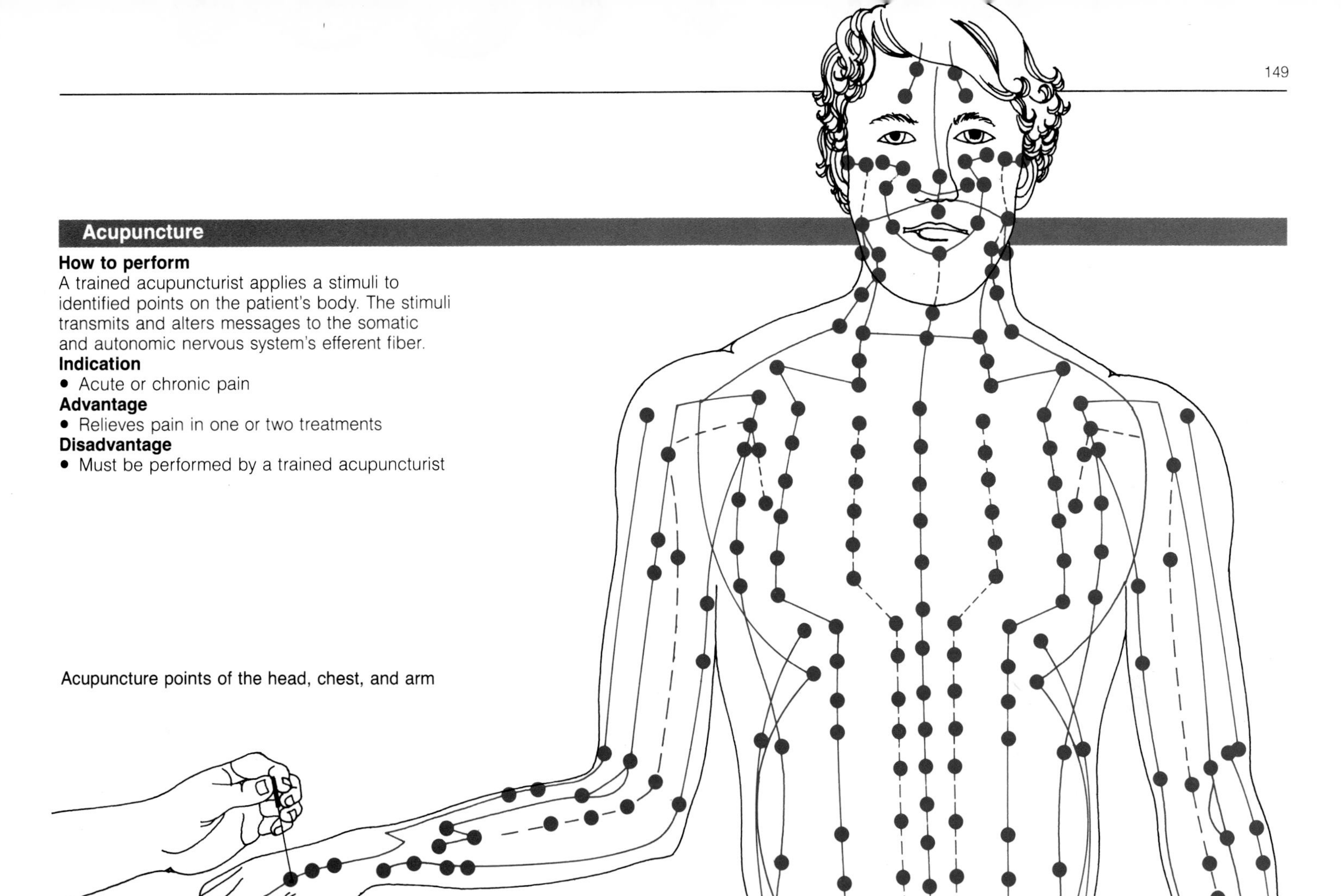

Acupuncture points of the head, chest, and arm

Biofeedback

How to perform
Seat patient in a comfortable chair, and apply three surface electrodes to his forehead, directly over the frontalis muscle. Attach electrode leads to a device that connects the signal from the muscle to an amplified tone machine. Keep the machine tone silent for the baseline reading. Then, turn on the tone and have the patient listen to his tension level. Encourage him to lower his tension level by identifying the tone made as the frontalis muscle relaxes. To lower the tone, he may use such pain-control techniques as guided imagery or distraction.

Indication
- Stress-related disorders, such as sleep onset insomnia, phobias, hypertension, migraine headache, and fecal incontinence

Advantage
- Provides accurate stress reading

Disadvantages
- Because all persons don't respond to the same stimuli, schedule, or technique, treatment must be individualized.
- May take several months to achieve results
- Requires special training and equipment as well as practice in deep relaxation
- May alter medication requirements, placing a patient with such a disease as hypertension or diabetes at risk

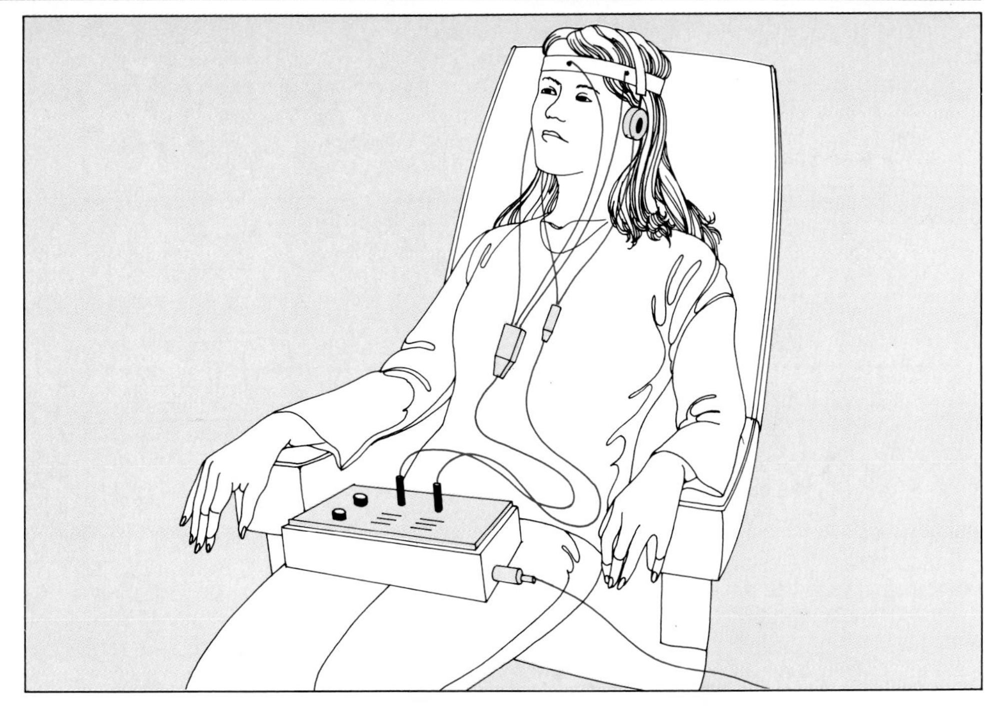

Postmortem care

If you're like most nurses, you don't take a patient's death in stride. But dealing with death is part of nursing. Make sure you know your responsibilities by reading the next few pages.

In this section, you'll learn:

- what steps to take immediately after a patient's death.
- how to notify the patient's family and provide emotional support after you tell them.
- how to prepare the body for the hospital morgue.
- when to call the coroner.

After a death in the family, family members may find comfort in religious beliefs. To help you take appropriate action in accordance with their beliefs, we provide a chart detailing practices for a few religions.

When a patient dies: Your responsibilities

Ed Sharpe, a retired civil engineer, has fought a long battle against lung cancer. Until recently, his disease was in remission. But several days ago, when his condition began deteriorating rapidly, he was admitted to your unit. The doctor suspects that Mr. Sharpe will not go home again.

You've done your best to make Mr. Sharpe comfortable and provide emotional support, even though he's not lucid most of the time. Although you know his condition's terminal, you're shocked and upset when you discover him dead.

No matter how often you face such a situation, dealing with a patient's death is never easy. But you can reduce the stress and anxiety such an event causes by knowing your professional responsibilities. The information on this page will help.

Of course, your professional responsibilities aren't limited to clinical duties. Equally important is the sensitivity you show the patient's survivors—his family and close friends. By showing concern for them, you communicate respect for your patient. You also have the satisfaction of knowing that you've done your best to help them through a crisis.

For details on your responsibilities, read the following.

Note: Be sure you're familiar with your hospital's resuscitative policy.

Initial steps

- If a doctor isn't available, call one to pronounce the patient dead and to complete the death certificate.
- If the patient practiced a religion that dispenses final sacraments or last rites, call the appropriate clergyman. (For guidelines on religious practices, see the chart on page 153.)
- Notify your supervisor (or other designated staff member, such as the admission clerk), according to hospital policy.
- Remind the doctor to notify the coroner, if the death is a coroner's case.
- Contact the family immediately. Unless family members knew the patient's death was imminent, don't tell them the news by phone. Instead, say something like, "Mrs. Sharpe? This is Lucy Wilkins at the hospital. Your husband's taken a turn for the worse. Can you come down as soon as possible?" Suggest that she have a family member or friend accompany her.

Preparing the body for the family

While you wait for the family to arrive, make Mr. Sharpe's body look as natural and peaceful as possible. Follow these guidelines:

- Close the eyes, if necessary, by gently pushing the upper lids down and holding them in place for several seconds.
- Unless the death is a coroner's case, remove invasive lines, tubes, drains, and other equipment. If necessary, apply pressure bandages to stop bleeding.
- If the death is a coroner's case, leave all invasive equipment in place. (For guidelines on preparing the body for the coroner, see the information on pages 152 and 153.)
- Cleanse blood and drainage from the skin, as necessary.
- If the patient wore dentures, put them in his mouth. They'll help his face assume a natural shape.
- If his mouth has dropped open, prop pillows behind his head to tip his chin toward his chest. Although his mouth may not close, this position makes an open mouth less apparent.
- Make sure the room has enough chairs for family members to sit on, if they wish. Provide privacy.

Supporting the family

Take the family to a quiet, private room to talk with the doctor. If possible, let the doctor break the news; this reassures the family that the patient had proper medical attention. If a family member asks you, "Is he dead?" before the doctor arrives, answer truthfully. Say something like, "Yes, he died a short while ago. Please have a seat and the doctor will talk with you."

After allowing family members time to cope with the situation, ask if they would like to see the body. If they would, be sure you have ammonia capsules in your pocket in case someone becomes faint. *Important:* Be alert for signs of a medical emergency triggered by stress; for example, a heart attack. Don't assume that unusual behavior is caused by grief alone.

Also, prepare the family for any equipment still attached to the body, and explain why it's in place.

Note: If the patient's death resulted from a mutilating accident—for example, a fire—prepare the family by gently describing his injuries.

Escort family members into the room, and stay with them for several minutes. Don't hesitate to reach out and touch them, if you sense they'd appreciate the gesture. Remind them they can touch the body; for example, you might ask, "Would you like to hold his hand?" Then, ask if they'd like to be left alone.

Suppose a family member asks you to remove a ring or other jewelry from the patient. If you do, *clearly* document what you gave to whom. *Note:* Wait until the family members leave the room before trying to remove a ring. If you have difficulty, they may become upset watching you struggle.

If a family member asks you to wait several hours before removing the body so other relatives can visit, discuss the request with your supervisor before agreeing. As you know, rigor mortis sets in within 4 hours, making preparation and removal of the body difficult.

Inquire about funeral arrangements; your supervisor needs to know who will remove the body. Use tact, especially if the family was unprepared for the death.

Before family members leave, give them the patient's personal belongings in your possession (except for belongings the coroner may need, if appropriate). Thoroughly document what you give to the family and what you send to the coroner. Finally, make sure each family member is accompanied home.

After the family leaves, finish cleaning the body and wrap it for the morgue. For details on this procedure, read the following photostory.

Performing postmortem care

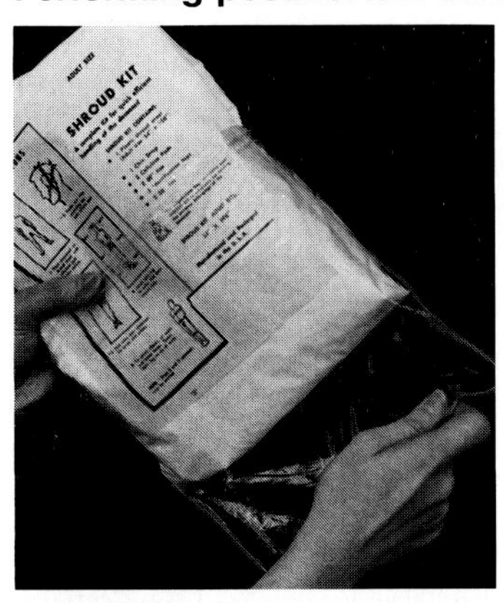

1 To prepare a patient for the morgue, obtain a stretcher and a shroud kit, like the one shown here. The kit contains a plastic sheet, chin strap, two cellulose pads, two 60″ (1.5-m) ties, three 36″ (91-cm) ties, and three identification tags. *Note:* If the patient dies of an infectious disease, check your hospital policy; you may have to obtain two kits and double-wrap the body, using isolation technique.

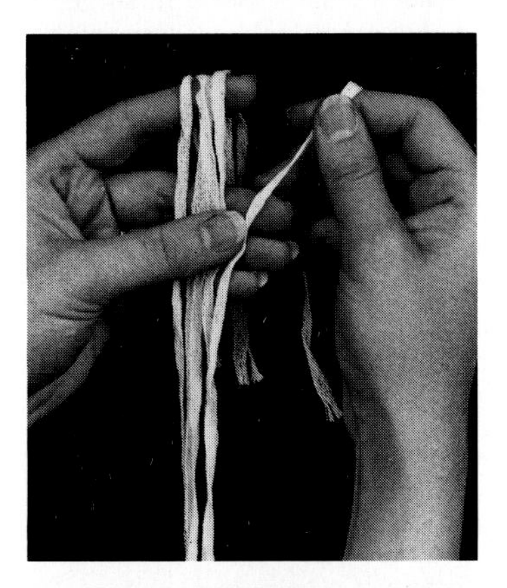

2 Unwrap the kit and separate the five ties, as the nurse is doing here. Lay the two long ties on the stretcher. When you lay the patient on the stretcher, one tie should be perpendicular to the shoulders (or neck) and the other, perpendicular to the waist. Place a short tie at knee level, and put the remaining two ties aside.

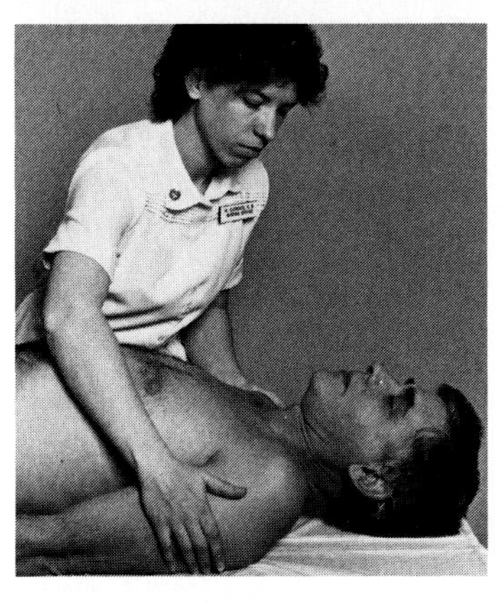

3 Now, lay the shroud sheet on the stretcher, on top of the ties. Ask a co-worker to help you move the patient from the bed to the stretcher. Center the patient on the stretcher, as shown.

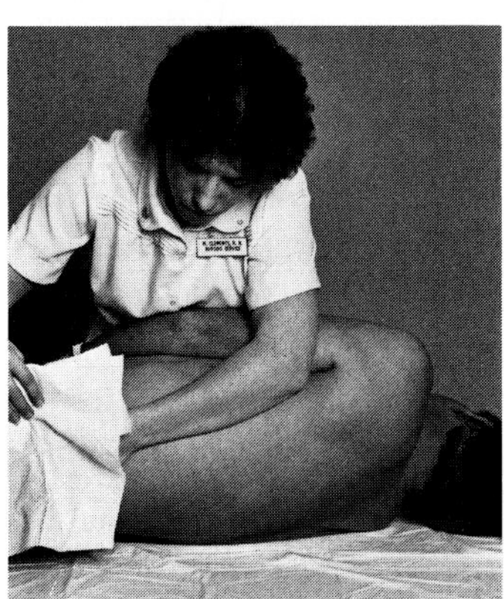

4 Place a cellulose pad under the patient's rectum, in case the anal sphincters relax.

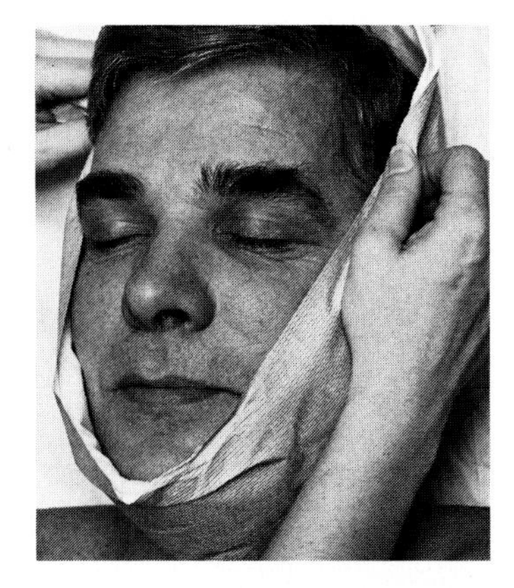

5 If the patient wore dentures, make sure they're in place. Then, pad his chin and lower jaw with a cellulose pad to prevent pressure marks when you tie the jaw shut. Apply the chin strap, as the nurse is doing here.

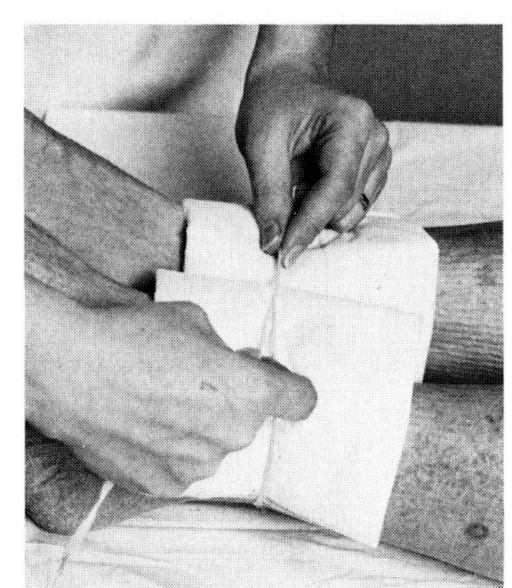

6 Place the patient's arms at his sides, and straighten his legs. To prevent tie marks, wrap several surgical pads around his ankles. Then, using a 36″ tie, fasten his ankles together.

Note: Don't cross his wrists over his chest and tie them, unless *required* by hospital policy; this leaves visible pressure marks, which may upset the family. If you must tie the wrists, first pad the skin.

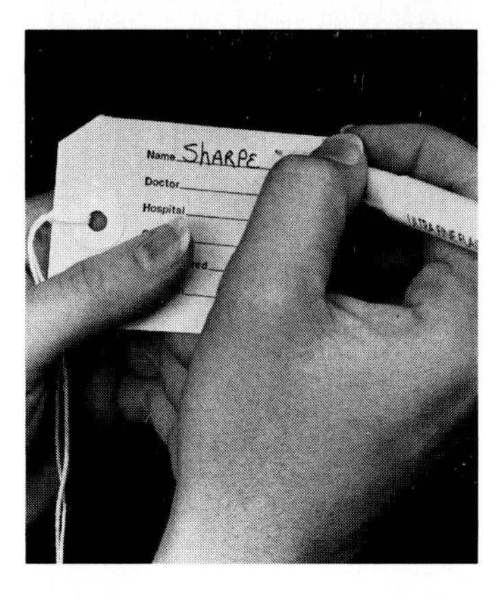

7 Fill out the tag marked *attach to toe,* as the nurse is doing here. Then, tie it to a great toe.

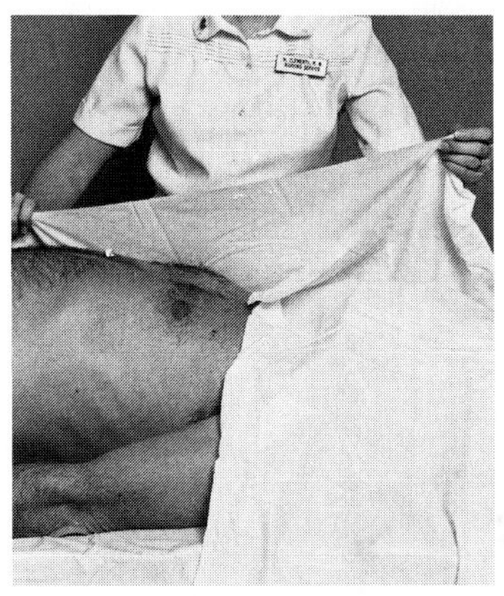

8 Now, fold the shroud over the patient, as follows: First, fold the shroud's top down over his head and its bottom up over his feet. Then, overlap the sides across his midline. *Note:* To avoid upsetting patients when the body's transported through the halls, some hospitals require that the head remain unwrapped until the body arrives at the morgue. Know your hospital's policy.

Postmortem care

Performing postmortem care continued

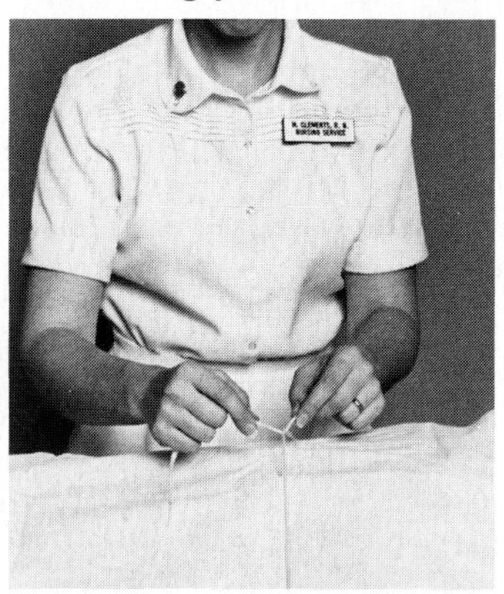

9 Secure the shroud with the ties. Tie one around the patient's shoulders or neck, one around his waist, and the third around his knees.

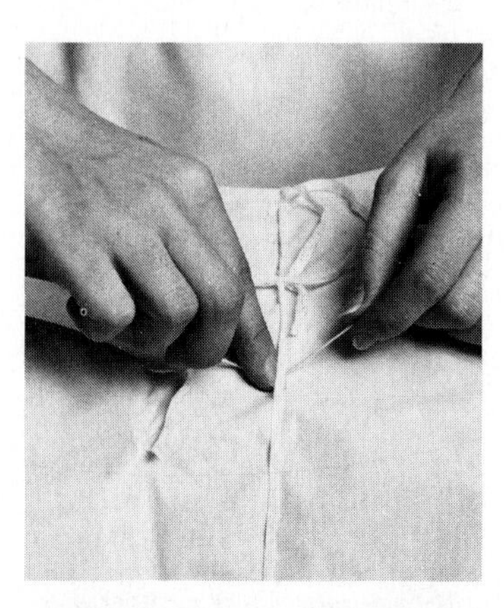

10 Fill out the tag marked *attach to outside.* Fasten it to the tie encircling the waist.

Important: If the patient died of an infectious disease, write the name of the disease in red on this tag.

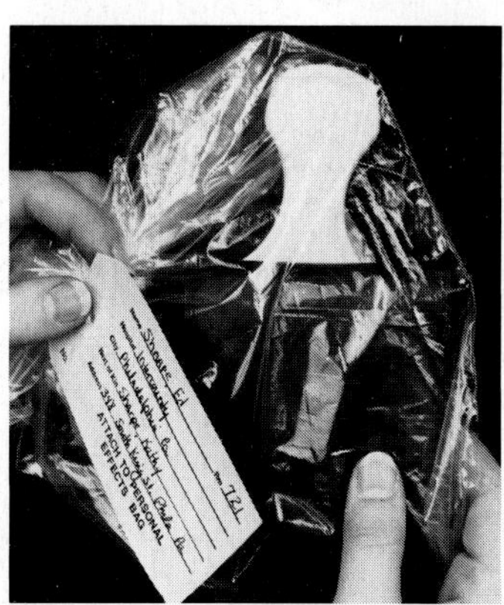

11 If the family hasn't taken all the patient's personal belongings, place them in a plastic bag. Fill out the tag marked *attach to personal effects bag,* and tie or tape it to the bag. Store your patient's belongings according to hospital policy. *Note:* You can use the kit's plastic wrapper to collect the patient's belongings.

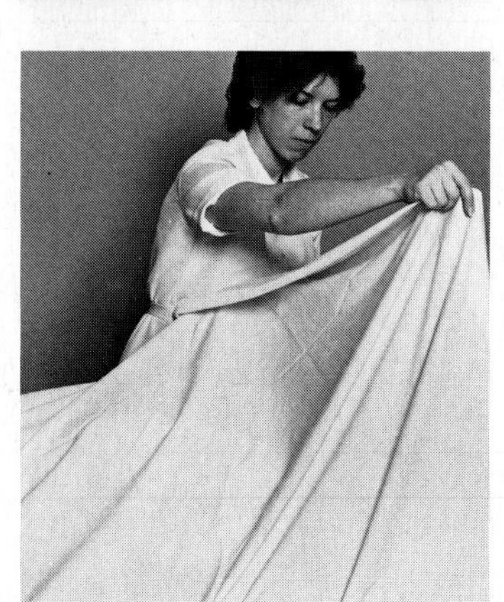

12 Cover the patient with a sheet, and take him to the morgue. Finally, document the event, according to hospital policy. Make sure the signed death certificate is sent to the medical records office.

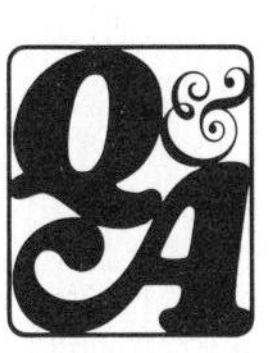

Knowing your legal responsibilities

Uncertain about your legal responsibilities following the death of a patient in your care? Read the following dialogue for general guidelines. But keep in mind that state laws vary. Know your state's requirements by using these resources:
- hospital policy on death and autopsy
- the coroner (or medical examiner) for your county or state
- your hospital's lawyer
- your supervisor.

Question:
When should I notify the coroner of a death?
Answer:
This depends on state law and the coroner's discretion. As a rule, you should notify the coroner when:
- the patient was involved (as a victim or a perpetrator) in any crime. (Always consider death by homicide a coroner's case.)
- the patient's committed suicide.
- the death was sudden and unattended by the patient's doctor.
- the patient lived out of state.
- the patient died within 24 hours of hospital admission (unless his condition was diagnosed as terminal on admittance).
- the circumstances surrounding the death were suspicious.

In some states, you must notify the coroner if the patient dies within 24 hours of a surgical procedure, after less than 24 hours of care by a doctor, or if he was a minor.

Question:
What if I suspect a death is a coroner's case, but I'm not sure?
Answer:
When in doubt, call the coroner with the facts. Be prepared to tell him the patient's name, address, age, and presumed cause of death; his medical history (including his doctor's name and medication history); and funeral home information.

Question:
What special care should I give the patient when the death is a coroner's case?
Answer:
Leave all invasive lines and other equipment in the patient, including I.V. lines, arterial lines, pulmonary artery lines, drains, pacemaker wires, and trach tubes. Tie or cover them to prevent drainage during body transportation. The coroner may permit you to remove an endotracheal tube, because it will deform the mouth.

If an I.V. line or other equipment is removed from the patient, circle the site with a felt-tipped pen and clearly document your action. Under some circumstances, the coroner may need to know that the puncture was caused by I.V. insertion, not illicit drug use.

Thoroughly document all care given to the patient before death; this information can be critical to the coroner's findings. In case of a suspicious death, for instance, the coroner needs to know whether a broken sternum resulted from cardiopulmonary resuscitation or from the event causing the death.

Question:
Can organs be retrieved from a body if the death is a coroner's case?
Answer:
Yes, if the coroner is notified beforehand. Under some circumstances, he may wish to be present at retrieval. Of course, before organ retrieval, all requirements for consent must be fulfilled. For details, see the information beginning on page 154.

Question:
Suppose the death isn't a coroner's case, but the doctor wants to perform an autopsy. Does this require written consent?
Answer:
Yes, written consent is necessary. Also, be sure the consent specifies any limitations, if appropriate.

Question:
Who can sign the consent form?
Answer:
In most cases, the person assuming responsibility for the patient has the authority to sign a consent form. But some states have specific laws about who can legally consent to an autopsy. For example, the patient's spouse may be required to sign, if he or she is available and competent. An adult child may be the second designee, and a parent, the third designee. Other states specify relatives who may sign, in no order of preference.

Some states allow the patient to make the decision before his death. But under most circumstances, health-care professionals are reluctant to discuss autopsy with a hospitalized patient.

Question:
Who should ask a family member to sign the consent form?
Answer:
Most states specify that this is the doctor's responsibility. You may witness a signature.

Question:
What if an autopsy is performed without consent?
Answer:
This may be considered intentional mutilation, which is a punishable crime and basis for civil liability.

Nurses' guide to religious practices

Religious group	Beliefs and practices surrounding death
Baha'i	Memorial service; no uniform ritual, readings, or prayers
Baptist	Clergy prays with family.
Black Muslim	Special procedure for washing and shrouding the dead
Buddhism	Contact priest; last-rite chanting at bedside; body cremated.
Christian Scientist	No last rites or autopsy; burial or cremation
Church of Christ	No last rites
Church of God	No last rites or cremation
Church of Jesus Christ of Latter-Day Saints (Mormons)	Baptism of dead; cremation discouraged; preaching of gospel to dead
Eastern Orthodox	Last rites in impending death; cremation discouraged
Episcopal	Last rites not mandatory; check with family.
Friends (Quakers)	Individual decision
Grace Brethren	No last rites; individual decision on burial
Greek Orthodox	Sacrament of Holy Communion considered last rites; autopsy and cremation discouraged
Hindu	Call priest in impending death. Don't remove the thread he'll probably tie around the patient's neck or wrist; it signifies a blessing. Priest pours water into corpse's mouth. Check with family about handling body.
Jehovah's Witnesses	No last rites
Judaism	In impending death, patient or fellow Jew may read psalms 23, 103, and 139 aloud. Last words should be, "Hear, O Israel, the Lord our God, the Lord is One." Burial within 24 hours. No burial on sabbath (Saturday). Attended by relative until buried.
Lutheran	Last rites optional
Muslim	Family washes and prepares patient for death; face body toward Mecca; no autopsy.
Nazarene	No last rites; stillborns are buried.
Orthodox Presbyterian	Reading of scripture and prayer
Roman Catholic	In impending death, call priest to perform Anointing of the Sick.
Russian Orthodox	No autopsy, embalming, or cremation; after death, arms are crossed with fingers set in cross; clothing worn by dead must be of natural fiber.
Seventh-Day Adventist	Dead are only asleep until Christ's return.
Unitarian/Universalist	Cremation preferred.

Organ donation

Medical advances in the past 2 decades have enabled doctors to successfully transplant the heart, lungs, kidneys, and the liver.

Of course, this expanding field of medicine carries with it a number of implications. As a nurse, you can recognize a potential organ donor, broach the subject of organ donation to the patient's doctor, and provide emotional support for family members while they make the difficult decision. Also, you may need to provide aggressive nursing care to maintain the prospective donor's organs until they're removed.

To learn more about your role in organ donation, read this and the following page carefully.

Learning about organ donation

Ronald Morgan is dying. The 48-year-old automobile mechanic suffered a massive cerebral hemorrhage, and his condition's deteriorating quickly. As you administer his afternoon medications, you realize that he's no longer responding to your commands and his breathing pattern's changing rapidly. Of course, you notify the doctor. When the doctor arrives, he advises the family that the patient probably won't live much longer.

After the doctor leaves, you ask the family members if you can do anything for them. Mr. Morgan's wife says, "No," but adds, "I wish we could do something. I hate to see Ron's life wasted by his dying so young."

If you've ever been involved in organ donation, you recognize that Mr. Morgan may be a potential donor. If you feel comfortable with his family members, your next responsibility is to help them understand how Mr. Morgan can improve the life of another.

Who can be an organ donor?

First, let's review the type of patient who can donate organs. For example, consider a patient between ages 1 and 60 who's dying of irreversible brain damage a potential donor. Although his condition may be critical, his transplantable organs—corneas, skin, heart, lungs, liver, and kidneys—remain in good condition. (*Note:* Age isn't a factor in corneal or skin transplantation.)

Patients considered unacceptable for organ donation include those with chronic hypertension or diabetes, untreated infections, septicemia, or cancer (except for primary brain tumor). In addition, patients with injuries to transplantable organs aren't considered potential donors.

Talking with the family

Before discussing organ donation with the family, examine your feelings about the subject. If you have qualms about the procedure or strong religious or philosophical beliefs against it, or you don't feel comfortable with the family members, ask the doctor to talk with them. Be sure to follow your hospital's policy.

In Mr. Morgan's case, you may raise the subject of organ donation by saying to his wife, "Although your husband may not have long to live, there's a way he can help others live longer." Then, briefly explain organ donation to her. Gauge the response of Mrs. Morgan and other family members. If they say they haven't given the idea much thought or object to your suggestion, don't pursue it. If you do, you'll only upset or alienate the family.

Suppose the family decides in favor of organ donation. Then, the doctor will have to obtain Mrs. Morgan's written permission. According to the Uniform Anatomical Gift Act (which all states have adopted in some form), the patient's next of kin must agree to the organ donation. In order of priority, the legal next of kin is the spouse, adult son or daughter, either parent, adult brother or sister, and then legal guardian. Even if the dying patient has signed a donor card, his next of kin can halt organ donation by refusing to agree to it.

Also, be sure to explain that you may have to maintain the patient's vital functions on a machine until the organs are removed.

Note: If foul play's suspected in a patient's death, the coroner or medical examiner must also grant permission for organ donation.

Determining when death occurs

The Uniform Anatomical Gift Act doesn't address organ donation's most controversial aspect: When should the patient be declared dead? This issue takes on increased significance because—except for skin and corneal transplantation—a prospective donor's vital functions must be artificially sustained until the donated organ's removed, or harvested.

Your hospital or the state in which it's located may have a brain-death law doctors must observe. If not, the decision's left to the doctor. He may base his decision on criteria listed by an ad hoc committee at Harvard Medical School. These criteria include:

- complete unresponsiveness to painful stimuli
- vital functions maintained by a respirator
- no cranial nerve reflexes
- EEG showing no electrical activity in the brain.

These conditions must persist for longer than 24 hours. Also, the doctor must rule out central nervous system intoxication and hypothermia.

Another way to detect brain death is by cerebral angiography, a test to determine the amount of blood flow to the brain. Absence of blood flow indicates brain death.

Remember, the patient's family may have difficulty accepting the brain-death determination. In fact, *you* may have difficulty with the ruling. For example, suppose you see a brain-dead patient move an arm or leg in response to stimuli. When you notice this movement, you may find it hard to believe that the patient has no brain function and that the response was only a spinal cord reflex.

What organs can be donated?

After a patient's listed as brain dead and permission for the organ donation has been obtained, the doctor orders a series of tests, which vary according to the organ being donated.

Organs used in transplantation include:

- *corneas.* The doctor has up to 8 hours after the patient's death to harvest corneas. Initially tried in 1908, corneal transplantation is now routine. First, the entire eye's removed. Then, the cornea is processed under sterile conditions and preserved.

Note: The doctor won't use the corneas of a patient who's had corneal disease or eye surgery.

- *skin.* Like the corneas, skin's viable for harvesting after death—up to 18 hours afterward, in fact. Also, as in corneal transplantation, no special tests are performed to match the donor and recipient. In most cases, skin's removed circumferentially from the donor's trunk and legs; then, it's processed and stored in a skin bank.
- *heart.* A heart donor's vital functions must be maintained until the doctor's determined that brain death has occurred. Usually, the donor's transported to the recipient's hospital, so the donated organ can be quickly exchanged. Doing so increases the chances of successful transplantation. Occasionally, an organ donation team goes to the donor's hospital, recovers and preserves the organ, returns to the recipient's hospital, and then transplants the organ.

Certain tests are performed before the donor's heart is removed. These tests include blood group typing, urine and blood cultures, complete blood count, fluid and electrolyte studies, chest X-ray, and EKG.

- *lungs.* Because chronic lung disease also affects heart function, the lungs and heart are usually transplanted together. Heart-lung transplantation is still in the infancy stage and is usually performed at a major medical center.

A heart-lung donor receives the same tests used for heart transplantation plus arterial blood gas measurements and sputum cultures.

- *liver.* Because of its complex makeup, the liver isn't transplanted as commonly as other organs. As in heart transplantation, a liver donor's vital functions must be artificially maintained until the organ's removed; in fact, his blood pressure and volume must be sufficient to withstand a 3-hour operation. After removal, the liver's processed and preserved, so it can be transported.

Optimally, the donor's liver should be smaller than the recipient's. Why? Because the recipient's diseased liver has shrunk from fibrosis. As a result, he has less space in his abdominal cavity than normal.

A liver donor receives the same tests as a heart donor plus liver function studies.

- *kidneys.* Cadaver donors supply most kidneys for transplantation. The donor's vital functions are artificially maintained until organ removal. A normal, healthy person can also donate a kidney. The success rate for cadaver kidneys is about 55%. The rate's higher for transplantation involving kidneys from living blood relatives, whose blood and tissue types are more compatible with the recipient's.

When a cadaver kidney's used, the donor first receives the same tests used for a heart donor. Then, after removal, the kidney's placed in a preservation machine, which keeps it viable for up to 72 hours.

Note: Most organ transplantations occur within 24 hours of removal from the donor.

Your role

Keep in mind that many areas or hospitals have transplantation teams that handle all aspects of organ donation. If your patient's next of kin consents to organ donation, you may contact one of these organizations.

Here are other general guidelines for you to follow:

- Use tact and compassion when discussing organ donation with your patient's family. If his next of kin consents to organ donation, explain that the patient may be taken to the ICU to maintain his vital functions until the organ's removed. Assure family members that the procedure won't disfigure the patient in any way and won't delay any funeral or burial plans they may have.
- Make sure the patient's next of kin has signed a consent form. Afterward, arrange for a medical social worker or a member of the clergy to contact the family and provide emotional support. *Note:* Many organizations inform the donor's family of the recipient's progress.
- Explain to the family that one doctor will probably declare the patient brain dead and another doctor will perform the transplant procedure.
- Assist with medical procedures required for organ donation, including obtaining blood and tissue specimens for analysis and maintaining the patient's blood pressure (by administering fluids or drugs I.V.), respiratory function, and fluid and electrolyte balance. You may have to assist with other procedures, depending on which organ your patient's donating.

Because you don't have to maintain a donor's vital functions for corneal and skin transplantation, you may assume a more active role in removing these organs. When caring for a cornea donor, follow these guidelines:

- Notify the doctor who will remove the eyes.
- Close the donor's eyes and place ice packs over them. Make sure the eyes are free of debris.
- Elevate the head of the bed to reduce the blood flow to the eyes.
- If the eyes are to be removed in the morgue, have the patient transported as soon as possible.

When caring for a skin donor, first cleanse the body. Then, wrap the body, following the procedure on pages 151 and 152. Make sure the body's transferred to the morgue as soon as possible to help preserve the skin.

Acknowledgements

We'd like to thank the following people and companies for their help with this PHOTOBOOK:

ACKRAD LABORATORIES
Garwood, N.J.

AMERICAN OPTICAL CORPORATION
Southbridge, Mass.

AMES DIVISION
Miles Laboratories, Inc.
Elkhart, Ind.

AUTO-SYRINGE, INC.
Hooksett, N.H.

CAMBRIDGE SCIENTIFIC INDUSTRIES, INC.
Cambridge, Md.

CHESEBROUGH-POND'S, INC.
Watertown, N.Y.

DELAWARE VALLEY TRANSPLANT PROGRAM
Philadelphia, Pa.
Stephen M. Sammut
Executive Director

HEALTHCO, INC.
Reading, Pa.

IMED CORPORATION
San Diego, Calif.

INDICATING CALIPER CO.
Oak Park, Ill.

INTERNATIONAL TECHNIDYNE CORP.
Edison, N.J.

MARKWELL MEDICAL INSTITUTE, INC.
Racine, Wis.

MEDA SONICS
Mountain View, Calif.

MEDTRONIC, INC.
Minneapolis, Minn.

MICRO ESSENTIAL LABORATORY, INC.
Brooklyn, N.Y.

ROCHE LABORATORIES
Nutley, N.J.

RON SONTAG PUBLIC RELATIONS, INC.
Waukesha, Wis.
Judith C. Amend

SCALE-TRONIX, INC.
White Plains, N.Y.

SONTEK INDUSTRIES, INC.
Lexington, Mass.

SORENSON RESEARCH CO., INC.
Subsidiary of Abbott Laboratories
Salt Lake City, Utah

WIGHTMAN MEDICAL, INC.
Doylestown, Pa.

Also the staffs of:

BRYN MAWR REHABILITATION HOSPITAL
Bryn Mawr, Pa.

GRAND VIEW HOSPITAL
Sellersville, Pa.

MEDICAL INTENSIVE CARE UNIT
Veterans Administration Hospital
Wilmington, Del.

THE EYE INSTITUTE
Pennsylvania College of Optometry
Philadelphia, Pa.

Selected references

Books

Brunner, Lillian S. THE LIPPINCOTT MANUAL OF NURSING PRACTICE, 3rd ed. Philadelphia: J.B. Lippincott Co., 1982.

Brunner, Lillian S., and Doris S. Suddarth. TEXTBOOK OF MEDICAL-SURGICAL NURSING, 4th ed. Philadelphia: J.B. Lippincott Co., 1980.

Burton, George G., et al., eds. RESPIRATORY CARE: A GUIDE TO CLINICAL PRACTICE. Philadelphia: J.B. Lippincott Co., 1977.

Del Regato, Juan A., and Harlan J. Spjut. ACKERMAN AND DEL REGATO'S CANCER: DIAGNOSIS, TREATMENT, AND PROGNOSIS, 5th ed. St. Louis: C.V. Mosby Co., 1977.

DIAGNOSTICS. Nurse's Reference Library™. Springhouse, Pa.: Intermed Communications, Inc., 1982.

Erickson, Milton H., et al. HYPNOTIC REALITIES: THE INDUCTION OF CLINICAL HYPNOSIS AND FORMS OF INDIRECT SUGGESTION. New York: Irvington Publishers, 1976.

Fletcher, Gilbert. TEXTBOOK OF RADIOTHERAPY, 3rd ed. Philadelphia: Lea & Febiger, 1980.

GIVING CARDIAC CARE. Nursing Photobook™ Series. Springhouse, Pa.: Intermed Communications, Inc., 1981.

Gutch, C.F., and Martha H. Stoner. REVIEW OF HEMODIALYZERS FOR NURSES AND DIALYSIS PERSONNEL, 3rd ed. St. Louis: C.V. Mosby Co., 1979.

IMPLEMENTING UROLOGIC PROCEDURES. Nursing Photobook™ Series. Springhouse, Pa.: Intermed Communications, Inc., 1981.

Leahy, Irene, et al. THE NURSE AND RADIOTHERAPY: A MANUAL FOR DAILY CARE. St. Louis: C.V. Mosby Co., 1978.

Levy, William S., and Gilbert H. Barnes. HYGIENIC PROBLEMS OF THE AMPUTEE. Washington, D.C.: American Orthotic and Prosthetic Association, 1961.

MANAGING I.V. THERAPY. Nursing Photobook™ Series. Springhouse, Pa.: Intermed Communications, Inc., 1980.

MANUAL FOR LOWER EXTREMITY AMPUTEES. West Orange, N.J.: Kessler Institute of Rehabilitation, Dept. of Physical Medicine.

Marino, Lisa. CANCER NURSING. St. Louis: C.V. Mosby Co., 1981.

Matsumoto, Teruo. ACUPUNCTURE FOR PHYSICIANS. Springfield, Ill.: Charles C. Thomas, Publishers, 1974.

Moss, William T., et al. RADIATION ONCOLOGY: RATIONALE, TECHNIQUE, RESULTS, 5th ed. St. Louis: C.V. Mosby Co., 1979.

Murdock, George. ADVANCES IN ORTHOTICS. Baltimore: Williams & Wilkins, 1977.

PERFORMING GI PROCEDURES. Nursing Photobook™ Series. Springhouse, Pa.: Intermed Communications, Inc., 1981.

PROCEDURES. Nurse's Reference Library™. Springhouse, Pa.: Intermed Communications, Inc., 1982.

PROVIDING RESPIRATORY CARE. Nursing Photobook™ Series. Springhouse, Pa.: Intermed Communications, Inc., 1979.

Ramsey, J.M. BASIC PATHOPHYSIOLOGY. Reading, Mass.: Addison-Wesley Pub. Co., 1982.

Shapiro, Barry A., et al. CLINICAL APPLICATION OF BLOOD GASES, 2nd ed. Chicago: Year Book Medical Pub., 1977.

Wilson, A. Bennet, Jr. LIMB PROSTHETICS, 5th ed. Melbourne, Fla.: Robert E. Krieger Pub. Co., 1976.

Wollard, Joy J. NUTRITIONAL MANAGEMENT OF THE CANCER PATIENT. New York: Raven Press, 1979.

Periodicals

Baker, J. *Radiotherapy: Implants and Applicators,* NURSING TIMES. Pp. 37-40, November 29, 1979.

Blackburn, G.L., et al. *Nutrition and Metabolic Assessment of the Hospitalized Patient,* JOURNAL OF PARENTERAL-ENTERAL NUTRITION. 1:1:11-22, 1977.

Bodnar, Donna M. *Rationale for Nutritional Requirements for Patients on Continuous Ambulatory Peritoneal Dialysis,* JOURNAL OF THE AMERICAN DIETETIC ASSOCIATION. 80:247-249, March 1982.

Boyd-Monk, Heather. *Screening for Glaucoma,* NURSING79. 9:42-45, August 1979.

Donaldson, Sarah. *Nutritional Consequences of Radiotherapy,* CANCER RESEARCH. 37:2407-2413, July 1977.

Doughty, Mary C., and Kathleen Gagnon Pierie. *Continuous Ambulatory Peritoneal Dialysis and the Blind Patient,* NEPHROLOGY NURSE. Pp. 11-14, January-February 1981.

Ekers, M., and S. Bhagwan. *EBA: A New Route for Vascular Rehabilitation,* NURSING82. 12:34-41, November 1982.

Grant, J.P., et al. *Current Techniques of Nutritional Assessment,* SURGICAL CLINICS OF NORTH AMERICA. 61:3, June 1981.

Hilderly, Laura. *The Role of the Nurse in Radiation Oncology,* SEMINARS IN ONCOLOGY. 7:1:39-47, March 1980.

Kilroy, June L. *Care and Teaching of Patients with Glaucoma,* NURSING CLINICS OF NORTH AMERICA. P. 393, September 1981.

Meakins, J.L., et al. *Delayed Hypersensitivity: Indicator of Acquired Failure of Host Defense in Sepsis and Trauma,* ANNALS OF SURGERY. 186:241-249, 1977.

Moncrief, J. *Continuous Ambulatory Peritoneal Dialysis,* DIALYSIS AND TRANSPLANTATION. 8:1077-1080, 1165, 1979.

Morgan, D.B., et al. *The Assessment of Weight Loss from a Single Measurement of Body Weight: The Problems and Limitations,* AMERICAN JOURNAL OF CLINICAL NUTRITION. 33:2101-2105, October 1980.

Mullen, J.L., et al. *Implications of Malnutrition in the Surgical Patient,* ARCHIVES OF SURGERY. 114:121-125, 1979.

Nolph, Karl D. *Continuous Ambulatory Peritoneal Dialysis,* AMERICAN JOURNAL OF NEPHROLOGY. 1:1-10, 1981.

Peck, Arthur, and John Boland. *Emotional Reactions to Radiation Treatment,* CANCER. 40:180-184, 1977.

Seltzer, M.H., et al. *Instant Nutritional Assessment in the Intensive Care Unit,* JPEN. 5:1:70-72, 1981.

Strosahl, Vickie S., and Paula V. Waldorf. *Visual Impairment: Not a Contraindication for Continuous Ambulatory Peritoneal Dialysis,* DIALYSIS AND TRANSPLANTATION. 10:5:371-378, May 1981.

Index

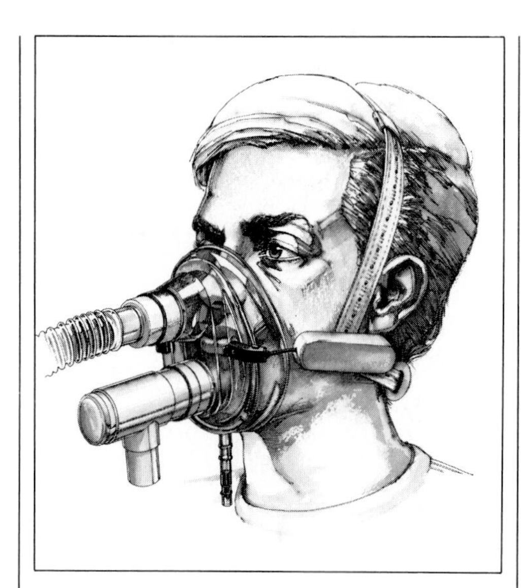

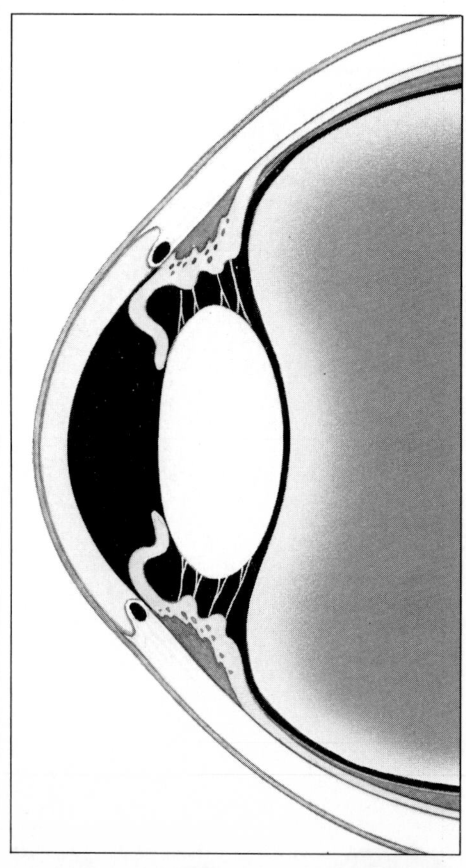

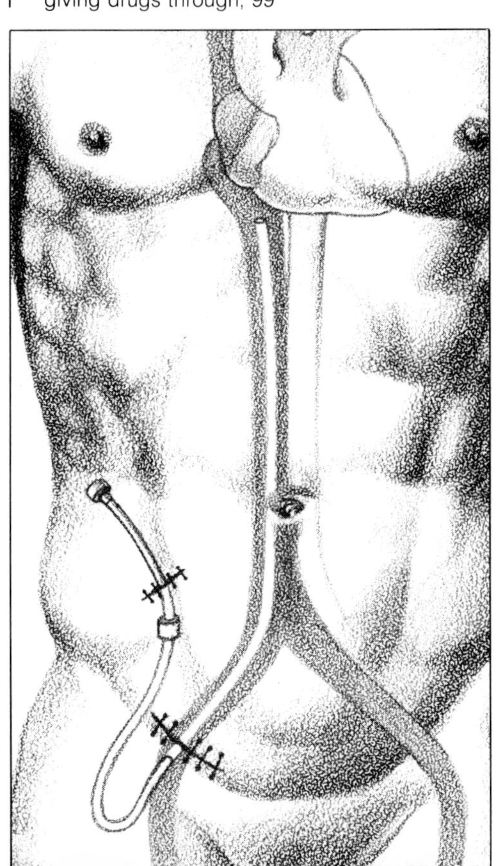

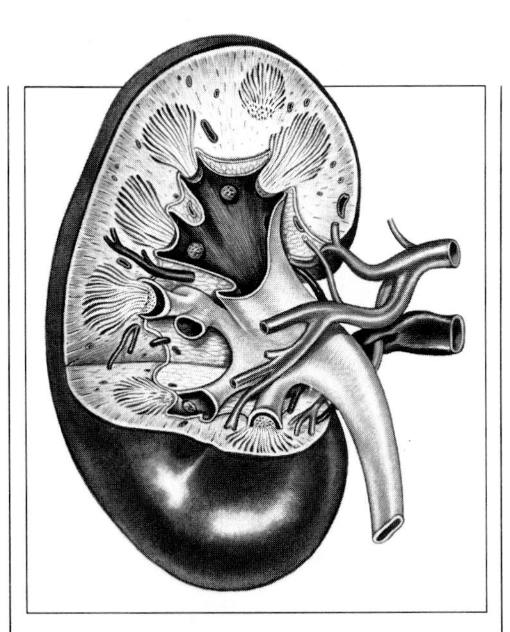

Index

R

S

T

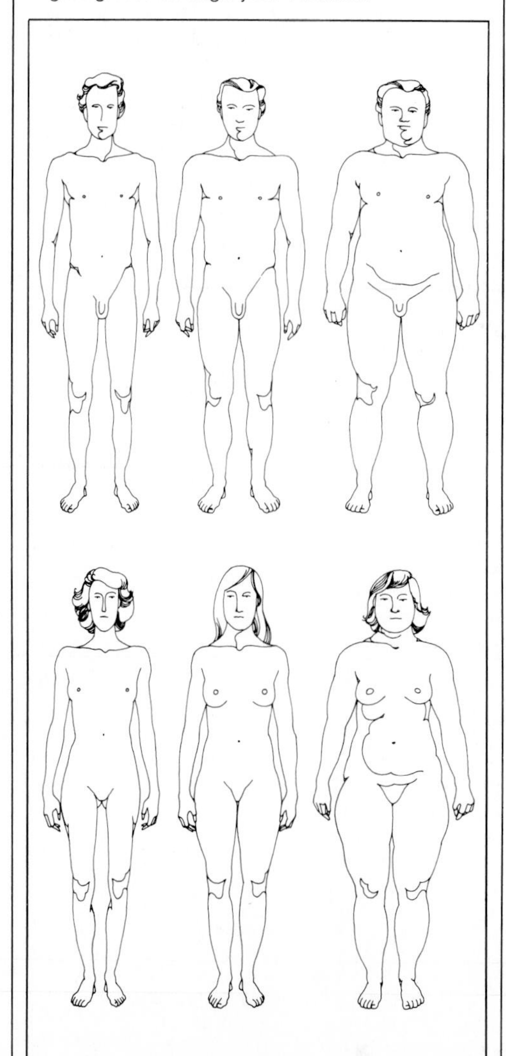

U

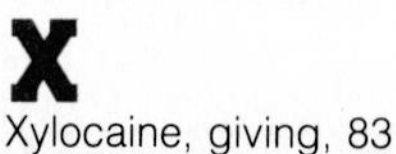

X